Perioperative Medicine: Care of Surgical Patients

Perioperative Medicine: Care of Surgical Patients

Editor: Bryson Cooper

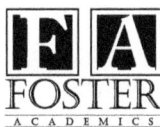

FA
FOSTER
ACADEMICS
www.fosteracademics.com

www.fosteracademics.com

FA FOSTER
ACADEMICS

Cataloging-in-Publication Data

Perioperative medicine : care of surgical patients / edited by Bryson Cooper.
    p. cm.
Includes bibliographical references and index.
ISBN 978-1-63242-790-8
1. Surgery, Operative. 2. Surgery--Complications--Prevention. 3. Therapeutics, Surgical. 4. Preoperative care.
5. Postoperative care. I. Cooper, Bryson.
RD54 .P47 2019
617--dc23

Foster Academics,
118-35 Queens Blvd., Suite 400,
Forest Hills, NY 11375, USA

ISBN 978-1-63242-790-8 (Hardback)

Contents

Permissions

List of Contributors

Index

Preface

Perioperative medicine refers to the medical care of surgical patients from the time of contemplation of surgery to full recovery. It covers the entire operative period but excludes the surgical procedure itself. Perioperative medicine includes the care of patients preparing for, having and recuperating from a surgery. It is usually provided by an intensivist, anesthesiologist or internal medicine generalist. Such care generally takes place in hospitals or surgical centers. Operative risks, patient specific risks, methods to reduce risks and management of risks are some of the focus areas which are related to the field of perioperative medicine. This book attempts to understand the multiple branches that fall under the discipline of perioperative medicine and how such concepts have practical applications. From theories to research to practical applications, case studies related to all contemporary topics of relevance to this field have been included in it. This book is a vital tool for all researching or studying perioperative medicine as it gives incredible insights into emerging trends and concepts.

This book unites the global concepts and researches in an organized manner for a comprehensive understanding of the subject. It is a ripe text for all researchers, students, scientists or anyone else who is interested in acquiring a better knowledge of this dynamic field.

I extend my sincere thanks to the contributors for such eloquent research chapters. Finally, I thank my family for being a source of support and help.

Editor

Strategies to promote reporting of Surgical Care Improvement Project (SCIP) measures

Rebecca M Speck[1,2], Mark D Neuman[1], Andrew R Bond[3] and Lee A Fleisher[1*]

Abstract

Background: The Surgical Care Improvement Project (SCIP) is a quality improvement initiative focused on reducing surgical complications. Reporting SCIP performance measures helps determine whether hospitals receive the full payment update from the Centers for Medicare and Medicaid Services. Strategies in use by hospitals to motivate departmental participation in SCIP reporting are poorly understood.

Methods: A 12-item pilot survey exploring strategies to promote reporting of SCIP measures was developed and mailed to department of anesthesiology chairs at 1,426 US hospitals. Descriptive statistics and χ^2 analysis were used to summarize respondent and survey data.

Results: In all, 29.5% of the sample responded to the survey, with 96.9% indicating SCIP participation; 62.5% participated primarily for voluntary reasons, and 4.2% reported an incentive from their hospital as the primary reason for participation.

Conclusions: Hospital strategies promoting physician participation in SCIP currently vary. A minority of survey respondents indicated that an incentive was used to encourage adherence to SCIP measures. Further research to optimize such strategies may support future efforts to improve perioperative care.

Keywords: Performance measures, Surgical Care Improvement Project

Background

In recent years, the use of financial incentives to drive improvements in the quality of health care has garnered significant attention in the US and abroad [1-3]. The Surgical Care Improvement Project (SCIP), initiated on 1 July 2006 [4], provides a mechanism for hospitals to receive financial incentives for efforts to reduce surgical complications, such as surgical site infections, perioperative myocardial infarction, and venous thromboembolism, through improved processes of perioperative care [5]. Current SCIP measures relate to the appropriate use of preoperative antibiotics (selection, timing, and discontinuation), routine venous thromboembolism prophylaxis (ordering and administration), appropriate hair removal practices, perioperative use of beta-blockers, and perioperative normothermia and normoglycemia in selected patients.

Medicare payment rules create financial incentives for hospitals to report data on SCIP measures, as hospitals that do not submit data on selected measures are subject to Medicare reimbursement reduction [6]. Per the Deficit Reduction Act of 2005, a payment reduction of 2.0 percentage points is implemented for hospitals that fail to report successfully [7]. According to the Centers for Medicare and Medicaid Services (CMS), as of March 2009, nearly 3,700 hospitals reported performance of SCIP measures [8], with only 30 general acute-care hospitals nationwide abstaining from collection and reporting of such data [9]. Of participating facilities, 97% have received the full annual payment incentive from Medicare each year [7].

Despite high rates of participation in SCIP, little is known regarding the mechanisms hospitals may employ to promote physician participation in reporting. Multiple potential strategies exist for a hospital to encourage

* Correspondence: lee.fleisher@uphs.upenn.edu
[1]Department of Anesthesiology and Critical Care, University of Pennsylvania, 3400 Spruce Street, Philadelphia, PA 19104, USA
Full list of author information is available at the end of the article

better practices at the level of the individual provider, including the re-engineering of clinical systems [10], provision of feedback or education to care providers [11], and creation of department-level or physician-level incentives for improved performance [12].

Efforts to understand the range of strategies used to promote physician adherence to reporting performance measures within US hospitals have implications for health policy, potentially offering insights to inform the design and dissemination of future quality improvement initiatives. To explore hospital strategies to promote anesthesiologist participation in SCIP, a pilot survey of anesthesiology department administrators at general acute-care hospitals in the US was undertaken. Respondents were surveyed on a range of hospital-level and department-level variables and on participation in SCIP, focusing on reasons for participation in the reporting of a SCIP measure relating to the dosing of preoperative antibiotics.

Methods

After obtaining approval from the University of Pennsylvania Institutional Review Board, a multiple-choice questionnaire was developed based on literature review, clinical experience, and consultation with experts in quality improvement. The final 12-item survey instrument included items relating to hospital characteristics (hospital affiliation, urban/rural location, state, bed number), anesthesia department business model (private practice, hospital employed, academic group practices, Department of Veterans Affairs, other governmental agency), participation in SCIP reporting, hospital practices for ordering of preoperative antibiotics, hospital practices for administration of preoperative antibiotics, and participation in pay-for-performance measures.

Respondents were offered four common reasons for SCIP participation, focusing on SCIP-INF-1, a measure relating to perioperative antibiotic administration; respondents indicated one 'primary' and one or more 'secondary' reasons for participation. The four reasons for SCIP participation were: (1) participation as part of a voluntary quality improvement initiative, (2) participation in preparation for pay-for-performance, (3) participation as mandated by the anesthesia department's service contract, and (4) participation in response to an incentive from the hospital.

Hospital data from the 2005 American Hospital Association (AHA) survey was used to identify hospitals of comparable size and to obtain hospital addresses. Our survey sample was restricted to acute-care facilities with at least 200 beds, yielding a total survey sample of 1,426 hospitals. The 12-item questionnaire was distributed through a single mailing via first-class US mail to all hospitals identified in our study population and was addressed to 'Chair, Department of Anesthesiology'. Completed questionnaires were returned via facsimile; no monetary or material

incentive was provided to survey subjects. All questionnaires were mailed in February 2008; a period of four months was allowed for survey responses.

One investigator entered all study data. The full 2006 AHA sample, the most recent available data at the time of analysis, was used as a comparison group for pilot survey respondents. The survey respondents and AHA sample were compared on US Census region, hospital bed size, rural status, and hospital ownership using Pearson's χ^2 test. To create categories comparable to those used in the AHA survey, survey respondents indicating their ownership status as 'University Affiliated' were grouped with private, not-for-profit facilities. Descriptive statistics determined the proportion reporting SCIP participation and the distribution of department business models identified by survey respondents. The distribution of reported reasons for SCIP participation was determined. All analyses were conducted using Stata 10.0 Software (StataCorp, College Station, TX, USA).

Results

Questionnaires were mailed to 1,426 US hospitals. Completed questionnaires were received from 421 (29.5%) of the study sample. Table 1 displays characteristics reported by survey respondents. Of all survey respondents, the largest proportion worked in hospitals located in the Northeastern USA (33.9%). The χ^2 analysis revealed significant differences between the present survey respondents and all US hospitals with 200 or more beds, as identified in the 2006 AHA survey. Overall, AHA survey data indicated a

Table 1 Descriptive characteristics of survey respondents

	Respondents, N (%)	2006 AHA sample, N (%)	P value
SCIP participation	408 (96.9%)	-	
Region			<0.0001
Northeast	140 (33.9)	296 (20.9)	
South	117 (28.3)	548 (38.7)	
Midwest	93 (22.5)	317 (22.4)	
West	63 (15.2)	254 (18.0)	
Hospital location			<0.0001
Rural	47 (11.7)	17 (1.2)	
Hospital ownership			0.003
Non-profit*	316 (75.2)	1,003 (70.0)	
For profit	45 (10.7)	177 (12.4)	
VA	16 (3.8)	63 (4.4)	
Other governmental	43 (10.2)	189 (13.2)	
Hospital size			0.07
Over 500 beds	97 (23.4)	277 (19.3)	
Under 500 beds	318 (76.6)	1,155 (80.7)	

*Includes 86 respondents indicating 'university-affiliated hospital'.
SCIP, Surgical Care Improvement Project.

greater proportion of hospitals located in the Southern USA (38.7%) and fewer in the Northeast (20.9%) than the respondents to the present survey ($P <0.0001$). The majority of respondents to the present survey reported working in a facility with 200 to 500 beds (76.6%), which did not differ significantly from respondents to the 2006 AHA survey (80.7%) ($P = 0.07$). The fraction of rural hospitals differed significantly from the AHA sample, in which only 1.2% of hospitals were located in rural areas ($P <0.0001$).

In terms of hospital ownership, survey respondents worked primarily at private, not-for-profit hospitals (n = 230, 54.8%) and university-affiliated hospitals (n = 86, 20.5%). Non-profit status was not specifically indicated by all who identified as a 'university-affiliated hospital', however, those facilities were considered to be non-profit entities for comparison with the 2006 AHA survey. The χ^2 analysis revealed significant differences between the distribution of our study sample and that of the 2006 AHA survey sample in regards to hospital ownership ($P = 0.003$).

The business model for the majority of respondents was a private practice group (64.4%). Fewer reported working directly for a hospital (12.4%), an academic group practice separate from a medical school or health system (11.6%), an academic group practice within a medical school or health system (5.2%), an independent contractor (1.9%), the US Department of Veterans Affairs (3.6%), or the US Military or Public Health Service (0.7%).

Most respondents participated in SCIP reporting for pre-operative antibiotic administration (n = 408, 96.9%). Table 2 lists the reasons indicated for SCIP participation. The majority of respondents (62.5%) indicated that participation in SCIP occurred for primarily voluntary reasons. A minority indicated an incentive from the hospital (4.2%) or a contractual mandate (2.5%) as the primary reason for participation. Considering primary and secondary reasons for SCIP participation, the proportions indicating a hospital incentive or a contractual mandate rose to 14.7% and 5.9%, respectively. Approximately one-fifth (20.2%) of

Table 2 Reasons for participation in the Surgical Care Improvement Project (SCIP)*

Reasons for SCIP participation	Primary reason		All reasons	
	N (%)	95% CI	N (%)	95% CI
Part of a quality improvement initiative-voluntary	255 (62.5)	57.8 to 67.2	299 (73.3)	69.0 to 77.6
Mandated by anesthesia service contract	10 (2.5)	0.9 to 3.9	24 (5.9)	3.6 to 8.2
Preparation for pay-for performance	37 (9.1)	6.3 to 11.9	171(41.9)	3.7 to 4.7
Incentive from hospital for participation	17(4.2)	2.2 to 6.1	60 (14.7)	11.3 to 18.2

*20.2% (85) of respondents provided no reason, and 21.8% (89) of respondents provided no primary reason. CI, confidence interval.

respondents did not select a primary or secondary reason for SCIP participation.

Discussion

Defining the strategies employed by hospitals to encourage adherence to reporting performance of quality measures is of relevance to current and planned efforts to improve perioperative care. CMS's ongoing initiative to link payment to SCIP reporting [13], its planned expansion to include additional SCIP measures for 2010 and 2011 [7], and the proposed role of SCIP measures as a model for a Medicare pay-for-performance program [14,15], all suggest that reporting of such measures will continue to grow in importance as a part of the structure of reimbursement for perioperative care in the US. As a result, policymakers and hospital administrators will have a growing need for information describing optimal strategies to encourage SCIP participation across a range of hospitals.

This pilot study of 1,426 anesthesia department chairs suggests that strategies to promote SCIP participation among anesthesiologists vary among hospitals. While the majority of our 421 respondents indicated voluntary participation in SCIP, we observed that a minority reported incentives or contractual mandates as primary or secondary reasons for SCIP participation. At these facilities, it appears likely that SCIP participation has been achieved without use of financial or other incentives (or contractual mandates) for the clinicians providing the data; while we did not collect data on actual adherence to SCIP measures, this finding offers a preliminary suggestion that anesthesiologists may be willing to participate in quality improvement initiatives on a voluntary basis.

These results should be interpreted in the context of multiple limitations. Our 29.5% response rate, combined with differences noted between respondent hospitals and those in the US at large, as indicated by the 2006 AHA survey, limits the degree to which our findings can be generalized to US hospitals at large. Eligible participants only received one mailing and no follow-up was completed. Further, as the study sample was constrained to hospitals over 200 beds our findings may not be applicable to smaller hospitals. We specified four potential reasons for SCIP participation *a priori*, yet some respondents likely participated in SCIP for other reasons, which we were unable to assess through the present survey instrument. Roughly 20% of survey respondents failed to provide a reason for their participation, which could indicate either the reason they participated was not offered as an answer option or that they did not know why they participated, limiting our ability to assess our principal hypothesis. Allowing respondents an answer option of 'other, please explain' would have given participants the opportunity to provide their alternative reasoning.

Further, although it cannot be determined from the present survey, the possibility exists that responses may have been influenced by the existence of a similar quality-reporting program whose goals overlap with those of SCIP. Specifically, the Physician Quality Reporting System (PQRS), Medicare's pay-for-reporting initiative, includes measures related to antibiotic dosing [16]; thus, participation in PQRS could have been conceivably confused by survey respondents for SCIP participation. Both SCIP and PQRS are measures of quality compliance with overlap in multiple content areas. The key difference is that in PQRS, financial incentives are targeted at individual physicians or physician practices, while SCIP offers incentives to hospitals. Whether there was any confusion, given the similarities of these two measures, is unknown. Lastly, as we were unable to confirm the identity of the individual completing the survey, we have limited insight into the degree to which survey responses reflect actual hospital practices.

Despite these limitations, our findings have relevance to current and planned perioperative quality improvement efforts. As regulators and payers seek to promote improvements in the quality of hospital care through an increasing number of reportable quality measures [7], effective implementation of such quality improvement initiatives will require an understanding of the considerations affecting individual hospitals' efforts to encourage individual physicians.

Conclusions

Our study offers preliminary insight into the range of strategies now in use in US hospitals to encourage physician participation in SCIP. The results of this pilot study suggest future hypotheses for exploration. For example, though we found high rates of departmental SCIP participation, we did not collect data on rates of adherence to specific SCIP measures, or the types of efforts departments engaged in to collect and report data to SCIP. Understanding variations in the mechanics of data collection and reporting may hold potential benefits by highlighting practices and procedures for data collection that may be more or less efficient and accurate than others. Further, it would be of interest to determine whether a direct feedback of that data, built into the data collection system, would motivate providers to improve quality. We encourage further research to support hospital administrators and quality advocates in improving the care delivered in the perioperative period.

Competing interests
The authors declare that they have no competing interests.

Acknowledgements
The authors acknowledge the assistance of Jill Panichelli MPH, Anje C Van Berckelaer MD, and Zachary F Meisel MD.

Author details
[1]Department of Anesthesiology and Critical Care, University of Pennsylvania, 3400 Spruce Street, Philadelphia, PA 19104, USA. [2]Department of Biostatistics and Epidemiology, University of Pennsylvania, 423 Guardian Drive, Blockley Hall, Philadelphia, PA 19104-6021, USA. [3]Department of Anesthesia, Brigham and Women's Hospital, 75 Francis StreetBoston, MA 02115, USA.

Authors' contributions
RS was involved with data analysis, manuscript preparation, and approval of the final manuscript. MN was involved with data analysis, manuscript preparation, review of original study data and data analysis, and approval of the final manuscript. AB was involved with study design, conduct of study, and approval of the final manuscript. LF was involved with study design, conduct of study, manuscript preparation, review of original study data and data analysis, and approval of the final manuscript. All authors read and approved the final manuscript.

References
1. Doran T, Fullwood C, Gravelle H, Reeves D, Kontopantelis E, Hiroeh U, Roland M: **Pay-for-performance programs in family practices in the United Kingdom.** *N Engl J Med* 2006, **355**:375–384.
2. Snyder L, Neubauer RL: **Pay-for-performance principles that promote patient-centered care: an ethics manifesto.** *Ann Intern Med* 2007, **147**:792–794.
3. Custers T, Hurley J, Klazinga NS, Brown AD: **Selecting effective incentive structures in health care: A decision framework to support health care purchasers in finding the right incentives to drive performance.** *BMC Health Serv Res* 2008, **8**:66.
4. Bratzler DW, Houck PM: **Antimicrobial prophylaxis for surgery: an advisory statement from the National Surgical Infection Prevention Project.** *Am J Surg* 2005, **189**:395–404.
5. *MedQic: SCIP Project Information.* http://qualitynet.org/dcs/ContentServer?c=MQParents&pagename=Medqic%2FContent%2FParentShellTemplate&cid=1137346750659&parentName=TopicCat.
6. Lin DM: In *Surgical Care Improvement Project: Improve Performance, Reduce Complications, and Comply With CMS.* Edited by Buckley L. Marblehead, MA: HCPro, Inc; 2007.
7. CMS Office of Public Affairs: *Proposals to improve quality of care in inpatient stays in acute care hospitals in FY 2010.* http://www.cms.hhs.gov/apps/media/fact_sheets.asp.
8. *Centers for Medicare and Medicaid: National Summary Statistics for RHQDAPU clinical process measures as reported on Hospital Compare March 2009.* http://www.cms.hhs.gov/HospitalQualityInits/downloads/HospitalNationalLevelPerformance.pdf.
9. QualityNet: *Hospitals that chose not to participate in APU for FY 2009.* http://www.qualitynet.org/dcs/ContentServer?c=Page&pagename=QnetPublic%2FPage%2FQnetTier4&cid=1228749194181.
10. Anthony D, Chetty VK, Kartha A, McKenna K, DePaoli MR, Jack B: *Re-engineering the hospital discharge: an example of a multifaceted process evaluation.* http://www.dtic.mil/cgi-bin/GetTRDoc?AD=ADA434087&Location=U2&doc=GetTRDoc.pdf.
11. Sautter KM, Bokhour BG, White B, Young GJ, Burgess JF Jr, Berlowitz D, Wheeler JR: **The early experience of a hospital-based pay-for-performance program.** *J Healthc Manag* 2007, **52**:95–108.
12. American Hospital Association: *Roundtable to discuss the Centers for Medicare & Medicaid Services' Hospital Value-based Purchasing Program Implementation Plan, Committee on Finance, United States Senate March 6, 2008.* http://www.aha.org/aha/testimony/2008/080306-tes-cms-vbp.pdf.
13. Buckley L: **CMS outlines value-based program.** http://www.healthleadersmedia.com/content/HOM-201274/CMS-Outlines-ValueBased-Program.html.
14. Jones RS, Brown C, Opelka F: **Surgeon compensation: "Pay for performance," the American College of Surgeons National Surgical Quality Improvement Program, the Surgical Care Improvement Program, and other considerations.** *Surgery* 2005, **138**:829–836.
15. Patterson P: **Surgical Care Improvement Project: four years later, what's the status?** *OR Manager* 2009, **25**:7 9.

Significant discrepancies exist between clinician assessment and patient self-assessment of functional capacity by validated scoring tools during preoperative evaluation

John Whittemore Stokes[1], Jonathan Porter Wanderer[2] and Matthew David McEvoy[2*]

Abstract

Background: Preoperative assessment of functional capacity is necessary to direct decisions regarding cardiac evaluation and may help identify patients at high risk for perioperative complications. Patient self-triage regarding functional capacity could be useful for discerning which patients benefit from a clinician evaluation at a Preoperative Evaluation Center prior to the day of surgery. We evaluated the feasibility of preoperative, patient self-triage regarding functional capacity.

Methods: Patients were recruited immediately prior to their preoperative evaluation. Study participants completed electronic versions of the Duke Activity Status Index (DASI) and the Patient-Reported Outcomes Measurement System (PROMIS)–Short Form 12a–Physical Function. DASI and PROMIS questionnaire responses were scored and evaluated for correlation with clinician assessments of functional capacity. Correlation was analyzed around the dichotomous outcome of <4 metabolic equivalents of task (METs) or ≥4 METs. Patients also evaluated the usability of the questionnaires.

Results: After IRB approval, 204 patients were enrolled and completed both DASI and PROMIS questionnaires. Clinicians assessed functional capacity at <4 METs for 109 patients (53.4 %) compared to 18 (8.8 %) patient self-assessments <4 METs as estimated by DASI. These results represent a significant discrepancy between assessments (Fisher's exact, two-tailed P value <0.0001). The standard T-score of PROMIS estimates of functional capacity correlated with DASI estimates (R^2 0.76). The mean and standard deviation for PROMIS T-scores were 43.3 and 9.86, respectively (mean 50.0; SD 10.0 for the general population).

Of the 203 patients who completed the entire study survey, 192 (94.6 %) stated that they did not require assistance from another person, and 187 (94 %) responded either "agree" or "strongly agree" to the DASI questionnaire being "easy to understand" and "easy to complete;" 186 (93 %) and 188 (94 %), respectively, responded similarly to the PROMIS questionnaire.

Conclusions: While both electronic questionnaires were easy to understand and complete for most study participants, there was a significant discrepancy between clinician assessments and patient self-assessments of functional capacity. Further study is needed to determine if either patient self-triage by means of activity questionnaires or clinician evaluation is valid and reliable in the preoperative setting.

Keywords: Functional capacity, Self-triage, Preoperative assessment, Perioperative risk, Electronic questionnaire

* Correspondence: matthew.d.mcevoy@vanderbilt.edu
[2]Multispecialty Adult Anesthesiology, Vanderbilt University Medical Center, 1301 Medical Center Drive, 4648 The Vanderbilt Clinic, Nashville, TN 37232-5614, USA
Full list of author information is available at the end of the article

Background

Valid and reliable assessment of functional capacity is an important component of the preoperative evaluation. Patient functional capacity directs decisions about preoperative cardiac evaluation and is useful for risk stratification prior to surgery (Fleisher et al. 2014). Poor performance on formal exercise tolerance testing reliably correlates to increased risk for perioperative complications in several different patient populations and treatment settings (Snowden et al. 2010; Wilson et al. 2010). However, because of expense and practical considerations, exercise tolerance testing is not routinely performed prior to non-cardiac surgery in the USA. Functional capacity is commonly assessed through obtaining the patient's history regarding their ability to perform certain physical activities. Clinician-elicited stair-climbing ability has been shown to correlate to perioperative cardiac events and other complications (Reilly et al. 1999), and categorical metabolic equivalents of task (METs) estimates, as determined through clinician history of physical capabilities, have been shown in a univariate analysis to be predictive of perioperative cardiac outcomes (Wiklund et al. 2001).

Activity questionnaires, such as the Duke Activity Status Index (DASI) (Hlatky et al. 1989) and the Patient-Reported Outcomes Measurement System (PROMIS)–Short Form 12a–Physical Function (www.nihpromis.org), are available to guide clinicians when estimating METs in the preoperative assessment of functional capacity (Fleisher et al. 2014). Patient-completed versions of the DASI questionnaire have been shown to correlate moderately well with physiologic measures of functional capacity or exercise tolerance in several clinical settings (Dunagan et al. 2013; Shaw et al. 2006; Struthers et al. 2008), and patient reported exercise capacity has been shown to be predictive of survival in vascular surgery patients (Boult et al. 2015). Patient self-assessment of functional capacity by means of electronic questionnaires would allow METs estimates to be known prior to in-person, preoperative evaluations, enabling preoperative triage of patients based on estimated functional capacity, a core component of preoperative evaluation (Fleisher et al. 2014).

In this study, we sought to evaluate the feasibility patient self-triage regarding functional capacity by investigating the correlation between clinician assessments and patient self-assessment of functional capacity, as assisted by electronic, patient-completed DASI and PROMIS questionnaires. In addition, we analyzed patient survey data regarding the usability of these two validated activity questionnaires.

Methods

Population and enrollment

The study was approved by the Vanderbilt University Institutional Review Board. All patients, age 18 years or older, who were scheduled for elective surgery at our institution and seen in the Preoperative Evaluation Center (PEC) prior to their surgery were eligible for enrollment. Patients undergoing moderate to high-risk surgeries or who have moderate to high-risk comorbidities are referred to our PEC by their surgeon. A member of the study team recruited patients immediately prior to the preoperative evaluation and obtained written informed consent. Baseline data was not available for power analysis prior to initiating enrollment; therefore, a convenience sample of patients was recruited during the month of March 2015.

Study questionnaire

Prior to initiation of the clinician encounter, participants were asked to independently complete electronic questionnaires on a tablet computer (iPad, Apple Inc.; Cupertino, CA). The DASI and the PROMIS questionnaires, in addition to questions to assess the comparative usability of these two formal activity questionnaires (see Additional files 1, 2, and 3), were administered using the research electronic data capture system (Harris et al. 2009). The study administrator was not present with the patients as they completed the questionnaire. Patients were asked to complete the questionnaire without assistance but were permitted help from an accompanying family member, friend, or care provider if necessary.

Clinician evaluation and functional capacity assessment

Following completion of the study questionnaire, each patient underwent preoperative clinical evaluation. The clinicians performed and documented the evaluation in accordance with the standard practice for all preoperative consultations in the PEC at our institution. Routine documentation of PEC evaluations includes estimating functional capacity in our electronic medical record as one of five categories: excellent (>7 METs); very good (5–7 METs); good (4 METs); fair (2–3 METs); and poor (1–2 METs). As a reference tool, clinicians are provided with a list of physical activities and the METs associated with those activities as described in the 2007 American College of Cardiology/American Heart Association Guidelines on Perioperative Cardiac Evaluation and Care for Noncardiac Surgery (Fleisher et al. 2007). Additionally, clinicians have structured documentation for reasons for physical limitations, including angina, dyspnea, claudication, and fatigue, as well as the ability to provide free text descriptions of other reasons for physical function limitations. The clinicians performing the preoperative assessments were blinded to the patient responses on the DASI and PROMIS forms.

Questionnaire scoring and data elements

At the conclusion of patient enrollment, the DASI and PROMIS questionnaire elements were scored. The DASI questionnaire was scored according to the published methodology to estimate functional capacity in terms of METs (Hlatky et al. 1989). Individual DASI questions carry different weight, and the questionnaire can be scored to produce a METs estimate from 2.74 to 9.89 METs. A raw score for the PROMIS questionnaire is generated from the responses to the five-point Likert options. Raw scores range from 6 to 60 and correlated to a standard T-score. The correlation of raw scores to standard T-scores is developed from population statistics of functional capacity.

Responses to the questions regarding the clarity and usability of the DASI and PROMIS electronic questionnaires were directly analyzed for comparative usability of these two formal activity questionnaires.

From the electronic medical record, we retrieved documented clinician estimates of functional capacity, as well as American Society of Anesthesiologists (ASA) physical status. The previously described categorical estimates of functional capacity were then compared to the results from patient-completed DASI and PROMIS electronic questionnaires. We also searched the medical record for study participants who had completed exercise tolerance testing or exercise stress testing.

Statistical analysis

To determine the correlation between clinician assessments and patient self-assessments of functional capacity, DASI METs estimates were compared to clinician categorical assessments of functional capacity using the dichotomous categories of ≥4 METs and <4 METs. Statistical correlation was analyzed using a two-tailed, Fisher's exact test. This METs threshold was chosen, as it is a branch point in the algorithm for preoperative evaluation of coronary artery disease, as described by the 2014 *American College of Cardiology/ American Heart Association Guideline on Perioperative Cardiovascular Evaluation and Management of Patients Undergoing Noncardiac Surgery* (Fleisher et al. 2014). The T-scores from the PROMIS questionnaire results were compared to the DASI METs estimates using linear regression analysis.

Results

After IRB approval, 211 patients consented for participation; 204 patients were eligible for inclusion in the final analysis of functional capacity assessments. Reasons for exclusion from the final analysis include failure to complete the survey (six patients) and absence of a documented clinician estimate of functional capacity (one patient). Of the six patients who did not complete the survey, two were due to clinician interruption, two were due to participant refusal to answer specific survey questions, one was due to inability to understand the questions, and one was due to accidental

closure of the electronic survey application. One patient completed both the DASI and PROMIS components of the survey and then accidentally closed the electronic survey application prior to completion of the final usability field; thus, only 203 participants are included in the final usability analysis.

Demographics

Of the 204 patients included in the final analysis of functional capacity assessments, the mean age was 56.8 (standard deviation 15.3); 32.2 % of the participants were classified as ASA I/II, 67.8 % ASA III/IV (Table 1).

Functional capacity estimates

Clinicians assessed functional capacity at <4 METs for 109 patients (53.4 %), while only 18 patients (8.8 %) assessed their functional capacity at <4 METs, as calculated by their responses on the DASI. These results represent a significant discrepancy between assessments around the clinically relevant point of 4 METs (Fisher's exact, two-tailed P value <0.0001). Graphical relationship between categorical clinician functional capacity assessments and DASI patient self-assessments is displayed in Figs. 1 and 2. The standard T-score of PROMIS estimates of functional capacity correlated linearly (R^2 0.76) with DASI estimates of functional capacity (see Fig. 3). The mean and standard deviation for PROMIS T-scores were 43.3 and 9.86, respectively (mean 50.0; SD 10.0 for the general population). No patients enrolled in our study had documentation of exercise testing; thus, comparison of clinician and patient assessments of functional capacity to physiologic measures of functional capacity was not possible.

Usability

Of the 203 included in the usability analysis, 192 (94.6 %) stated they did not require assistance from another person. One hundred eighty-seven (94 %) responded either "agree" or "strongly agree" to the DASI questionnaire being "easy

Table 1 Patient characteristics

Age	(Mean ± SD)
	56.8 ± 15.3
Gender	N (%)
Male	85 (41.7)
Female	119 (58.3)
ASA classification	N (%)
ASA 1	1 (0.5)
ASA 2	63 (31.7)
ASA 3	129 (64.8)
ASA 4	6 (3.0)

This table describes the demographics of the study population by age, gender, and American Society of Anesthesiologists (ASA) classification

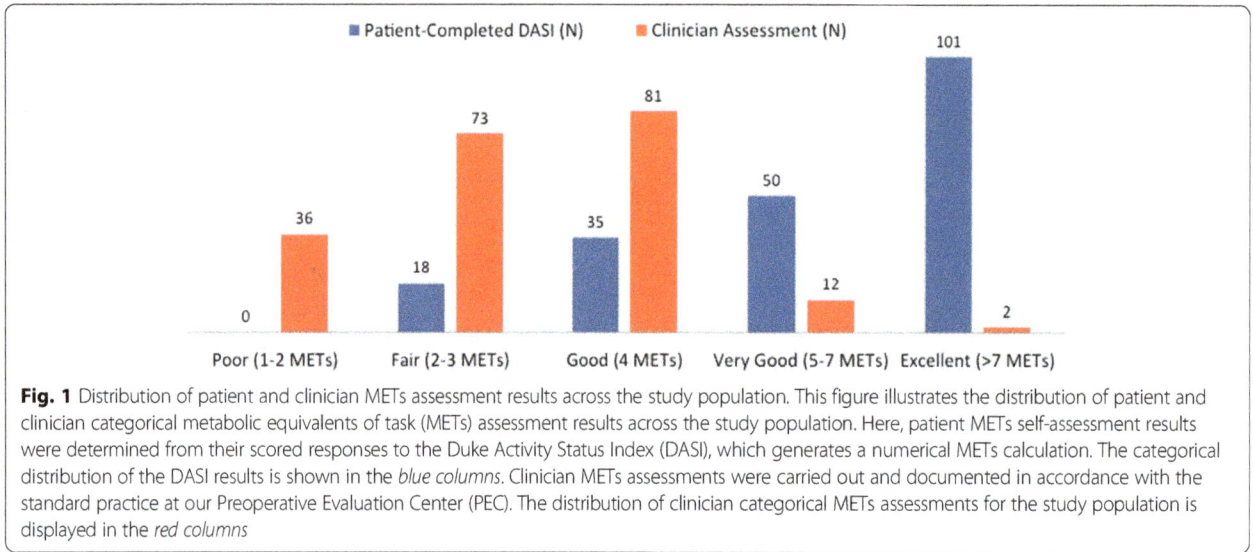

Fig. 1 Distribution of patient and clinician METs assessment results across the study population. This figure illustrates the distribution of patient and clinician categorical metabolic equivalents of task (METs) assessment results across the study population. Here, patient METs self-assessment results were determined from their scored responses to the Duke Activity Status Index (DASI), which generates a numerical METs calculation. The categorical distribution of the DASI results is shown in the *blue columns*. Clinician METs assessments were carried out and documented in accordance with the standard practice at our Preoperative Evaluation Center (PEC). The distribution of clinician categorical METs assessments for the study population is displayed in the *red columns*

to understand" and "easy to complete," and 186 (93 %) and 188 (94 %), respectively, responded similarly for the PROMIS questionnaire. See Table 2 for further usability data.

Discussion

The assessment of functional capacity is an integral component of the preoperative evaluation. We sought to determine whether patient self-assessment of functional capacity using electronic activity questionnaires is feasible and valid in the setting of preoperative evaluations. In our patient population, while both electronic questionnaires were easy to understand and complete for most study participants, there was a significant discrepancy between clinician assessments and patient assessments from formal valid questionnaires, particularly around the dichotomous result of whether or

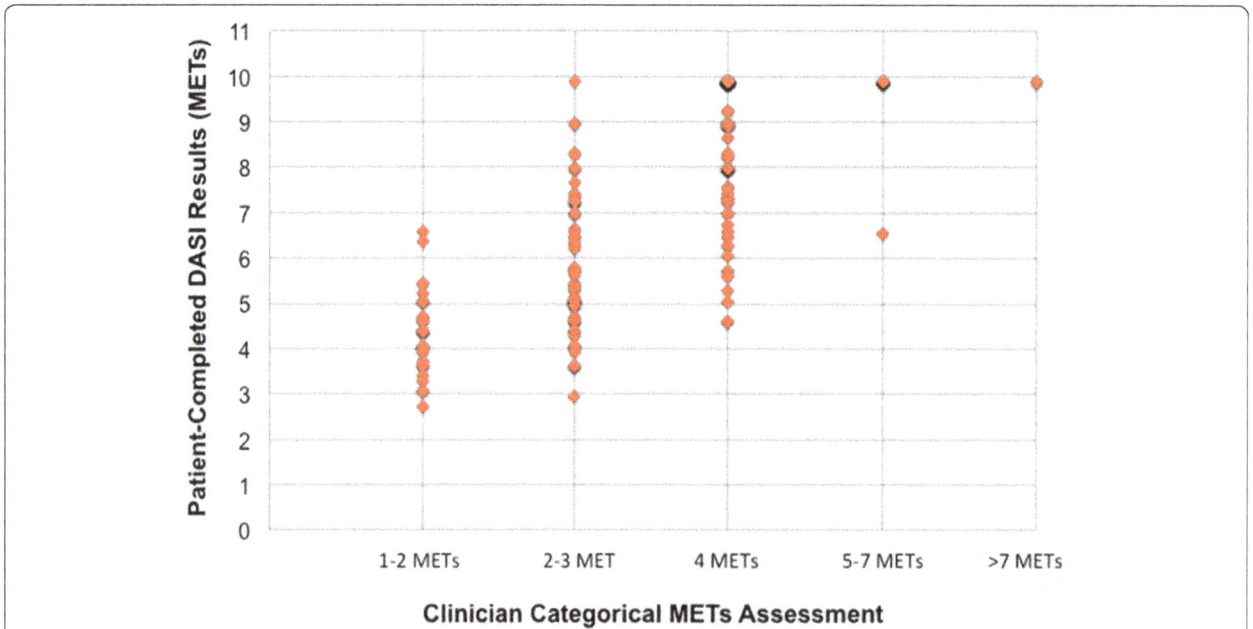

Fig. 2 Clinician vs. patient self-assessment (DASI results). This graph displays the discrepancy between clinician categorical assessments of functional capacity and patient self-assessments of functional capacity. Once again, patient self-assessments of functional capacity were determined from their scored responses to the Duke Activity Status Index (DASI), which generates calculated functional capacity in terms of metabolic equivalents of task (METs). At our Preoperative Evaluation Center, clinician functional capacity assessments are routinely documented in terms of the categorical groupings displayed on the x-axis. In this figure, the DASI patient self-assessments are plotted against clinician assessments of functional capacity. A lack of correlation is evident in this figure, particularly around the clinically significant value of four METs of physical work

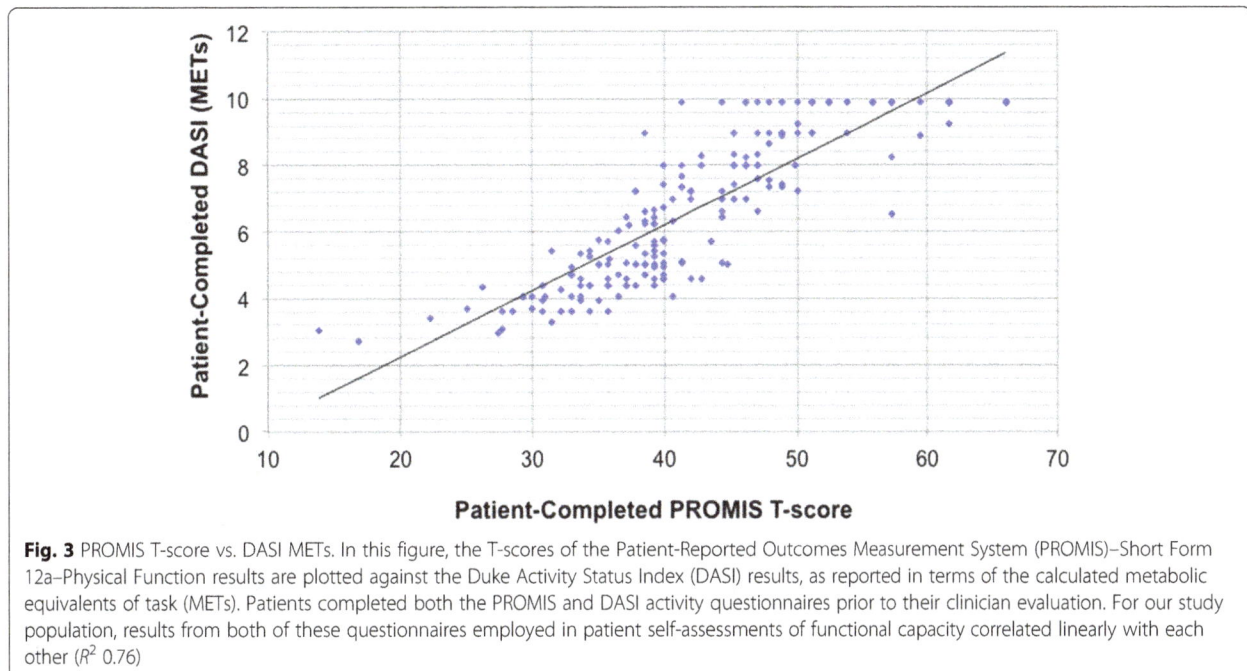

Fig. 3 PROMIS T-score vs. DASI METs. In this figure, the T-scores of the Patient-Reported Outcomes Measurement System (PROMIS)–Short Form 12a–Physical Function results are plotted against the Duke Activity Status Index (DASI) results, as reported in terms of the calculated metabolic equivalents of task (METs). Patients completed both the PROMIS and DASI activity questionnaires prior to their clinician evaluation. For our study population, results from both of these questionnaires employed in patient self-assessments of functional capacity correlated linearly with each other (R^2 0.76)

not a patient can achieve four or more METs of physical work.

METs assessment discrepancy

The significant discrepancy between clinician and patient assessments of functional capacity in our patient population highlights that a clinician-elicited history regarding physical capabilities may be very different than physical capabilities that are purely patient-reported. This distinction was evident even in the initial validation of the DASI (Hlatky et al. 1989). The DASI was developed in two phases, a development phase in which an interviewer asked the subjects questions regarding physical function, and a validation phase in which the subjects independently completed the initial version of the

DASI. In both phases, subjects underwent exercise tolerance testing after either the interview or completion of the DASI questionnaire. Both phases showed statistically significant correlation of "patient-reported" functional capacity to physiologic measures of functional capacity; however, the correlation was better in the development phase (Spearman's correlation 0.81) than in the validation phase (Spearman's correlation 0.58) (Hlatky et al. 1989). It may be that the personal interaction between interviewer and interviewee increases the accuracy of patient-reported physical capabilities. McGlade et al. (2001) demonstrated that patient-completed DASI scores correlated with a next of kin's DASI assessment of functional capacity; however, patients slightly overestimated their capabilities as compared to their next of kin (McGlade et al. 2001). In our study, participants were often accompanied by a spouse, friend, child, or other care provider, who may have added to the interaction through verbal or non-verbal communication with the clinician, which could increase the accuracy of clinician functional capacity assessments.

Reliability of patient-reported health information

Several studies have evaluated the ability of patients to identify clinical risk factors in the setting of chronic diseases and demonstrated that patient-completed surveys regarding diagnosed medical conditions are probably at least as reliable as the medical record (Tisnado et al. 2006; Okura et al. 2004). It has also been shown that Revised Cardiac Risk Index (Lee et al. 1999) scores calculated from patient survey data correlate well with scores calculated from clinician documentation of risk factors (Manaktala et al. 2013). However, these studies

Table 2 Electronic activity questionnaire usability results

	DASI	PROMIS
	n (%)	n (%)
Independent completion	192 (94.6)	192 (94.6)
Easy to understand	187 (93.5)	186 (93.0)
Easy to complete	187 (93.5)	188 (94.0)
Which was easier to complete?	139 (68.1)	64 (31.5)
	Mean ± SD	Mean ± SD
Completion time (min:s)	01:55 ± 02:08	02:29 ± 1:42

This table displays the results of the responses to survey questions regarding the usability of the two activity questionnaires employed for patient self-triage of functional capacity, the Duke Activity Status Index (DASI), and the Patient-Reported Outcomes Measurement System (PROMIS)–Short Form 12a–Physical Function. The majority of study participants found these questionnaires easy to understand and easy to complete using a first generation iPad. The average time to complete both surveys was less than 3 min

SD standard deviation

did not evaluate the reliability of patient-reported functional capacity, which may be different than other types of patient-reported health information.

Patients may have an increased tendency to over-estimate their physical capabilities when completing an activity questionnaire. Dunagan et al. (2013) showed slight over-estimation of METs level by the DASI questionnaire when compared to exercise tolerance testing in the setting of cardiac rehabilitation, although this over-estimation did not represent a significant difference in their sample (Dunagan et al. 2013). Formal activity questionnaires are traditionally validated by having participants complete the questionnaire and then subsequently asking patients to undergo a physiologic measure of functional capacity, such as exercise tolerance testing (Hlatky et al. 1989; Struthers et al. 2008). In the absence of being required to demonstrate physical capabilities, as was the case in our study, participants may have an increased tendency to exaggerate physical capabilities. McGlade et al. (2001) found that of 68 patients who answered affirmatively to DASI question number four regarding stair climbing, 13 patients were unable to demonstrate the ability to climb a flight of stairs (McGlade et al. 2001). The authors concluded that rather than asking patients if they are capable of a physical task, it may be more useful to ask them to demonstrate their ability to do so (McGlade et al. 2001).

It is also possible that clinician underestimation of functional capacity contributed to the discrepancy demonstrated in our study. Anecdotally, the authors have observed that clinicians often use one or two history questions in the assessment of a patient's functional capacity. Thus, a negative response to a single question may lead a clinician to underestimate a patient's functional capacity when a patient is capable of achieving four METs of physical work during activities not addressed by the clinician.

Additionally, while the clinician functional capacity tool employed at our PEC includes phrases to describe physical activity that are very similar or equivalent to the language used in DASI questions, the categorical METs assessments assigned to a particular group of activities does not necessarily correspond to the DASI scoring formula. Thus, it is possible for clinician and patient-completed DASI METs estimates to be discrepant, even if patients described their physical capabilities to clinicians in complete concordance with how they responded to DASI questions.

Usability

While there is poor correlation between clinician and questionnaire estimates of functional capacity, the majority of our study participants found the electronic questionnaires easy to understand and easy to complete. Patients were able to complete these surveys on a touch-screen, tablet computer independently and in a timely manner. Our patient-entered responses to the usability of the electronic questionnaires suggest that this modality would be acceptable for application in patient-self triage if self-assessment of functional capacity using a formal activity questionnaire was validated as an accurate method of determining functional capacity in the preoperative setting.

Limitations

As there were no physiologic measures of functional capacity obtained on patients enrolled in our study, we cannot comment on the validity of either clinician assessments or patient assessments of functional capacity relative to performance on physiologic measures of functional capacity, such as cardiopulmonary exercise testing. Without physiologic measures of functional capacity, we cannot determine whether the discrepancy between clinician and questionnaire estimates of functional capacity represents patient over-estimation or clinician underestimation of functional capacity. Similarly, without data regarding the surgical outcomes of the study participants, we cannot determine whether clinician or patient assessments of functional capacity are more clinically relevant for predicting surgical complications or major adverse cardiac events, nor can we determine the relative clinical significance patient responses to particular survey questions, such as stair-climbing ability. Whether or not patients can accurately report their functional capacity or clinicians accurately assess functional capacity, both assessments may still be useful in screening for high-risk patients (Reilly et al. 1999; Wiklund et al. 2001; Boult et al. 2015).

Directions for future study

Electronic versions of formal activity questionnaires have theoretical potential to enable patient self-triage regarding functional capacity. As it is unclear which patients may benefit from a clinician evaluation at a PEC prior to the day of surgery, implementation of patient self-assessments using such tools could improve the efficiency and quality of preoperative evaluations while reducing costs by limiting unnecessary evaluations and testing in patients who have good functional capacity. However, further work is needed to determine whether patients accurately assess their own functional capacity in the preoperative setting using electronic versions of formal activity questionnaires. Future study is also needed to determine whether self-assessment of functional capacity by means of electronic questionnaires can predict perioperative complications or major adverse cardiac events. Finally, since functional capacity is commonly assessed by clinicians, more study is needed to determine whether clinicians accurately and reliably assess a patient's functional capacity through routine history questions.

Conclusions

Our patient population found electronic versions of both the DASI and PROMIS activity questionnaires easy to understand and complete, suggesting a potential for application of similar tools for patient self-triage prior to preoperative evaluations. However, we found a significant discrepancy between clinician and patient self-assessment of functional capacity. Before preoperative, patient self-triage regarding functional capacity is implemented, more study is needed to determine whether patients accurately assess their own functional capacity using activity questionnaires. Additionally, our results highlight the importance of the distinction between clinician-elicited and patient-reported functional capacity, as the two may not be equivalent.

Additional files

Additional file 1: Usability Survey. This file represents the survey completed by participants to assess the usability of the two formal activity questionnaires employed in this study for patient self-triage regarding functional capacity. (DOCX 73 kb)

Additional file 2: Patient-Reported Outcomes Measurement System (PROMIS)–Short Form 12a–Physical Function. This file is a text version of the PROMIS–Short Form 12a–Physical Function formal activity questionnaire. (PDF 46 kb)

Additional file 3: Duke Activity Status Index (DASI). This file is a text version of the Duke Activity Status Index (DASI) formal activity questionnaire. (PDF 43 kb)

Abbreviations
ASA, American Society of Anesthesiologists; DASI, Duke Activity Status Index; METs, metabolic equivalents of task; PEC, Preoperative Evaluation Center; PROMIS, Patient-Reported Outcomes Measurement Information System

Acknowledgements
We would like to thank Martha Tanner for her assistance in final preparation and formatting of the manuscript.

Funding
Dr. Wanderer is supported by the Foundation for Anesthesia Education and Research (FAER) and the Anesthesia Quality Institute (AQI), Mentored Research Training Grant in Health Services Research (MRTG-HSR).

Authors' contributions
JS helped has seen the original study data, reviewed the analysis of the data, conduct the study, enrolled participants, analyzed the data, and wrote the manuscript. JW has seen the original study data, reviewed the analysis of the data, designed the study, advised in the data analysis, edited the manuscript, and is the author responsible for archiving the study files. MM has seen the original study data, reviewed the analysis of the data, participated in study design, data analysis, and edited the manuscript. All authors read and approved the manuscript.

Authors' information
Dr. McEvoy receives funding for research from the GE Foundation and Edwards Life Sciences. This project did not have funding or involvement from either of these entities. Neither entity is referenced in the manuscript. Dr. Wanderer is supported by the Foundation for Anesthesia Education and Research (FAER) and the Anesthesia Quality Institute (AQI), Mentored Research Training Grant in Health Services Research (MRTG-HSR).

Competing interests
The authors declare that they have no competing interests.

Author details
[1]Vanderbilt University School of Medicine, 2215 Garland Avenue (Light Hall), Nashville, TN 37232, USA. [2]Multispecialty Adult Anesthesiology, Vanderbilt University Medical Center, 1301 Medical Center Drive, 4648 The Vanderbilt Clinic, Nashville, TN 37232-5614, USA.

References
Boult M et al. Self-reported fitness of American Society of Anesthesiologists class 3 patients undergoing endovascular aortic aneurism repair predicts patient survival. J Vasc Surg. 2015;62:299–303.

Dunagan J, Adams J, Cheng D, Barton S, Bigej-Cerqua J, Mims L, Molden J, Anderson V. Development and evaluation of a treadmill-based exercise tolerance test in cardiac rehabilitation. Proceedings (Baylor Univ Med Center). 2013;26:247.

Fleisher LA, Beckman JA, Brown KA, Calkins H, Chaikof EL, Fleischmann KE, Freeman WK, Froehlich JB, Kasper EK, Kersten JR, Riegel B, Robb JF, Smith SC Jr, Jacobs AK, Adams CD, Anderson JL, Antman EM, Buller CE, Creager MA, Ettinger SM, Faxon DP, Fuster V, Halperin JL, Hiratzka LF, Hunt SA, Lytle BW, Nishimura R, Ornato JP, Page RL, Riegel B, Tarkington LG, Yancy CW. ACC/AHA 2007 guidelines on perioperative cardiovascular evaluation and care for noncardiac surgery: a report of the American College of Cardiology/American Heart Association Task Force on Practice Guidelines (Writing Committee to Revise the 2002 Guidelines on Perioperative Cardiovascular Evaluation for Noncardiac Surgery) developed in collaboration with the American Society of Echocardiography, American Society of Nuclear Cardiology, Heart Rhythm Society, Society of Cardiovascular Anesthesiologists, Society for Cardiovascular Angiography and Interventions, Society for Vascular Medicine and Biology, and Society for Vascular Surgery. J Am Coll Cardiol. 2007;17:1707–32.

Fleisher LA, Fleischmann KE, Auerbach AD, Barnason SA, Beckman JA, Bozkurt B, Davila-Roman VG, Gerhard-Herman MD, Holly TA, Kane GC, Marine JE, Nelson MT, Spencer CC, Thompson A, Ting HH, Uretsky BF, Wijeysundera DN. 2014 ACC/AHA guideline on perioperative cardiovascular evaluation and management of patients undergoing noncardiac surgery: a report of the American College of Cardiology/American Heart Association Task Force on Practice Guidelines. J of the Am Col of Cardiol. 2014;64:e77–137.

Harris PA, Taylor R, Thielke R, Payne J, Gonzalez N, Conde JG. Research electronic data capture (REDCap)—a metadata-driven methodology and workflow process for providing translational research informatics support. J Biomed Inform. 2009;42:377–81.

Hlatky MA, Boineau RE, Higginbotham MB, Lee KL, Mark DB, Califf RM, Cobb FR, Pryor DB. A brief self-administered questionnaire to determine functional capacity (the Duke Activity Status Index). Am J of Cardiol. 1989;64:651–4.

Lee TH, Marcantonio ER, Mangione CM, Thomas EJ, Polanczyk CA, Cook EF, Sugarbaker DJ, Donaldson MC, Poss R, Ho KKL, Ludwig LE, Pedan A, Goldman L. Derivation and prospective validation of a simple index for prediction of cardiac risk of major noncardiac surgery. Circulation. 1999;100:1043–9.

Manaktala S et al. Validation of pre-operative patient self-assessment of cardiac risk for non-cardiac surgery: foundations for decision support. AMIA Annu Symp Proc. 2013;2013:931–8.

McGlade DP et al. The use of a questionnaire and simple exercise test in the preoperative assessment of vascular surgery patients. Anaesth Intensive Care. 2001;29:520–6.

Okura Y et al. Agreement between self-report questionnaires and medical record data was substantial for diabetes, hypertension, myocardial infarction and stroke but not for heart failure. J Clin Epidemiol. 2004;57:1096–103.

Patient Reported Outcomes Measurement Information System SF 12a. National Institutes of Health. www.nihpromis.org. Accessed January 27, 2015.

Reilly DF, McNeely MJ, Doerner D, Greenberg DL, Staiger TO, Geist MJ, Vedovatti PA, Coffey JE, Mora MW, Johnson TR, Guray ED, Van Norman GA, Fihn SD. Self-reported exercise tolerance and the risk of serious perioperative complications. Arch of Intern Med. 1999;159:2185–92.

Shaw LJ, Olson MB, Kip K, Kelsey SF, Johnson BD, Mark DB, Reis SE, Mankad S, Rogers WJ, Pohost GM, Arant CB, Wessel TR, Chaitman BR, Sopko G, Handberg E, Pepine CJ, Merz CNB. The value of estimated functional capacity in estimating outcome: results from the NHBLI-Sponsored Women's Ischemia Syndrome Evaluation (WISE) study. J Am Col Cardiol. 2006;47:s36–43.

Snowden CP, Prentis JM, Anderson HL, Roberts DR, Randles D, Renton M, Manas DM. Submaximal cardiopulmonary exercise testing predicts complications and hospital length of stay in patients undergoing major elective surgery. Annals of Surg. 2010;251:535–41.

Struthers R, Erasmus P, Holmes K, Warman P, Collingwood A, Sneyd JR. Assessing fitness for surgery: a comparison of questionnaire, incremental shuttle walk, and cardiopulmonary exercise testing in general surgical patients. Br J Anaesth. 2008;101:774–80.

Tisnado DM et al. What is the concordance between the medical record and patient self-report as data sources for ambulatory care? Med Care. 2006;44:132–40.

Wiklund RA, Stein HD, Rosenbaum SH. Activities of daily living and cardiovascular complications following elective, noncardiac surgery. Yale J Bio Med. 2001;74:75.

Wilson RJT, Davies S, Yates D, Redman J, Stone M. Impaired functional capacity is associated with all-cause mortality after major elective intra-abdominal surgery. Brit J of Anaesth. 2010;105:297–303.

The incidence of un-indicated preoperative testing in a tertiary academic ambulatory center

Onyi C. Onuoha[1*], Michael B. Hatch[1], Todd A. Miano[2] and Lee A. Fleisher[3]

Abstract

Background: Despite existing evidence and guidelines advocating for appropriate risk stratification, ambulatory surgery in low-risk patients continues to be accompanied by a battery of routine tests prior to surgery. Using a single-center retrospective cohort study, we aimed to quantify the incidence of un-indicated preoperative testing in an academic ambulatory center by utilizing recommendations by the recently developed American Society of Anesthesiology (ASA) "Choosing Wisely" Top-5 list.

Methods: We utilized data from the EPIC medical records of 3111 patients who had ambulatory surgery at the Hospital of the University of Pennsylvania during a 6-month period. Data were abstracted from laboratory studies— complete blood count, electrolyte panel, coagulation studies, and cardiac studies—stress test, and echocardiogram obtained within 30 days prior to surgery. Preoperative tests obtained from each patient were categorized into "indicated" (ASA ≥ 3) and "un-indicated" (ASA 1 and 2) tests, and percentages were reported.

Results: During the study period, 52.9 % (95 % confidence interval (CI) 37.6–66.4) of all patients had at least one un-indicated laboratory test performed preoperatively. Further analysis revealed variation in the incidence of preoperative ordering between tests; 73 % of all complete blood counts (CBCs), 70 % of all metabolic panels, and 49 % of all coagulation studies were considered un-indicated by "Top-5 List" criteria. Stated differently, of the patients included in the sample, 51 % of patients received an un-indicated CBC, 41 % an un-indicated metabolic panel, and 16 % un-indicated coagulation studies. Twelve percent of "any un-indicated preoperative test" were obtained from ASA 1 healthy patients. Of the 587 patients less than 36 years old, 331 (56 %) had at least one test that was deemed un-indicated. Forty-one patients had either an echocardiogram or stress test ordered and performed within 30 days of surgery. Of these, eight (19.5 %) studies were un-indicated as determined by chart review.

Conclusions: The incidence of ordering "at least one un-indicated preoperative test" in low-risk patients undergoing low-risk surgery remains high even in academic tertiary institutions. In the emerging era of optimizing patient safety and financial accountability, further studies are needed to better understand the problem of overuse while identifying modifiable attitudes and institutional influences on perioperative practices among all stakeholders involved. Such information would drive the development of feasible interventions.

Keywords: Preoperative testing, Ambulatory, Low risk, Un-indicated, Routine, ASA (American Society of Anesthesiology), Laboratory test (complete blood count, metabolic panel, coagulation studies)

* Correspondence: Onyi.Onuoha@uphs.upenn.edu
This work has been presented at the following meeting: 9th Annual Pennsylvania Anesthesiology Resident Research Conference (PARRC), May 2014 at The University of Pittsburgh School of Medicine, Pittsburgh, PA. Won "Best Original Poster."
[1]Department of Anesthesiology and Critical Care, Perelman School of Medicine at the University of Pennsylvania, 3400 Spruce Street Dulles 680, Philadelphia, PA 19104, USA
Full list of author information is available at the end of the article

Background

With the release of the "Choosing Wisely" Top-5 lists of activities to avoid in 2013[1] (Onuoha et al. 2014a), the American Society of Anesthesiologists (ASA) identified five diagnostic tests or treatments that are commonly practiced in the perioperative setting but offer limited to no benefits to patients according to evidence-based studies and may incur significant costs to the health system[1] (Onuoha et al. 2014a; Onuoha et al. 2014b). Two of these items were preoperative recommendations focusing on unnecessary preoperative testing. They include the following:

Don't obtain baseline laboratory studies in patients without significant systemic disease (ASA I or II) undergoing low-risk surgery - specifically complete blood count, basic or comprehensive metabolic panel, coagulation studies when blood loss (or fluid shifts) is/are expected to be minimal[1], (Onuoha et al. 2014a; Onuoha et al. 2014b)

Don't obtain baseline diagnostic cardiac testing (trans-thoracic/esophageal echocardiography – TTE/TEE) or cardiac stress testing in asymptomatic stable patients with known cardiac disease (e.g. CAD, valvular disease) undergoing low or moderate risk non-cardiac surgery[1] (Austin et al. 2014; Benarroch-Gampel et al. 2012)

The ubiquitous use of routine testing in un-indicated patients has remained a hot topic for much over a decade (Benarroch-Gampel et al. 2012; Roizen 1997; Vogt and Henson 1997). In addition, the number of surgical procedures now performed on an outpatient basis continues to increase (Fleisher LA 2013; Richman 2010). It is estimated that about 30 million people undergo surgery annually in the USA, of which approximately 60–70 % are ambulatory procedures (Benarroch-Gampel et al. 2012; Fleisher LA 2013; Richman 2010). Ambulatory procedures are often performed in low-risk patients—healthy individuals or those with stable chronic medical conditions—and restricted to procedures of short duration with a low risk of intraoperative surgical complications (Benarroch-Gampel et al. 2012). Despite existing evidence-based guidelines advising the contrary, a battery of preoperative tests continue to be performed in low-risk patients undergoing low-risk ambulatory surgery (Benarroch-Gampel et al. 2012; Brown and Brown 2011; Fleisher LA 2013; Richman 2010; Schein et al. 2000; Soares Dde et al. 2013; Vogt and Henson 1997). Routine preoperative tests when performed in low-risk patients rarely change management and as much as 93 % of these tests are not indicated

(Brown and Brown 2011). In a study by Benarroch-Gampel et al. (2012), the authors showed that although rates of testing were lower in patients with no comorbidities, rates remained high, with 54 % of patients receiving at least one preoperative test. The overall incidence of complications was less than 1 %, and after controlling for patient comorbidities and the operative procedure, neither testing nor the presence of abnormal results were associated with postoperative complications. With the combination of routine preoperative testing in the setting of an increasing prevalence of ambulatory surgery, the elimination of un-indicated tests in low-risk patients would promote patient safety, better quality of care, and result in substantial cost savings (Brown and Brown 2011; Fleisher LA 2013; Schein et al. 2000).

While most of the body of research driving evidence-based guidelines originate from academic tertiary institutions, it is not clear whether such institutions adhere to these guidelines, and hence, display a lower incidence of overuse of preoperative tests in low-risk patients undergoing ambulatory surgery than stated in the literature. To establish and quantify the incidence of the ordering of un-indicated preoperative tests in an academic tertiary ambulatory center, we conducted a retrospective cohort study of all patients who underwent outpatient surgery at the Perelman Center for Advanced Medicine (PCAM), Hospital of the University of Pennsylvania during a 6-month period.

Methods

We obtained approval from the Institutional Review Board of the Perelman School of Medicine, University of Pennsylvania.

Data sources

Data was abstracted from the EPIC[2] medical records of 3918 patients who underwent ambulatory surgery at PCAM between the months of November 2012 and April 2013.

Participants

We restricted our sample to patients scheduled for ambulatory surgery only in this dedicated facility. Ambulatory surgery was defined as a "same day or 23-hour-stay elective procedure." Scheduled outpatient procedures upgraded to inpatient status due to intraoperative events were included in the study sample since unplanned intraoperative events have no effect on the initial preoperative testing decisions. In addition, we excluded procedures that used only local anesthesia or conscious sedation without an anesthesiologist or mid-level anesthesia provider, yielding a final cohort of 3111 patients.

Study variables

(a) Surgical risk

The preoperative period was defined as 30 days prior to the scheduled procedure. We defined all outpatient procedures taking place in the ambulatory setting as "low-risk surgery" as referenced in recommendation #1 of the Top-5 list (Onuoha et al. 2014a; Onuoha et al. 2014b). Preoperative patient and surgical characteristics were abstracted and included: age, gender, height, weight, surgical procedure performed, surgeon, surgical service/clinic, date of procedure, comorbidities, and ASA physical status score. We also obtained specific laboratory and imaging studies obtained within the 30-day preoperative period: complete blood count (CBC), metabolic panel (basic metabolic panel (BMP) or comprehensive metabolic panel (CMP)), coagulation studies (prothrombin time (PT), activated partial thromboplastin time (aPTT)) and cardiac studies (transesophageal/transthoracic echocardiography (TTE/TEE), stress test—exercise, persantine, dobutamine echocardiography).

(b) Patient health status

Patient health status was defined using the ASA physical status (PS) score assigned by the clinical anesthesiologist on the day of surgery. Patients assigned ASA 1 or 2 were defined as patients "without significant systemic disease" as referenced in recommendation #1 of the "Top-5 List"[1] (Onuoha et al. 2014a; Onuoha et al. 2014b). For the purpose of this study, significant systemic disease was defined as an ASA classification of 3 and above[3] (Daabiss 2011; Hata and Moyers 2009; Vogt and Henson 1997).

(c) Defining "Indicated" vs "Un-indicated Testing"

Preoperative BMP, CMP, and CBCs performed were categorized into "indicated" (obtained on a patient with ASA PS ≥3) and "un-indicated" (obtained on a patient with ASA PS <3). Coagulation studies were un-indicated if a patient was classified as ASA PS <3 *and* was not on any anticoagulant therapy. For cardiovascular function studies, a retrospective chart review was completed to establish the indication and rationale for the test performed within 30 days of the procedure. The review involved identifying both the ordering clinician and listed indications from related clinic notes, and reviewing the documentation of telephone encounters to further understand the rationale for the order placement. Of note, our data collection process through EPIC enabled us capture only studies ordered within the University of Pennsylvania Health System (UPHS). Hence, we were unable to capture radiographic studies ordered and performed outside UPHS.

Data analysis

Our primary endpoint was the percentage of patients with *at least one* un-indicated laboratory test, in accordance with the previous literature (Katz et al. 2011), Katz et al. (2011) found that the number of inappropriate tests per patient follows a geometric distribution. The geometric distribution has a proportion (p) as its sole parameter. If the counts of un-indicated tests follow this distribution, knowing the percentage of patients with at least one un-indicated test provides just as much information as the number per patient (Katz et al. 2011). We examined this assumption with the chi-square goodness of fit test.

There are 12 surgical specialties that operate at PCAM ambulatory surgical center. We expected practice patterns to vary among the different specialties and the probability of un-indicated testing to be correlated within a specialty. We accounted for this correlation by using time series analysis (Dexter et al. 2005a; Dexter et al. 2005b). We tabulated the number of patients with at least one un-indicated test among successive batches of 4-week periods for each specialty and subsequently applied the Freeman-Tukey transformation to each of the $n = 6$ batches (Mosteller and Youtz 1961). Differences between specialties were examined using a one-way analysis of variance (ANOVA) on the mean of the transformed proportions (Austin et al. 2014). Confidence intervals (CIs) were calculated for each specialty using the Student 1-sample t test (Dexter et al. 2005a). We finally applied the inverse transformation to express the estimates as proportions (Dexter et al. 2005a). Five surgical specialties accounted for >80 % of all procedures performed. We collapsed the remaining surgical specialties into one category to avoid unstable estimates due to low numbers (Dexter et al. 2005a). We hypothesized the incidence of un-indicated testing to be ≥50 %.(Benarroch-Gampel et al. 2012; Katz et al. 2011; Mantha et al. 2005). We thus estimated the sample size required to obtain a lower bound of the 95 % CI ≥ 47 % to be 2915 patients. All data analyses were conducted using Stata/IC 12.1 for Mac (StataCorp, College Station, TX).

Results

Patient characteristics are shown in Table 1. The majority of patients were female and classified as having "mild systemic disease."

Table 1 Demographics: patient and surgical characteristics

Characteristic		Total N = 3111
		N (%)
Age years (range, mean, SD)	12.3 to 94.8	51.6 ± 16.5
Age (years)	≤35	587 (18.9)
	36—55	1153 (37.1)
	56—75	1143 (36.7)
	>75	228 (7.3)
Gender	Male	1106 (36)
	Female	2005 (64)
ASA physical status	1	348 (11.2)
	2	1972 (63.4)
	3	782 (25.1)
	4	9 (0.3)

Surgical specialties and incidence of un-indicated testing

Surgical specialty	Frequency (percent)[c]	95 % confidence interval[b]
Endocrine oncologic	338/753 (55.1)	49.4–61.4
Gynecological	419/537 (78.0)	72.6–82.4
Otology	154/408 (37.5)	33.2–43.0
Plastic	199/408 (48.8)	43.3–53.3
Urology	220/467 (47.1)	41.1–53.9
Other[a]	241/538 (44.8)	42.2–48.0
All specialties	1648 /3111 (52.9)	37.6–66.4

Incidence of un-indicated testing among surgical specialties
[a]Colorectal, gastrointestinal, oral maxillofacial surgery, head and neck surgery, orthopedic, trauma, transplant
[b]Freeman-Tukey transformation among $n = 6$ batches of 4-week periods. Ninety-five percent confidence intervals calculated from the Student 1-sample t test among batches, with the inverse transformation taken
[c]Ordering rates were significantly different among specialties (Freeman-Tukey transformed ANOVA, p value = 0.001)

Preoperative testing—laboratory (lab) data

During the study period, 52.9 % (95 % CI 37.6–66.4) of all patients had at least one un-indicated lab test (CBC, metabolic panel, or coagulation study) performed preoperatively. The wide CI around this estimate is due to substantial heterogeneity in ordering across surgical specialties (Table 1). Further analysis revealed variation in

the incidence of ordering between different tests. Seventy-three percent of all CBCs, 70 % of all metabolic panels, and 49 % of all coagulation studies were considered un-indicated. Stated differently, of the patients included in the sample, 51 % of patients obtained an un-indicated CBC, 41 % an un-indicated metabolic panel, and 16 % un-indicated coagulation studies (Fig. 1). In this cohort, 15 % (455) of the patients received all three laboratory test types and in each instance, the test was considered un-indicated. Of these 455 patients, 10 % were healthy ASA 1 patients. Un-indicated testing was present even among the youngest and healthiest of patients. Of the 587 patients less than 36 years old, 331 (56 %) had at least one test that was considered un-indicated and 12 % of patients with "any un-indicated preoperative test" were classified as ASA 1 patients (Fig. 2). Sixty-five percent of the orders were placed by a surgeon, 34 % by a nurse practitioner or physician assistant, and 1 % had no indicated ordering clinician.

Geometric distribution

We found the distribution of the number of un-indicated tests per patient to depart significantly from the geometric distribution ($p = 0.001$, chi-square goodness of fit test). The departure was due to a lower-than-expected number of patients with only a single un-indicated test and a higher number of patients with two or more un-indicated tests (Fig. 3).

Preoperative testing—cardiac imaging studies

Only 41 (1.3 %) patients in the sample had either an echocardiogram or stress test ordered and performed within 30 days of surgery. Of the 41 studies ordered within UPHS, 22 were ordered for reasons not related to surgery. For instance, 4 patients received surveillance echocardiograms for potentially cardiotoxic chemotherapeutic agents, 2 for an unrelated hospital admission, and 2 as surveillance studies for a history of a heart transplant. Of the 19 studies ordered for preoperative evaluation, a retrospective chart review revealed 11 were due to either known cardiac conditions deemed unstable by

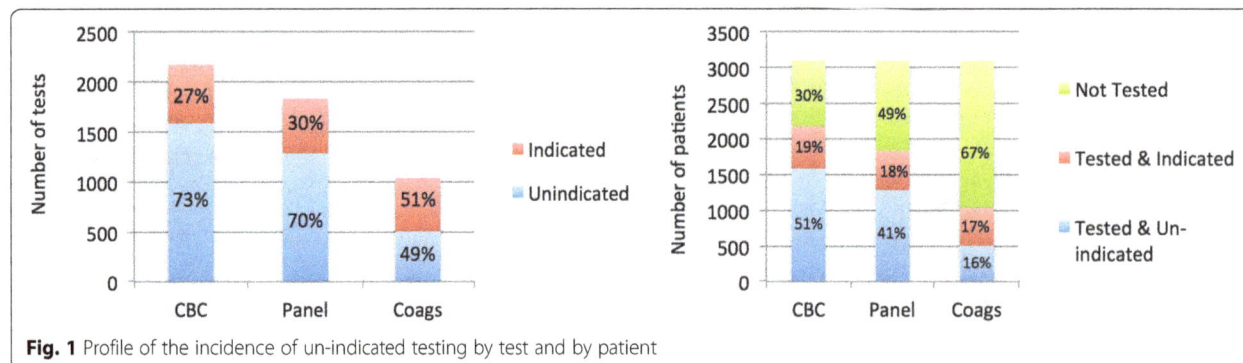

Fig. 1 Profile of the incidence of un-indicated testing by test and by patient

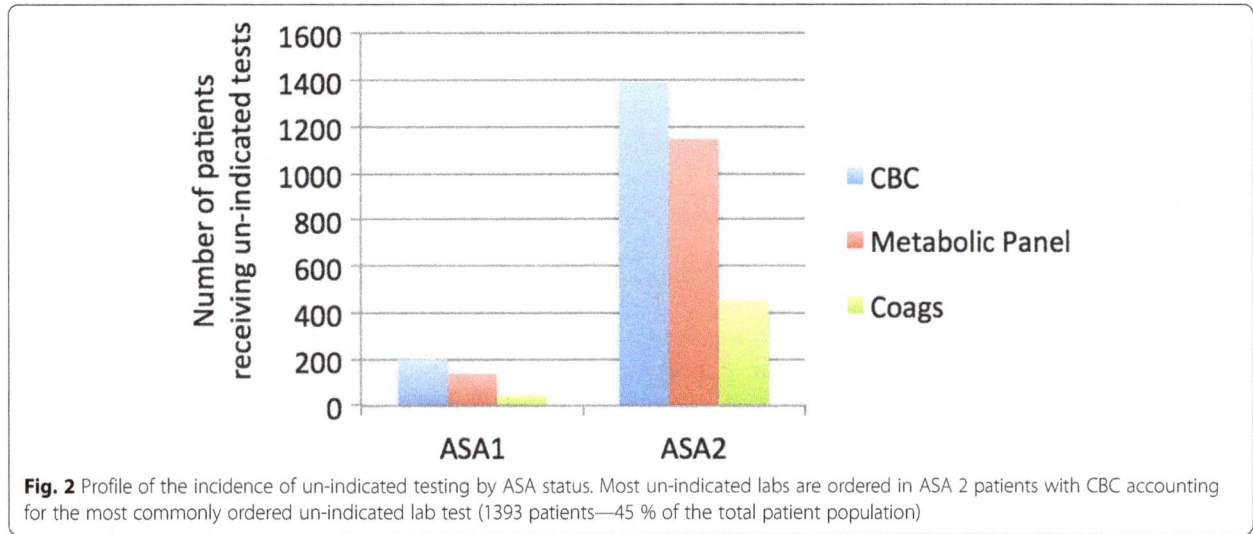

Fig. 2 Profile of the incidence of un-indicated testing by ASA status. Most un-indicated labs are ordered in ASA 2 patients with CBC accounting for the most commonly ordered un-indicated lab test (1393 patients—45 % of the total patient population)

the ordering clinician, new electrocardiogram (EKG) findings or cardiovascular symptomatology in patients without preexisting cardiac disease. Eight studies were considered "un-indicated"—that is, they were ordered in the absence of cardiac disease or documented new cardiac symptoms.

Discussion

Our study demonstrates a high incidence of obtaining "at least one un-indicated preoperative test" in low-risk patients undergoing ambulatory surgery despite multiple studies and guidelines (Committee on Standards and Practice Parameters et al. 2012; Czoski-Murray et al. 2012) addressing the lack of an indication for routine preoperative testing in this patient population. The issue

of overuse transcends all types of practices and is pervasive even in the academic tertiary setting where most of the studies demonstrating the futility of low-value testing tend to be published. Our findings compare to other studies consistently showing a greater than 50 % risk of receiving at least one un-indicated laboratory test during preoperative evaluation (Benarroch-Gampel et al. 2012; Katz et al. 2011; Mantha et al. 2005).

During the past three decades, routine preoperative testing has been challenged by several academic publications with concerns about the sizeable cost of testing, false positive tests leading to unnecessary work-ups or treatments, and the unknown benefit of routine testing to patients (Kumar and Srivastava 2011). Obviously, the goal of preoperative testing should be to detect

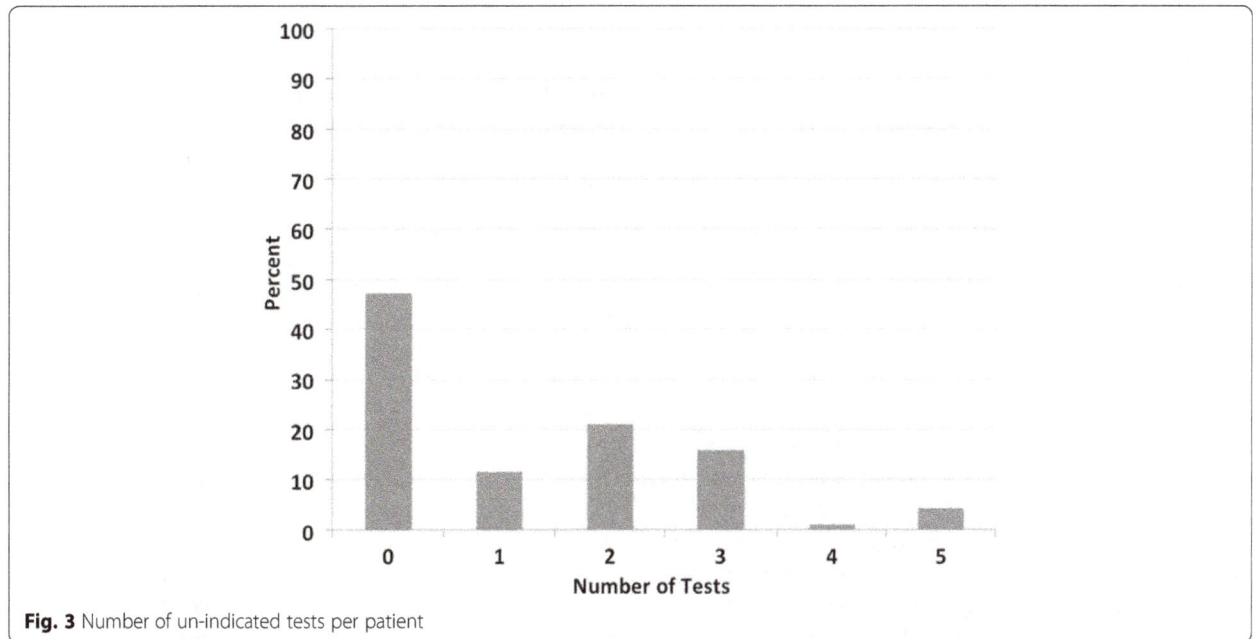

Fig. 3 Number of un-indicated tests per patient

abnormalities that will alter management and ensure better patient outcomes (Benarroch-Gampel et al. 2012; Keay et al. 2012; Schein et al. 2000). However, several studies including randomized clinical trials continue to show no difference in outcomes when comparing routine to no preoperative testing (Benarroch-Gampel et al. 2012; Keay et al. 2012; Schein et al. 2000; Sheffield et al. 2013). Finding changes in tests of clinically healthy or stable patients usually does not alter clinical management during the perioperative period (Soares Dde et al. 2013). Instead, un-indicated investigations detect minor abnormalities of no clinical relevance which may be unsafe for patients causing unnecessary delay, further scrutiny of false positive or inconsequential findings, and cancellation of surgery and medico-legal liability if not addressed (Kumar and Srivastava 2011).

Onuoha et al. (2014b) in conjunction with the ASA conducted a survey of clinical anesthesiologists and results indicated that the utilization of low-value services are often driven by external factors other than patient safety such as the lack of control by anesthesiologists over preoperative testing, surgeon preference, patient preference or demand, medico-legal concerns, or postoperative needs. Additional predictors include facility preference, practice tradition, concerns about surgical delay or cancellation, institutional policies and procedures, and the lack of both clear guidelines or the awareness of current evidence with respect to preoperative testing (Benarroch-Gampel et al. 2012; Brown and Brown 2011; Soares Dde et al. 2013). In a survey of anesthesiologists, the most notable but modifiable challenge was the lack of communication and collaboration by all stakeholders involved in the perioperative care of the patient (Onuoha et al. 2014b).

Clinical and research implications

With multiple studies establishing the persistent use of un-indicated preoperative testing, further studies are needed to not only identify modifiable attitudes and institutional influences on perioperative practices but also to develop and test feasible interventions that could curtail these practices. Most of the studies addressing preoperative testing originate in the anesthesia literature; however, approximately 80 % of preoperative tests are ordered by surgeons (Benarroch-Gampel et al. 2012; Onuoha et al. 2014b; Soares Dde et al. 2013). According to Soares Dde et al. (2013), when anesthesiologists take responsibility for preoperative tests, more appropriate tests are ordered via clinical profile, and consequently, surgery cancellations due to inadequate evaluation are reduced. Prior studies have also indicated a potential cost reduction of billions of dollars in preoperative testing without negatively affecting patient care when anesthesiologists assess patients and order tests prior to surgery

(Fleisher 2000; Foss and Apfelbaum 2001; Soares Dde et al. 2013). Although preoperative clinics by anesthesiologists are effective (Foss and Apfelbaum 2001; Katz et al. 2011; Pollard 2002), many patients are not seen in them due to the unavailability of such clinics in several institutions. Hence, the effort to curtail un-indicated preoperative testing will require collaboration between anesthesia and surgical and primary care providers with associated mid-level providers, including nurse practitioners, nurse anesthetists, and physician assistants, to develop clinical pathways as to when preoperative tests are required. Increasing the awareness of the current evidence and guidelines through education of all departments and the institution of constant reminders in the electronic medical ordering system could be the first step. The creation and adherence to clear succinct evidence-based guidelines by a task force in the perioperative setting can be spearheaded by anesthesiologists and would at least begin to address the enforcement of existing practice parameters.

Limitations of the study

Despite our findings, this study should be considered in the context of important limitations. First, the design of the study as a retrospective review makes it difficult to understand the decision making process when medical indications for preoperative testing are not documented clearly in the electronic medical record. Additionally, it is possible that testing may have been ordered as part of a diagnostic work-up of a presenting symptom rather than part of the preoperative screening process. We believe the contribution of error from this source to be negligible since over 90 % of the orders were placed as "outpatient orders." Furthermore, as noted in the results, we found the distribution of the number of un-indicated tests per patient to depart significantly from the geometric distribution. Thus, in our institution, providers tend to order multiple un-indicated tests per patient, which suggests ordering is driven more by practice patterns than individual patient evaluation. Second, the use of the ASA PS classification as the sole measure of a patient's health status may be an imperfect measure. In this study, an anesthesiologist assigned the ASA classification while the surgical staff placed the orders in question. Thus, the possibility exists that surgeons, in placing the preoperative screening orders, were considering factors in addition to those recognized by the anesthesiologist. Nevertheless, multiple studies including surveys by surgeons continue to show a routine instead of selective pattern to ordering preoperative tests (Benarroch-Gampel et al. 2012; Brown and Brown 2011; Schein et al. 2000; Soares Dde et al. 2013; Vogt and Henson 1997). A third limitation relates to the external validity and generalizability of our findings. PCAM at the Hospital of the University of Pennsylvania is a single-site institution and does not account for both the geographic or practice variability that can exist in other institutions. Involving multiple clinical sites in different parts of the country would provide better insight into the presence and enormity of this public health issue. These limitations notwithstanding, our findings carry important implications for current clinical practice, future research, and health policy in what is becoming an emerging era of optimizing patient safety and financial accountability. It also validates a pressing issue already described in several outpatient centers across the country.

Conclusions

In summary, we demonstrated a high prevalence of ordering un-indicated preoperative tests in low-risk ambulatory surgery across multiple surgical specialties in an academic tertiary setting. Our findings emphasize the need for a collaborative effort among all perioperative providers to address this significant burden on the health care system. The creation and adherence to clear guidelines by a task force spearheaded by anesthesiologists would at least begin the process of implementing existing practice parameters.

Endnotes

[1]American Society of Anesthesiologists: Five things physicians and patients should question. Choosing Wisely: An initiative of the ABIM Foundation. Created by Onuoha OC, Arkoosh VA, Fleisher LA. 2013. http://www.choosingwisely.org/doctor-patient-lists/american-society-of-anesthesiologists/.

[2]Epic Software. http://www.epic.com/software-index.php Accessed on 13 October, 2014.

[3]American Society of Anesthesiologists: ASA Physical Status Classification System. https://www.asahq.org/resources/clinical-information/asa-physical-status-classification-system Accessed on 13 October, 2014.

Abbreviations

ANOVA: analysis of variance; aPTT: activated partial thromboplastin time; ASA: American Society of Anesthesiologists; BMP: basic metabolic panel; CBC: complete blood count; CI: confidence interval; CMP: comprehensive metabolic panel; EKG: electrocardiogram; PCAM: Perelman Center for Advanced Medicine; PS: physical status; PT: prothrombin time; TEE: transesophageal echocardiography; TTE: tranthoracic echocardiography; UPHS: University of Pennsylvania Health System.

Competing interests

The author declares that they have no competing interests.

Authors' contributions

OO helped design and conduct the study, including data acquisition from the Penn Data store, and data analysis, and helped in writing and revising the manuscript. MH helped in the coordination of the study, data acquisition, data analysis, and writing of the manuscript. TM helped analyze the data (performed the statistical analysis) and write the manuscript. LF helped design the study and write and revise the manuscript. All authors read and approved the final manuscript.

Acknowledgements

The authors wish to acknowledge the Perelman School of Medicine Data Store. In addition, TM is supported by a research training grant from the National Heart, Lung, and Blood Institute (1F32HL124914-01).

Author details

[1]Department of Anesthesiology and Critical Care, Perelman School of Medicine at the University of Pennsylvania, 3400 Spruce Street Dulles 680, Philadelphia, PA 19104, USA. [2]Center for Clinical Epidemiology and Biostatistics, Perelman School of Medicine, University of Pennsylvania, Philadelphia, Pennsylvania, USA. [3]Department of Anesthesiology and Critical Care, Perelman School of Medicine, Senior Scholar, Leonard Davis Institute, University of Pennsylvania, Philadelphia, Pennsylvania, USA.

References

Austin TM, Lam HV, Shin NS, Daily BJ, Dunn PF, Sandberg WS. Elective change of surgeon during the OR day has an operationally negligible impact on turnover time. J Clin Anesth. 2014;26:343–9.

Benarroch-Gampel J, Sheffield KM, Duncan CB, Brown KM, Han Y, Townsend CM, et al. Preoperative laboratory testing in patients undergoing elective, low-risk ambulatory surgery. Ann Surg. 2012;256(3):518–28.

Brown SR, Brown J. Why do physicians order unnecessary preoperative tests? A qualitative study. Fam Med. 2011;43(5):338–43.

Committee on Standards and Practice Parameters, Apfelbaum JL, Connis RT, Nickinovich DG, American Society of Anesthesiologists Task Force on Preanesthesia Evaluation, Pasternak LR, et al. Practice advisory for preanesthesia evaluation: an updated report by the American Society of Anesthesiologists Task Force on preanesthesia evaluation. Anesthesiology. 2012;116(3):522–38.

Czoski-Murray C, Lloyd JM, McCabe C, Claxton K, Oluboyede Y, Roberts J, et al. What is the value of routinely testing full blood count, electrolytes and urea, and pulmonary function test before elective surgery in patients with no apparent clinical indication and in subgroups of patients with common comorbidities: a systematic review of the clinical and cost-effective literature. Health Technol Assess. 2012;16(50):1–159.

Daabiss M. American Society of Anaesthesiologists physical status classification. Indian J Anaesth. 2011;55(2):111–5.

Dexter F, Marcon E, Epstein RH, Ledolter J. Validation of statistical methods to compare cancellation rates on the day of surgery. Anesth Analg. 2005a;101:465–73.

Dexter F, Epstein RH, Marcon E, Ledolter J. Estimating the incidence of prolonged turnover times and delays by time of day. Anesthesiology. 2005b;102:1242–8. discussion 6A.

Fleisher LA. Effect of preoperative evaluation and consultation on cost and outcome of surgical care. Current Opinion in Anesthesiology. 2000;13:209–13.

Fleisher LA. Preoperative consultation before cataract surgery: are we choosing wisely or is this simply low-value care? JAMA Intern Med. 2014;174(3):389-90. jamainternalmedicine.com.

Foss JF, Apfelbaum J. Economics of preoperative evaluation clinics. Curr Opin Anaesthesiol. 2001;14(5):559–62.

Hata TM, Moyers JR. Preoperative patient assessment and management. In: Barash PG, Cullen BF, Stoelting RK, Cahalan MK, Stock MC, editors. Clinical Anesthesia. 6th ed. Philadelphia: Lippincott Williams & Wilkins; 2009. p. 569–97.

Katz RI, Dexter F, Rosenfeld K, Wolfe L, Redmond V, Agarwal D, et al. Survey study of anesthesiologists' and surgeons' ordering of unnecessary preoperative laboratory tests. Anesth Analg. 2011;112(1):207–12.

Keay L, Lindsley K, Tielsch J, Katz J, Schein O. Routine preoperative medical testing for cataract surgery. Cochrane Database Syst Rev. 2012;3:CD007293. doi: 10.1002/14651858.CD007293.pub3.

Kumar A, Srivastava U. Role of routine laboratory investigations in preoperative evaluation. J Anaesthesiol Clin Pharmacol. 2011;27(2):174–9.

Mantha S, Roizen MF, Madduri J, Rajender Y, Shanti Naidu K, Gayatri K. Usefulness of routine preoperative testing: a prospective single observer study. J Clin Anesth. 2005;17:51–7.

Mosteller F, Youtz C. Tables of the Freeman-Tukey transformations for the binomial and Poisson distributions. Biometrika. 1961;48:433–40.

Onuoha OC, Arkoosh VA, Fleisher LA. "Choosing Wisely" in anesthesiology: Top-5 List—addressing the gap between evidence and practice. ASA Newsletter. 2014a;78(1):44–5.

Onuoha OC, Arkoosh VA, Fleisher LA. Choosing wisely in anesthesiology: the gap between evidence and practice. JAMA Intern Med. 2014b;174(8):1391–5.

Pollard JB. Economic aspects of an anesthesia preoperative evaluation clinic. Curr Opin Anaesthesiol. 2002;15(2):257–61.

Richman DC. Ambulatory surgery: how much testing do we need? Anesthesiol Clin. 2010;28:185–97.

Roizen MF. Preoperative evaluation: a shared vision for change. J Clin Anesth. 1997;9:435–6.

Schein OD, Katz J, Bass EB, Tielsch JM, Lubomski LH, Feldman MA, et al. The value of routine preoperative medical testing before cataract surgery. N Engl J Med. 2000;342:168–75.

Sheffield KM, McAdams PS, Benarroch-Gampel J, Goodwin JS, Boyd CA, Zhang D, et al. Overuse of preoperative cardiac stress testing in medicare patients undergoing elective noncardiac surgery. Ann Surg. 2013;257(1):73–80.

Soares Dde S, Brandao RR, Mourao MR, Azevedo VL, Figueiredo AV, Trindade ES. Relevance of routine testing in low risk patients undergoing minor and medium surgical procedures. Braz J Anesthesiol. 2013;63(2):197–201.

Vogt AW, Henson LC. Unindicated preoperative testing: ASA physical status and financial implications. J Clin Anesth. 1997;9:437–41.

4

Perioperative intravenous fluid prescribing: a multi-centre audit

Benjamin Harris[1]* , Christian Schopflin[2], Clare Khaghani[3], Mark Edwards[4] and on behalf of collaborators from the Southcoast Perioperative Audit and Research Collaboration (SPARC)[1]

Abstract

Background: Excessive or inadequate intravenous fluid given in the perioperative period can affect outcomes. A number of guidelines exist but these can conflict with the entrenched practice, evidence base and prescriber knowledge. We conducted a multi-centre audit of intraoperative and postoperative intravenous fluid therapy to investigate fluid administration practice and frequency of postoperative electrolyte disturbances.

Methods: A retrospective audit was done in five hospitals of adult patients undergoing elective major abdominal, gastrointestinal tract or orthopaedic surgery. The type, volume and quantity of fluid and electrolytes administered during surgery and in 3 days postoperatively was calculated, and electrolyte disturbances were studied using clinical records.

Results: Data from four hundred thirty-one patients in five hospitals covering 1157 intravenous fluid days were collected. Balanced crystalloid solutions were almost universally used in the operating theatre and were also the most common fluid administered postoperatively, followed by hypotonic dextrose-saline solutions and 0.9 % sodium chloride. For three common uncomplicated elective operations, the volume of fluid administered intraoperatively demonstrated considerable variability. Over half of the patients received no postoperative fluid on day 1, and even more were commenced on free oral fluids immediately postoperatively or on day 1. Postoperative quantities of sodium exceeded the recommended amounts for maintenance in half of the patients who continued to receive intravenous fluids. Potassium administration in those receiving intravenous fluids was almost universally inadequate. Hypokalaemia and hyponatraemia were the common findings.

Conclusions: We documented the current clinical practice and confirmed that early free oral fluids and cessation of any intravenous fluids is common postoperatively in keeping with the aims of enhanced recovery after surgery programmes. Excessive sodium and water and inadequate potassium in those given intravenous fluids postoperatively is common and needs to be investigated. The variation in intraoperative fluid volume administration for three common procedures is considerable and in keeping with other international studies. Future trials of fluid therapy should include the intraoperative and postoperative phases.

Keywords: Intravenous fluids, Electrolytes, Perioperative, Anaesthesia, Surgery, Postoperative

Background

The fundamental goal of any intravenous fluid therapy is to restore and maintain normal fluid and electrolyte physiology in situations where patients are unable to control their own fluid intake, while minimising the risk of fluid-related complications. Excessive or inadequate intravenous fluid therapy in surgical patients is associated with adverse outcomes and can cause significant harm (Minto and Mythen 2015; Lobo et al. 2001).

Most of the intravenous fluid that surgical patients receive during their admission is delivered in the postoperative stage and most of the responsibility for prescribing these intravenous fluids lies with junior surgical staff (Walsh and Walsh 2005). The National Confidential Enquiry into Perioperative Deaths (1999) attributed significant perioperative morbidity and mortality to errors in fluid and electrolyte administration (Callum et al. 1999). Despite this, the evidence base around

* Correspondence: benjamin.harris1@btinternet.com
[1]Academic Department of Critical Care, Queen Alexandra Hospital, Southwick Hill Road, Cosham, Portsmouth PO6 3LY, UK
Full list of author information is available at the end of the article

fluid administration in the postoperative period is still very limited (Gonzalez-Fajardo et al. 2009).

There have been a number of guidelines and recommendations regarding perioperative intravenous fluid therapy in recent years, and these aim to provide a basis for good practice and provide a resource for quality improvement (National Institute for Health and Care Excellence 2013; Powell-Tuck et al. 2011). They highlight those areas of the hospital, such as general surgical wards, where errors are more likely than in operating theatres and patients may be at greatest risk of inappropriate and potentially harmful intravenous fluid therapy (Minto and Mythen 2015; National Institute for Health and Care Excellence 2013). Intravenous fluid guidelines have to combine physiological principles with entrenched historical and variable practice, an inadequate and often contradictory evidence base, a multitude of intravenous solutions that often vary in availability between individual hospitals and a deficiency of prescribing knowledge among many medical staff. While there is some debate about the content of these guidelines (Woodcock 2014; Soni 2009) and a recognition that deviations from guidelines may be an appropriate response to a patient's clinical situation, for the majority of elective cases, the guideline recommendations represent an appropriate standard of care against which to audit.

It has been suggested that despite the guidelines and the evidence, intraoperative and postoperative fluid prescribing practice is both variable and suboptimal (Minto and Mythen 2015; National Institute for Health and Care Excellence 2013; Powell-Tuck et al. 2011). We conducted a multi-centre audit of intraoperative and postoperative intravenous fluid therapy in adult elective major surgery patients to investigate the following: current intraoperative intravenous fluid administration practice, current postoperative intravenous fluid administration practice (both compared to recent guidelines) and frequency of postoperative electrolyte disturbances. The data produced will be used for future quality improvement projects.

Methods

We undertook a multi-centre retrospective observational audit across five Wessex deanery hospitals. This included four district general hospitals and one university teaching hospital. Appropriate approval was obtained via individual hospital audit departments, and the investigation was co-ordinated by one local lead investigator in each hospital. We aimed to investigate 100 cases in each hospital. Inclusion criteria were adult patients who underwent elective major surgery during the year 2013 as defined by the BUPA complexity categories. These ascend in surgical complexity order from major, major+

and complex major operation (CMO) (BUPA Schedule of Procedures 2005). Specialities included orthopaedic, upper and lower gastrointestinal, urological and gynaecological surgeries. All patients irrespective of postoperative destination were included. Exclusion criteria were non-elective surgery, minor or intermediate surgery, day case surgery and patient age less than 18 years.

A list of all patients meeting the inclusion criteria was obtained in each hospital, and the first 100 patients in chronological order (January 2013 onwards) were selected. In high-volume centres, the target of identifying 100 patients was reached within the first 4 months of the year. In lower volume centres, to identify the required 100 subjects, operations up to October 2013 were included. Once 100 patients were identified in each centre, collection of identifying details ceased and the medical notes were requested. Hospital C was a very high volume centre, and in order to improve the overall number of patients in the audit, an additional 50 patients were identified in hospital C and their notes requested.

From the medical notes, where available, patient and procedure characteristics including age, weight (actual body weight recorded on the pre-operative assessment or anaesthetic paperwork prior to the operation) and operation type were recorded. For each patient, we collected data on volume and fluid type administered, quantities of sodium, chloride and potassium administered per kilogram body weight per day, calculated fluid balance based on input/output charts (fluid prescription charts and output charts recording urine, drain and other losses) and serum electrolyte measurements. We defined hyponatraemia as a serum sodium of less than 135 mmol.l^{-1} and hypokalaemia as a serum sodium of less than 3.5 mmol.l^{-1}. Data collection covered the period from the day of the operation up to and including postoperative day 7, and the day after intravenous fluids were completely ceased or the day of discharge if this came first. The 'standards' used for this audit were the GIFTASUP guidelines (Powell-Tuck et al. 2011) that advocate early resumption of oral intake, early cessation of intravenous fluids and careful attention to fluid balance. The volume and type of intravenous fluid together with the quantity of electrolytes administered perioperatively was compared with the recommended values (Powell-Tuck et al. 2011). These recommendations are, for the maintenance of homeostasis, approximately 1500–2500 ml water per day (interpreted by us as 25–30 ml.kg.day^{-1} of water) (Powell-Tuck et al. 2011). For sodium and potassium, requirements for maintenance should be close to the reference nutrient intake (RNI) (Powell-Tuck et al. 2011). Values of 50–100 mmol per day for sodium and potassium 40–80 mmol per day are recommended (interpreted by us as 0.8–1.2 mmol.kg.day^{-1}).

These quantities are very similar to other more recent intravenous fluid guidelines (National Institute for Health and Care Excellence 2013).

Each hospital was assigned a random letter (A–E) with the identity of each hospital known only to the principal investigator. No patient identifiable data was recorded and kept, and all recorded data was anonymised and encrypted using commercially available software. Data in figures is expressed either as absolute numbers with percentages or as measures of central tendency (mean or median). Measures of spread used were standard error of the mean or interquartile range, and this is indicated in the figure legends. We did not undertake any further statistical tests so as not to deviate from the observational nature of the audit.

Results

Data were collected for 431 subjects. Although we requested the notes of the first 100 (150 in hospital C) patients in each hospital, during the analysis period, a number of patient notes that were requested were not available due to administrative reasons. These included being lost or in use at a different hospital department. Therefore, the final number of patient records analysed was 431 (Fig. 1).

The median age was 78 years (range 20–93 years) and median weight was 79 kg (range 36–210 kg). Forty-three percent of the patients underwent orthopaedic surgery, 23.5 % upper gastrointestinal and 33.5 % lower gastrointestinal, gynaecological or urological surgery. Table 1 summarises the number of cases according to speciality, category of surgical complexity and postoperative destination.

Fluid volume and electrolyte quantities

The audit set out to record fluid and electrolyte quantities for each postoperative day up to and including postoperative day 7. However, the quality of fluid prescription charts and fluid balance documentation was subjectively noted by the data analysing team to become progressively less complete or even present in the medical notes as length of stay progressed. Early on in the data collection process (after analysing approximately 20 notes in each centre), it was therefore decided to limit further data collection to 3 days postoperatively only due to the paucity of data. We did continue to collect the date when free oral fluids were started because this information was easier to find in the narrative medical notes. Overall, 1157 intravenous fluid days have been included in the analysis over postoperative days 1, 2 and 3.

Type of intravenous fluid

During the entire time period studied, the balanced crystalloid solutions were the most common intravenous fluid (57.6 % of all fluid administered by volume). Figure 2 demonstrates that during the intraoperative period, for all types of surgery, by far the most commonly used intravenous fluids were the balanced crystalloids. In the postoperative period, balanced crystalloids were still the most common but the use of hypotonic dextrose-saline and 0.9 % sodium chloride increased markedly.

When the balanced intravenous solutions are subdivided into Hartmann's and Plasma-Lyte (the only two balanced solutions used in this audit), Hartmann's was the most commonly used balanced solution intraoperatively and on postoperative day 1 (Fig. 3). This was the same for postoperative days 2 and 3 (data not shown).

Immediate postoperative destination and type of fluid

The type of fluid given on postoperative day 1 demonstrated a similar pattern for all clinical areas. The only difference was more hypotonic dextrose-saline was used in the intensive care unit (ICU) compared to wards or ward-based high dependency unit (HDU) (see Fig. 4).

Hospital code	A	B	C	D	E	TOTAL
No. eligible patients identified	100	100	100+50	100	100	550
Target for full analysis	100	100	150	100	100	550
Practical difficulties obtaining notes	⇩	⇩	⇩	⇩	⇩	⇩
Number of notes actually analysed	87	89	130	43	82	431

Fig. 1 Flow chart demonstrating the target number of patients at each hospital and the number successfully included in the audit

Table 1 The number of patients in each surgical speciality, BUPA complexity category and immediate postoperative destination clinical area

		Surgical speciality			
		Lower GI, gynaecology and urology	Orthopaedics	Upper GI	Total
BUPA category and postoperative clinical area	CMO	57	110	63	230
	ICU	12 (21 %)	3 (2.7 %)	36 (57 %)	
	HDU/ward	45 (79 %)	107 (97.2 %)	27 (43 %)	
	Major+	79	73	10	162
	ICU	28 (35 %)	2 (3 %)	4 (40 %)	
	HDU/ward	51 (65 %)	71 (97 %)	6 (60 %)	
	Major	8	3	28	39
	ICU			1 (4 %)	
	HDU/ward	8 (100 %)	3 (100 %)	27 (96 %)	
	Total	144	186	101	431

BUPA category codes are defined in the text of the "Methods" section
Abbreviations: *GI* gastrointestinal, *CMO* complex major operation,

Volume of intraoperative fluid

In keeping with the surgical severity in the group studied, almost all patients received some intravenous fluid during their time in the operating theatre. Three common procedures were laparoscopic right hemicolectomy ($n = 36$), total hip replacement ($n = 58$) and total knee replacement ($n = 70$). The volume of fluid administered intraoperatively (where recorded) for these index procedures demonstrated considerable variability (Fig. 5).

Volume of postoperative fluid

On postoperative days 1 and 2, over half of the patients received no intravenous fluid at all (Fig. 6). This proportion increased on day 3 to nearly three quarters. A small

minority of patients received >35 ml.kg^{-1} intravenous fluid on all three postoperative days. There appeared to be no correlation between volume of fluid prescribed and body weight as shown in Fig. 7.

Free oral fluid orders

The day when 'free oral fluids' were ordered by the surgical team is listed in Table 2. We recognise this as the day that intravenous fluids should be stopped as the patient is able to take oral fluids. This day was accurately recorded in the clinical notes in 67 % ($n = 289$) of all subjects. Where recorded, free fluids were ordered immediately postoperatively or on postoperative day 1 in the majority of patients (Table 2).

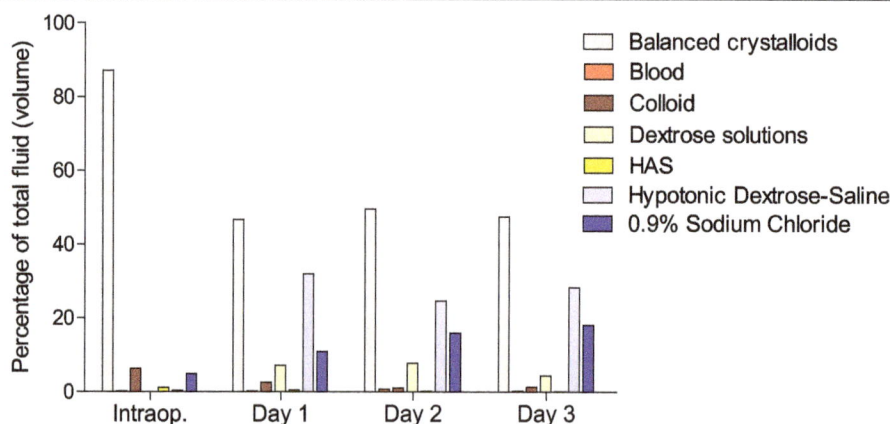

Fig. 2 Type of intravenous fluid administered in different phases of the perioperative pathway. Balanced crystalloid solutions were the most common fluid administered at all stages of the perioperative pathway expressed as the percentage of the total volume of intravenous fluid used. Balanced crystalloids (Hartmann's and Plasma-Lyte), hypotonic dextrose-saline solutions (0.18 and 0.45 % dextrose-saline), dextrose solutions (5 and 10 % dextrose) and HAS (human albumin solution)

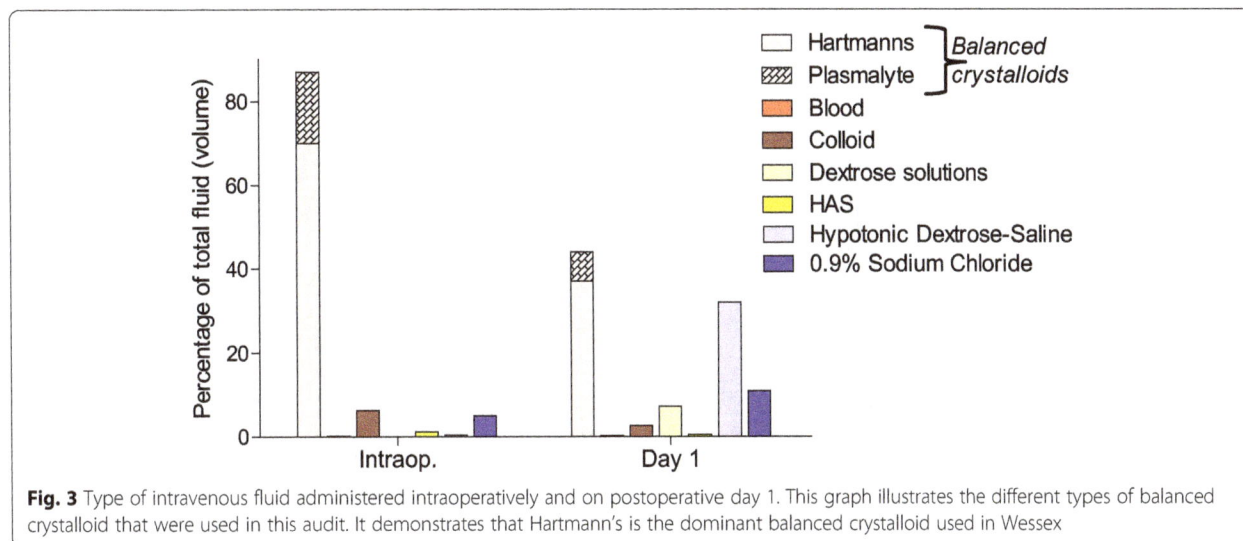

Fig. 3 Type of intravenous fluid administered intraoperatively and on postoperative day 1. This graph illustrates the different types of balanced crystalloid that were used in this audit. It demonstrates that Hartmann's is the dominant balanced crystalloid used in Wessex

Postoperative dose of electrolytes

The quantity of sodium, potassium and chloride administered on postoperative day 1 was calculated from the known volume and type of fluid administered. Of patients who received intravenous fluid on postoperative day 1 ($n = 248$), quantities of sodium and chloride exceeded maintenance requirements in approximately half of those studied (Table 3). Almost all received less potassium than their maintenance requirements with a third of patients receiving none (Table 3). We subsequently examined patients with an apparent ongoing intravenous fluid requirement in more depth by analysing only those patients that were receiving intravenous fluids on day 2 as well as day 1 ($n = 96$). We found similar trends in day 1 sodium and potassium dosing (Table 4).

Electrolyte disturbances

Table 5 lists the percentage of patients with hypokalaemia in the various perioperative phases. The incidence of hyponatraemia increased after surgery (Fig. 8). It appeared most marked on postoperative day 2 in those given dextrose solutions (5 or 10 % dextrose) on postoperative day 1 compared to those given other types of fluid although the pre-operative serum sodium was lower in this group (Fig. 8).

Discussion

This was a large retrospective audit of current intravenous fluid prescribing practice in the five hospitals in the Wessex region. We found that early cessation of intravenous fluids in the postoperative elective surgical patient was common and in keeping with the approach

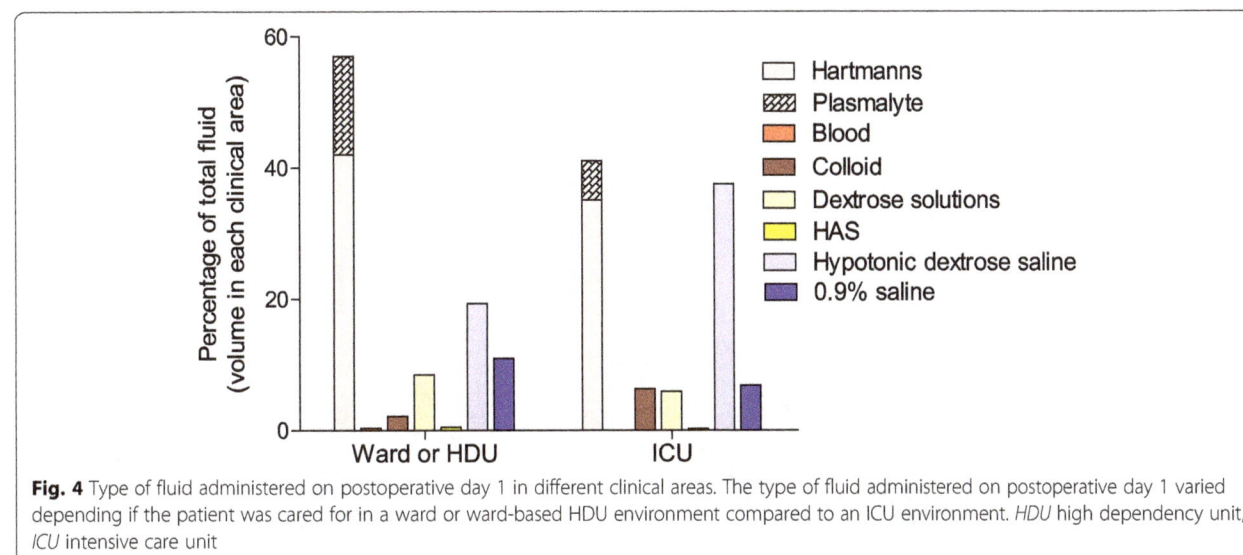

Fig. 4 Type of fluid administered on postoperative day 1 in different clinical areas. The type of fluid administered on postoperative day 1 varied depending if the patient was cared for in a ward or ward-based HDU environment compared to an ICU environment. *HDU* high dependency unit, *ICU* intensive care unit

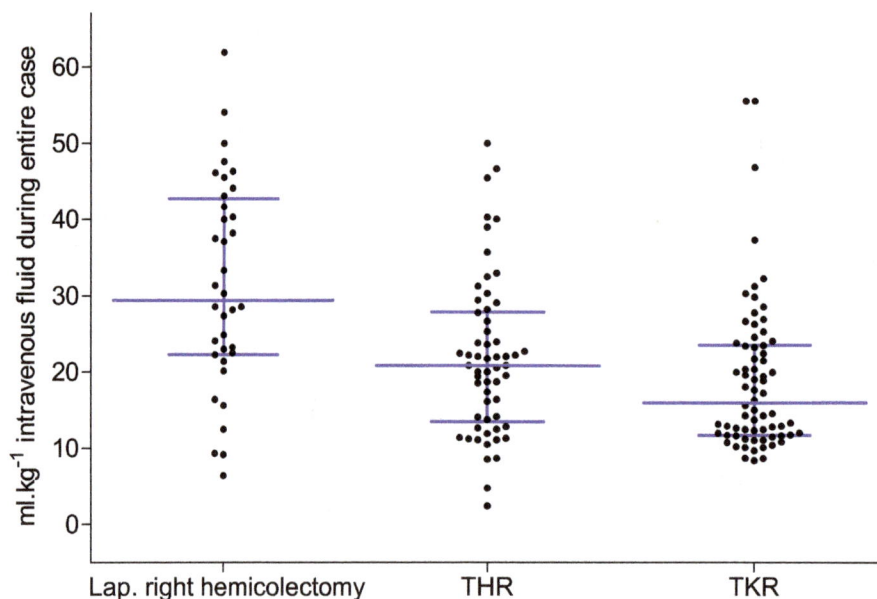

Fig. 5 Volume of intraoperative fluid administered for three common surgeries. Volume of fluid administered expressed as ml.kg^{-1} during the entire operation. *Error bars* represent the interquartile range. The *wide horizontal line* represents the median. *Abbreviations: THR* total hip replacement, *TKR* total knee replacement

promoted by enhanced recovery after surgery programmes. In those patients that continue to receive intravenous fluids, a considerable proportion appear to receive excessive or inadequate quantities of various electrolytes in relation to reference requirements. A small but important proportion appears to receive excessive volumes of water. The type of intravenous fluid administered varies according to the stage of the patient pathway. There was considerable variation in the volume of fluid administered in the operating theatre for three common elective procedures. Electrolyte disturbances were frequent and became more common as the postoperative days passed.

Strengths of this audit

This is a large, multi-centre audit across five hospitals serving a wide geographical area with a sample population typical of most regions across the country. The included surgical procedures are common and relevant to a wide audience. The data collected has allowed a detailed analysis of the current practice, and the findings are in keeping with previous work (Minto and Mythen

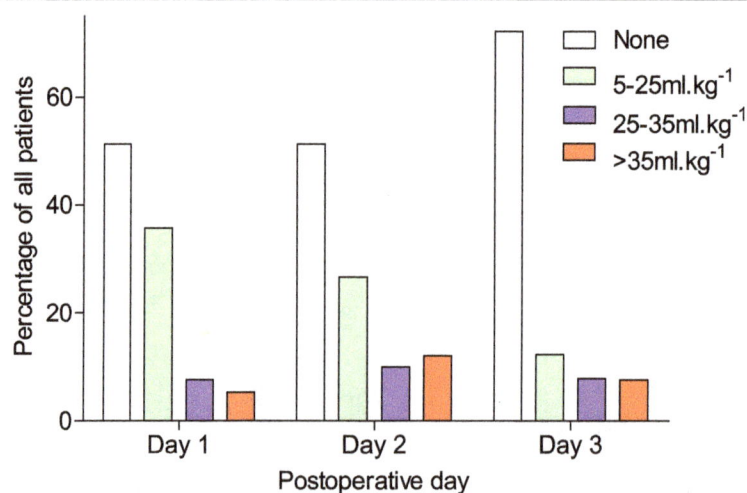

Fig. 6 Intravenous fluid received on postoperative days 1, 2 and 3. Percentage of all patients who received different volumes of intravenous fluid expressed as ml.kg.day^{-1}

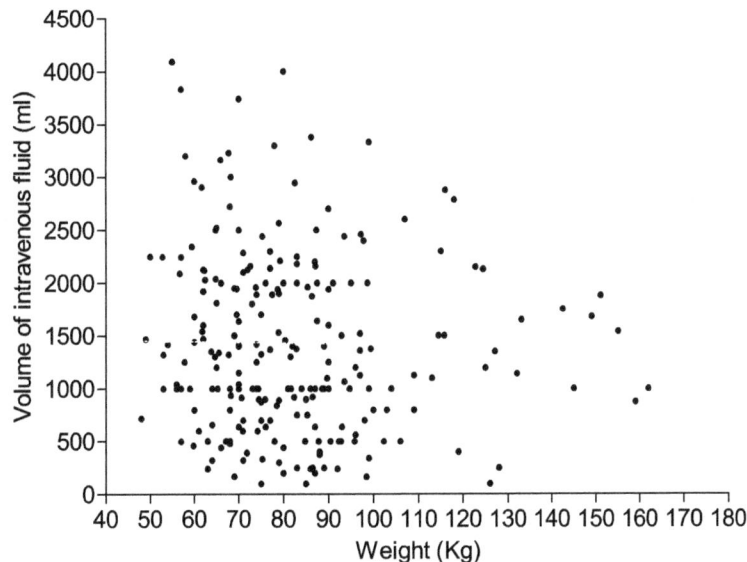

Fig. 7 Volume of intravenous fluid given on postoperative day 1 compared to body weight. In those patients receiving intravenous fluid on postoperative day 1, there was no relationship between volume received and body weight

2015; Callum et al. 1999; Lilot et al. 2015). The majority of recent major trials regarding intravenous fluids focus on intraoperative fluid management. However, only a small proportion of the perioperative journey is spent in the operating theatre under the direct care of an anaesthetist. Our work addresses both the intraoperative and postoperative periods.

Limitations of this audit
Heterogeneity
The patients included are a very heterogeneous group, with a wide range of age, body weight, mode of anaesthesia and operation type.

Data capture
For administrative and logistical reasons at the different institutions, we could not obtain 100 % of the notes identified leading to a potential for selection bias. Hospital C contributed relatively more patients potentially skewing the overall results.

Table 2 Postoperative day that 'free oral fluids' were ordered by the surgical team

Perioperative day	Number of patients (%)
Immediately postoperative	185 (42.9)
Day 1	65 (15.1)
Day 2	15 (3.5)
Day 3	10 (2.3)
Day 4 or after	14 (3.2)
Not recorded in notes	142 (32.9)

Data limitations
The majority of medical records in this audit were paper based and often subjectively of poor quality which may affect the results. We did not collect detailed data on individual patient perioperative risk scores in the form of ASA (American Society of Anaesthesiologists) grade or other perioperative risk scoring systems. We considered ASA grade to be insufficiently robust to determine perioperative risk, and other risk scoring systems were rarely used by anaesthetists in this audit.

When calculating intraoperative fluid administration data for the three common procedures, our ability to determine that these were uncomplicated was based on discharge summaries and anaesthetic charts. Neither of these two methods may have recorded all the technical difficulties or other 'complications' during the surgery that may have mandated higher than average intravenous fluid administration volumes. In addition, the length of time spent in the operating theatre was not recorded so we were unable to present intraoperative fluid

Table 3 Quantity of sodium, potassium and chloride given in intravenous fluids on postoperative day 1

	Quantity administered in mmol.kg^{-1}			
	None (%)	0.1–0.7 (%)	0.8–1.2 (%)	≥1.3 (%)
Sodium	7	24	*14*	55
Chloride	7	28	*17*	48
Potassium	30	68	*2*	0

For all patients receiving intravenous fluid on postoperative day 1 (n = 248), the percentage of those in each electrolyte dose range is listed. The dose range of 0.8–1.2 mmol.kg^{-1} is expressed in italics because this represents maintenance requirements

Table 4 Quantity of sodium, potassium and chloride given on postoperative day 1 in those with an ongoing need for intravenous fluids (n = 96)

	Quantity administered in mmol.kg−1			
	None (%)	0.1–0.7 (%)	*0.8–1.2 (%)*	≥1.3 (%)
Sodium	4	14	*9*	72
Chloride	4	15	*10*	69
Potassium	25	67	*6*	0

For all patients receiving intravenous fluid on postoperative day 1, the percentage of those in each electrolyte dose range is listed. An ongoing need for intravenous fluids was defined as those receiving intravenous fluid on postoperative days 1 and 2, therefore demonstrating an ongoing need during day 1. The dose range of 0.8–1.2 mmol.kg^{-1} is expressed in italics because this represents maintenance requirements

administration volumes as ml.kg.h^{-1}. Also, these patients were not matched in terms of perioperative risk score (e.g. ASA), co-morbidities, surgical complexity or operative time, although we did exclude non-elective patients and those with significant blood loss. Fluid balance charts were studied to help assess appropriateness of intravenous fluids. These were subjectively noted to be often of poor quality and do not record all losses, such as fluid sequestration in sepsis, so they do not provide all the information needed to assess whether the fluid administered is clinically appropriate. Fluid prescription charts were better in terms of completion.

Study design
Volumes of fluid and quantities of sodium were calculated to be excessive in reference to the maintenance requirements in a large number of patients in the postoperative period. An unknown proportion might have been septic, bleeding or hypovolaemic requiring additional replacement over and above the maintenance requirements. A detailed notes review would be required to assess how clinically appropriate the fluid volume and sodium quantity given in each case was. Enhanced recovery pathways and fluid prescription guidelines often vary between individual hospitals and even individual surgical teams in the same institution. This may explain some of the variation in practice.

Meaning of this audit
One of the principles of enhanced recovery after surgery protocols is an early return to oral intake to improve patient comfort, gut function and limit the detrimental effects of intravenous fluid (Guidelines for the Implementation of Enhanced Recovery Protocols 2009). Intravenous fluid guidelines (National Institute for Health

and Care Excellence 2013; Powell-Tuck et al. 2011) also make reference to promoting the early return to oral intake. Over 50 % of the patients had a free oral fluid order on the day of their operation or postoperative day 1, indicating an attempt to return them to normal oral fluid intake. Of the patients, 32 % had no record of any free fluid order being made possibly because it was obvious that the patient could drink freely or that the hospitals have adopted an enhanced recovery approach and assumed free oral fluids can be given unless specifically documented otherwise. Poor medical record keeping is another possibility. At least some of these 32 % of patients would have been allowed to drink free oral fluids; therefore, the lack of documentation is unlikely to underestimate the already large number of patients with an early (day of operation or postoperative day 1) free fluid order.

The balanced crystalloid solutions were the most common postoperative fluid, with hypotonic crystalloids (dextrose-saline solutions) and 0.9 % sodium chloride as the next most common. There is increasing recognition that the traditional postoperative regime of 0.9 % sodium chloride and 5 % dextrose risks sodium, chloride and salt overload (De Silva et al. 2010). Sodium chloride (0.9 %), even when not given in excessive quantities, is associated with a variety of detrimental effects such as hyperchloraemic acidosis, reduced renal blood flow, increased chance of renal failure and increased in-hospital mortality after major abdominal surgery (Lobo 2012). Data from Wessex in 2007 found that over 70 % of postoperative fluid prescriptions were 0.9 % sodium chloride or 5 % dextrose (De Silva et al. 2010). This figure was reduced to 40 % in 2009 after a targeted education intervention (De Silva et al. 2010). It appears that this downward trend has continued as evidenced by our work.

Differences in intraoperative and postoperative fluid types is partially explained by the prescriber (anaesthetists in theatre vs junior doctors or non-anaesthetists postoperatively) and the different physiology occurring at the different time points.

Even the use of the balanced crystalloids can result in sodium overload and some hospitals and the NICE (National Institute for Health and Care Excellence 2013) advocate hypotonic dextrose-saline solutions as a means of giving water with minimal sodium to meet the maintenance requirements. It is not surprising that the greater use of hypotonic dextrose-saline solutions was seen in patients that went to the ICU postoperatively compared

Table 5 Percentage of patients with hypokalaemia in the various perioperative phases

Pre-operative value	Postoperative day 1	Postoperative day 2	Postoperative day 3
1.5 %	4 %	6 %	10 %

Percentage of patients (who had serum potassium measured) with a serum potassium less than 3.5 mmol.l^{-1} at the various perioperative stages

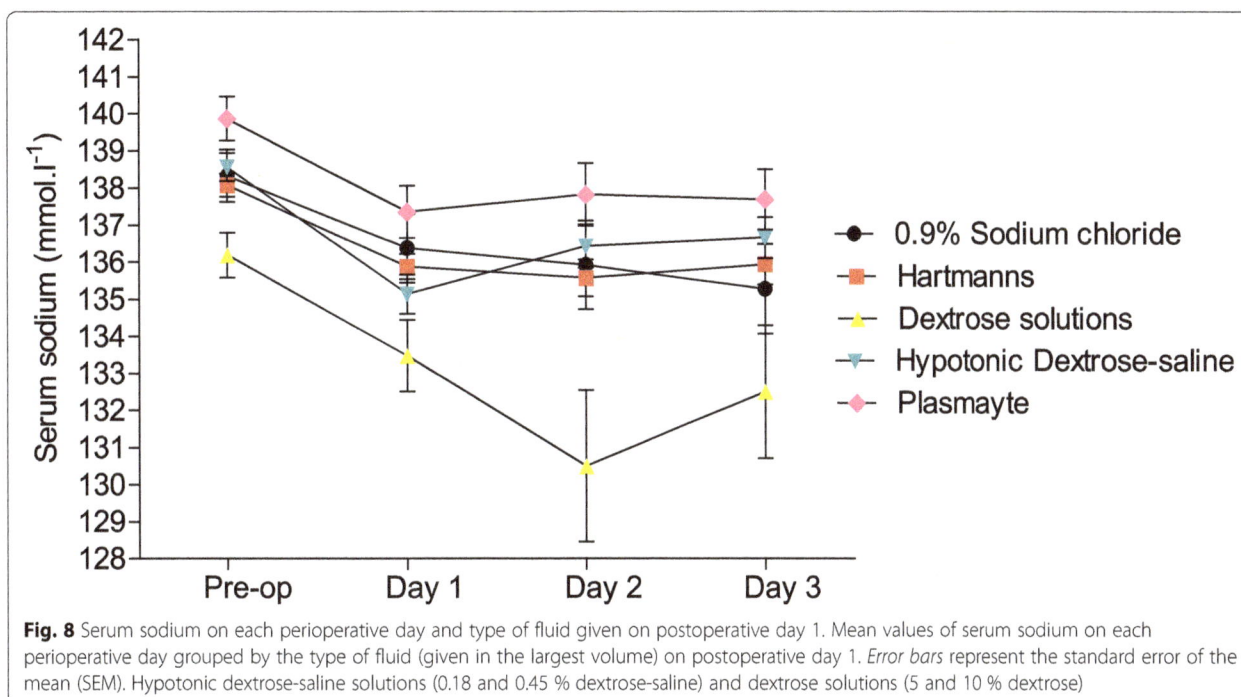

Fig. 8 Serum sodium on each perioperative day and type of fluid given on postoperative day 1. Mean values of serum sodium on each perioperative day grouped by the type of fluid (given in the largest volume) on postoperative day 1. *Error bars* represent the standard error of the mean (SEM). Hypotonic dextrose-saline solutions (0.18 and 0.45 % dextrose-saline) and dextrose solutions (5 and 10 % dextrose)

to HDU or ward, perhaps indicating better intravenous fluid prescribing practice or awareness of guidelines.

The inadequate doses of intravenous potassium required to meet the maintenance seen in our audit are in keeping with previous work (Lu et al. 2013) and our anecdotal observations. Although it is possible that some patients received potassium supplementation by other means (i.e. orally), the increasing incidence of hypokalaemia as the postoperative period progresses suggests that inadequate intravenous (and other) potassium supplementation is a true finding and is a problem that requires addressing. There are a number of potential reasons behind this but fear of intravenous potassium and the belief that the balanced crystalloid solutions contain adequate potassium for all patients are possible explanations. Hypokalaemia in the postoperative patient has been associated with slower return of gut function as well as other complications, and there is a suggestion that preventing hypokalaemia in the postoperative stage may improve outcomes (Lu et al. 2013).

Postoperative hyponatraemia was common and is multifactorial. It is not possible to determine the causes without a detailed notes analysis of the affected patients. As Fig. 8 demonstrates, mean serum sodium declined by 2.6 mmol.l^{-1} in the 356 subjects in whom pre- and postoperative day 1 serum sodium values were available. This is despite the vast majority of intraoperative intravenous fluid therapy consisting of balanced crystalloid solutions. Therefore, the decline in mean serum sodium compared to pre-operative values is most likely to represent the physiological stress response to surgery. This is

a spectrum of changes that occur throughout various body systems (neuroendocrine, metabolic, immunological and haematological) in response to surgical incision and trauma. Neuroendocrine changes are particularly relevant to perioperative fluids because the release of catecholamines and cortisol, vasopressin and aldosterone result in retention of sodium and water (often water in excess of sodium hence hyponatraemia), loss of potassium, reduced creatinine clearance and urine output. These effects can last well beyond the operative period into the postoperative phase.

Hyponatraemia can cause a variety of neurological and other symptoms but, more importantly, has been associated with increased risk of in-hospital and long-term mortality in a variety of patient groups (Lu et al. 2013). The mean drop in serum sodium from postoperative day 1 to postoperative day 2 was 0.21 mmol.l^{-1}. When only looking at those patients who received any dextrose solutions on postoperative day 1, the mean drop was 2.9 mmol.kg^{-1}. This raises the possibility that the use of dextrose solutions on postoperative day 1 is associated with subsequent hyponatraemia (compared to other fluids) and should be avoided. It should be noted that the pre-operative mean serum sodium was lower in this group. With the relatively small number of subjects, the retrospective nature of the audit and the large number of contributory factors, it is not possible to suggest causation. From our limited data, it would appear that the use of hypotonic dextrose-saline on postoperative day 1 was not associated with hyponatraemia and therefore, the recommendation made in several fluid guidelines

(National Institute for Health and Care Excellence 2013; Woodcock 2014) that this is the preferred fluid is reasonable based on the results of this audit.

The range of intraoperative fluid doses for three index procedures was wide and in keeping with a recent two-centre observational study in America of fluid administration for uncomplicated elective abdominal surgery with minimal blood loss (Lilot et al. 2015). This found wide variability of crystalloid administration both within and between anaesthesia providers (Lilot et al. 2015). In that study, for most procedures, 50 % of patients received 4–10 $ml.kg^{-1}.h^{-1}$ of crystalloid (corrected for urine output and estimated blood loss) but 50 % fell outside of this wide range with some patients receiving as much as 35 $ml.kg^{-1}.h^{-1}$ (Lilot et al. 2015). Although a patient's fluid requirements will vary and depend on a number of factors, it would be surprising to see such a wide range of physiological needs during similar surgical episodes, raising the possibility that variation is due to variation in individual anaesthetists' fluid approach.

The lack of correlation between the volume of postoperative day 1 fluids and body weight is interesting. In terms of absolute volumes given, if clinicians were calculating fluid doses on a millilitre per kilogram basis, we might expect absolute volumes to increase with body weight. We saw the opposite of this with smaller patients getting larger volumes of fluids. This suggests that practitioners are thinking in terms of 'number of bags' for a 'standard' patient and not taking into account weight.

Unanswered questions and future research
Most intravenous fluid trials take place in the operating theatre. We have demonstrated the type of intravenous fluid prescribed varies depending on whether the patient is in the postoperative ward or in theatre. The type of prescriber is likely to be different as well. Some previous intravenous fluid research has excluded the first postoperative day from any analysis because fluid prescriptions during this period may have been complicated by surgery-induced fluid and electrolyte shifts and any postoperative fluid prescriptions completed by the anaesthetist (Walsh and Walsh 2005). Being a continuum, any future research should cover the intraoperative and postoperative phases, something that has been recognised as important by an international trial looking at fluid therapy during and after major abdominal surgery Myles PS & Wallace SK (2015). Interestingly, prostatectomies in the American study (Lilot et al. 2015) had a much narrower range of fluid administered because a fluid protocol exists. A similar fluid protocol intervention may be needed in Wessex.

Education of junior doctors can make an impact on their prescribing choices (De Silva et al. 2010) but there is always a risk that any relatively short lived intervention only lasts a limited period of time before traditional practice starts to re-establish itself. The variation in intraoperative fluid volumes observed in theatre means that there is a quality improvement work that might be required in this environment as well.

Conclusions
Our aims were to accurately document the current clinical practice of perioperative intravenous fluid prescribing and identify key areas for improvement. There is some evidence of good practice in terms of early cessation of intravenous fluid, reduced use of 0.9 % sodium chloride compared with previous audits and early free fluid orders. However, there is clearly a need for effective implementation of intravenous fluid therapy guidelines to assist prescribers in the postoperative period prescribe appropriate quantities of sodium, potassium and water relevant to the clinical need. The wide variation of intraoperative volume for three common elective procedures is of concern and needs to be investigated further. We have identified that the suboptimal use of intravenous fluid therapy is relatively common and a potential cause of excessive complications. It is of concern that a basic principle such as appropriate potassium supplementation appears to be inadequate. The publication of prominent guidelines for all involved in fluid prescribing can only help raise basic standards, while acknowledging that fluid physiology is a complex and evolving area not fully understood even by those with expertise in this field.

Abbreviations
IV: intravenous; kg: kilogram; l: litre; $mmol.l^{-1}$: millimoles per litre.

Competing interests
The authors declare that they have no competing interests.

Authors' contributions
BH participated in the design of the study, recruited the contributors and organised the data collection and project management, collated and analysed the majority of the data and drafted the manuscript. BH is also the chair of the Southcoast Perioperative Audit and Research Collaboration (SPARC). CS participated in the design of the study, recruited the contributors and organised the data collection, collected the data, and contributed to the data analysis and drafting of the manuscript. CS is also the vice-chair of the Southcoast Perioperative Audit and Research Collaboration (SPARC). CK recruited the contributors, collected the data, organised the project logistics and helped proof read the manuscript. CK is also the vice-chair of the Southcoast Perioperative Audit and Research Collaboration (SPARC). ME led the design of the study, assisted in gaining the appropriate approvals, provided leadership, analysed the data and contributed to the drafting of the manuscript as well as is the consultant advisor of the Southcoast Perioperative Audit and Research Collaboration (SPARC). SPARC is the collaborative group composed of the above authors and a number of additional contributors listed below. SPARC contributed to the data collection and organisation. All of the above authors have read and approved the final manuscript.

Authors' information

BH, CS and CK are all anaesthetic speciality training registrars in the Wessex deanery. They are the founder members of the trainee-led audit and research network SPARC (Southcoast Perioperative Audit and Research Collaboration) that aims to promote multi-centre collaborative audit and research led by speciality trainees. ME is a consultant in anaesthesia and perioperative medicine.

Acknowledgements

The following individuals are members of SPARC and were the major contributors to this study as local lead investigators: Sophia Henderson, Ilana Delroy-Buelles, Phil McGlone, Louise Young and Rob Wiltshire. The following individuals are members of SPARC and were the major contributors to this study as local investigators: Chris White, Chris Redburn, Honor Hinxman, Jamie Briggs, Helen Gordon and Keith Ritchie. The following individuals are members of SPARC and were the minor contributors to this study as local investigators: Andrea Ackerman, Andrew Nash, Angus Sutherland, James Gaynor, Kate Shepherd, Kavil Shah, Laura Wood, Louise Bates, Lucy White, Nick Goddard, Paul Stevens, Robert Lowe, Rob Charnock and Tom Hutley. We would like to thank Professor Mike Grocott, Dr. Mark Edwards, Dr. Richard Thomas, Dr. Matthew Wood and Dr. Kayode Adeniji for their significant support towards initiating and promoting SPARC in the Wessex deanery. Dr Matthew Wood (Clinical Director Portsmouth Anaesthetics) supported the project by kindly paying for the administration costs of obtaining clinical records in Portsmouth Hospital from the anaesthetic department audit budget (less than £150). Dr. Richard Thomas donated £500 from the Royal Hampshire County Hospital trainee-support budget to cover general administrative costs of running SPARC but not specifically for this project. No other grants or awards were received or used to support or fund this project.

Author details

[1]Academic Department of Critical Care, Queen Alexandra Hospital, Southwick Hill Road, Cosham, Portsmouth PO6 3LY, UK. [2]Anaesthetic Department, Queen Alexandra Hospital, Southwick Hill Road, Cosham, Portsmouth PO6 3LY, UK. [3]Anaesthetic Department, Royal Hampshire County Hospital, Romsey Road, Winchester, , Hampshire SO22 5DG, UK. [4]Anaesthetic Department Mail Point 24, University Hospital Southampton NHS Foundation Trust, Tremona Road, Southampton SO16 6YD, UK.

References

BUPA Insurance Ltd. Schedule of Procedures. London, UK. 2014. http://codes.bupa.co.uk/procedures. [accessed 15/12/15].

Callum KG, Gray AJG, Hoile RW, Ingram GS, Martin IC, Sherry KM, et al. Extremes of age: the 1999 report of the National Confidential Enquiry into Perioperative Deaths. London: National Confidential Enquiry into Perioperative Deaths; 1999.

De Silva NA, Scibelli T, Itobi E, Austin P, Abu-Hilal M, Wootton SA, et al. Improving peri-operative fluid management in a large teaching hospital. Proc Nutr Soc. 2010;69:499–507.

Gonzalez-Fajardo JA, Mengibar L, Brizuela JA, Castrodeza J, Vaquero-Puerta C. Effect of postoperative restrictive fluid therapy in the recovery of patients with abdominal surgery. Eur J Vasc Endovasc Surg. 2009;37(5):538–43.

Kahn S, Gatt M, Horgan A, Anderson I, MacFie J. Association fo Surgeons of Great Britain and Ireland: Guidelines for implementation of enhanced recovery protocols. (2009). http://www.asgbi.org.uk/download.cfm?docid=BE0B52EE-AE0E-42C1-A10EDDE7BABDC57A. [Accessed 15/12/15]

Lilot M, Ehrenfeld JM, Lee C, Harrington B, Cannesson M, Rinehart J. Variability in practice and factors predictive of total crystalloid administration during abdominal surgery: retrospective two-centre analysis. BJA. 2015;114(5):767–76.

Lobo DN. Intravenous 0.9 % saline and general surgical patients: a problem, not a solution. Ann Surg. 2012;255(5):830–2.

Lobo DN, Dube MG, Neal KR, Simpson J, Rowlands BJ, Allison SP. Problems with solutions: drowning in the brine of an inadequate knowledge base. Clin Nutr. 2001;20(2):125–30.

Lu G, Yan Q, Huang Y, Zhong Y, Shi P. Prevention and control system of hypokalaemia in fast recovery after abdominal surgery. Curr Ther Res. 2013;74:68–73.

Minto G, Mythen MG. Perioperative fluid management: science, art or random chaos? Br J Anaesth. 2015;114(5):717–221.

Myles PS, Wallace SK. REstrictive versus LIbEral Fluid therapy in major abdominal surgery: RELIEF study. (2015). ClinicalTrials.gov Identifier: NCT01424150. https://clinicaltrials.gov/ct2/show/NCT01424150. Accessed 25th July 2015.

National Institute for Health and Care Excellence (2013) Intravenous fluids for adults in hospital. NICE guideline (CG174). London, UK.

Powell-Tuck J, Gosling P, Lobo DN, Allison SP, Carlson GL, Gore M, et al. British Consensus Guidelines on Intravenous Fluid Therapy for Adult Surgical Patients. The British Association for Parenteral and Enteral Nutrition. 2011. http://www.bapen.org.uk/pdfs/bapen_pubs/giftasup.pdf. Accessed 4th August 2015.

Soni N. British Consensus Guidelines on Intravenous Fluid Therapy for Adult Surgical Patients (GIFTASUP)—Cassandras's view. Anaesth. 2009;64:235–8.

Walsh SR, Walsh CJ. Intravenous fluid-associated morbidity in postoperative patients. Ann R Coll Surg Engl. 2005;87(2):126–30.

Woodcock T. GIFTAHo; an improvement on GIFTASuP? New NICE guidelines on intravenous fluids. Anaesth. 2014;69(5):410–5.

5

Fluid resuscitation practice patterns in intensive care units of the USA: a cross-sectional survey of critical care physicians

Timothy E. Miller[1], Martin Bunke[2], Paul Nisbet[3] and Charles S. Brudney[1*]

Abstract

Background: Fluid resuscitation is a cornerstone of intensive care treatment, yet there is a lack of agreement on how various types of fluids should be used in critically ill patients with different disease states. Therefore, our goal was to investigate the practice patterns of fluid utilization for resuscitation of adult patients in intensive care units (ICUs) within the USA.

Methods: We conducted a cross-sectional online survey of 502 physicians practicing in medical and surgical ICUs. Survey questions were designed to assess clinical decision-making processes for 3 types of patients who need volume expansion: (1) not bleeding and not septic, (2) bleeding but not septic, (3) requiring resuscitation for sepsis. First-choice fluid used in fluid boluses for these 3 patient types was requested from the respondents. Descriptive statistics were performed using a Kruskal-Wallis test to evaluate differences among the physician groups. Follow-up tests, including t tests, were conducted to evaluate differences between ICU types, hospital settings, and bolus volume.

Results: Fluid resuscitation varied with respect to preferences for the factors to determine volume status and preferences for fluid types. The 3 most frequently preferred volume indicators were blood pressure, urine output, and central venous pressure. Regardless of the patient type, the most preferred fluid type was crystalloid, followed by 5 % albumin and then 6 % hydroxyethyl starches (HES) 450/0.70 and 6 % HES 600/0.75. Surprisingly, up to 10 % of physicians still chose HES as the first choice of fluid for resuscitation in sepsis. The clinical specialty and the practice setting of the treating physicians also influenced fluid choices.

Conclusions: Practice patterns of fluid resuscitation varied in the USA, depending on patient characteristics, clinical specialties, and practice settings of the treating physicians.

Keywords: Fluid resuscitation, Intensive care unit, Sepsis, Bleeding, Colloids, Crystalloids, Albumin, Survey

Background

Fluid resuscitation is a cornerstone of intensive care treatments, and fluid therapy is one part of a complex strategy in hemodynamic resuscitation (Myburgh and Mythen 2013). There is considerable debate about the effects of fluid type, timing of administration, appropriate amount of fluid, and techniques for determining fluid responsiveness (Cherpanath et al. 2014; van Haren and Zacharowski 2014). The principles of fluid exchange and how they influence clinical decisions regarding fluid type have been a major topic of interest. With approximately 1.7 million inpatient stays associated with sepsis during 2009, sepsis has become the sixth most common reason for hospitalization in the USA (Elixhauser et al. 2006). Thus, it is of interest to understand how physicians approach fluid resuscitation in sepsis relative to nonseptic conditions. Since 1896, Starling's Principle of Fluid Exchange stated that fluid movement across the capillary wall depends on the balance between the hydrostatic pressure gradient that pushes water outward into the interstitial space and the colloid oncotic pressure that pulls water inward into the vessel (Aditianingsih and George 2014). As we come to better understand that successful fluid resuscitation depends on the disease "context"

* Correspondence: scott.brudney@duke.edu
[1]Department of Anesthesiology, Duke University Medical Center, Durham, NC 27710, USA
Full list of author information is available at the end of the article

(i.e., the physiological state of the patient), it becomes apparent that the classic Starling's Principle does not apply to all situations and needs to be adapted to encompass conditions involving systemic inflammation and vascular barrier damage (Jacob and Chappell 2013).

In recent years, new research efforts increasingly recognize the endothelial glycocalyx layer (EGL) as a crucial determinant of vascular barrier function (Weinbaum et al. 2007; Becker et al. 2010). The EGL acts as a filter that generates an effective colloid oncotic pressure with the presence of a protein-free layer in the subglycocalyx space of the EGL. Large molecules, (e.g., albumin in colloid solutions) are retained inside the vessel, generating colloid oncotic pressure in the intravascular compartment (Myburgh and Mythen 2013; Aditianingsih and George 2014; Jacob and Chappell 2013). Small molecules (e.g., electrolytes in crystalloid solutions) traveling freely through the vessel wall can draw water into the interstitial space. Animal and human studies suggest that the EGL is damaged in numerous systemic inflammatory states, including trauma (Johansson et al. 2011) and sepsis (Steppan et al. 2011), and may become compromised, leading to interstitial edema (Weinbaum et al. 2007; Ait-Oufella et al. 2010). In other words, colloids may behave more like crystalloids in sepsis, and several large studies have failed to show any benefit from colloids in this context. On the other hand, if a patient has an intact EGL and an intravascular volume deficit, then volume therapy with a colloid fluid restores the intravascular volume as predicted by Starling, and far higher volumes of crystalloids are required to achieve the same result (Rehm et al. 2000). In this context, at least theoretically, colloids may have advantages over crystalloids (Roger et al. 2014).

In addition, there is still on-going debate over whether liberal or restricted fluid volume strategies would yield more favorable clinical outcomes in critically ill patients (Polderman and Varon 2015). What is generally accepted is that fluid administration should be managed to achieve zero or negative fluid balance by the time patients recover from all 4 phases of fluid resuscitation [(1) salvage/rescue, (2) optimization, (3) stabilization, (4) deescalation] (Vincent and De Backer 2013; Myburgh 2015; Hoste et al. 2014; Rewa and Bagshaw 2015). The context of where the patients are in their course of critical illness is important (Vincent and De Backer 2013). The FIRST (James et al. 2011) and CRISTAL (Annane et al. 2013) trials enrolled patients undergoing resuscitation for highly severe trauma and severe hypotensive, hypovolemic shock, respectively, which presumably mean those patients were in the *salvage/rescue phase*. On the other hand, the SAFE (Finfer et al. 2004), CHEST (Myburgh et al. 2012), and ALBIOS (Caironi et al. 2014) trials enrolled patients who were mostly in the *optimization phase* with lower fluid volume needs and

likely longer time interval from shock onset. Likewise, other trials (Navarro et al. 2015; Opperer et al. 2015) conducted in the perioperative disease context were likely in the *optimization phase*.

It is important to assess how fluids are currently being used in the USA for sepsis and other critical care conditions. The objectives of this study were the following: (A) to examine the use of different types of fluids for resuscitation (i.e., crystalloids, plasma-derived colloid [albumin], synthetic colloids [hydroxyethyl starches, HES]) in critically ill patients in adult intensive care units within the USA; (B) to determine whether certain patient characteristics and/or practice settings have an influence on the type of fluid utilized for resuscitation; and (C) to determine whether the fluid selected for resuscitation varies by clinical specialties of the treating physicians.

Methods
Study design

This study is cross-sectional and collected survey data from physicians practicing in medical and surgical ICUs of the USA. A 10-min online survey was administered to 502 physicians to investigate the patterns of fluid utilization in the ICU. Initial survey questions were developed by 2 of the authors (TM and CSB), finalized through discussion and input from all authors then pretested to ensure the quality of the survey. The 25-item self-administered questionnaire (Additional file 1) obtained information on preferences for fluid use in hemodynamic management and volume status indicators used most often to determine volume expansion needs. The survey questions were designed to assess clinical decision-making for 3 types of patients: "patient type 1" needs volume expansion but is not bleeding and not septic, "patient type 2" needs volume expansion in the presence of blood loss when blood transfusion is not indicated (adequate Hb) and the patient is not septic, and "patient type 3" needs volume expansion for resuscitation in sepsis. First-choice fluid used in fluid boluses for these 3 different types of patients was requested from the respondents. In addition, physicians were presented with the 3 patient scenarios sequentially and asked to identify their first choice of fluid from a list of 5 colloid and crystalloid solutions for volume expansion for each patient type. The 5 types of fluids were crystalloids, 5 % albumin, 25 % albumin, 6 % HES 450/0.70 and 6 % HES 600/0.75 (first-generation HES), and 6 % HES 130/0.4 (third-generation HES). For simplification, we will refer to "6 % HES 450/0.70 and 6 % HES 600/0.75" as *HES 450/600* and "6 % HES 130/0.40" as *HES 130* throughout the rest of this manuscript. Physicians rated the frequency with which they preferred various products for volume expansion using a 5-point scale, from "always" to "never," and they were also asked to indicate the bolus volume (milliliter) of the crystalloids and colloids that they typically use for volume expansion. In addition, they were asked to rate the importance of certain colloid characteristics (e.g., more sustained volume expansion, faster volume expansion) and nononcotic properties of albumin (e.g., transport of metabolites, free radical scavenging) on the treatment decision-making process using a 5-point scale, from "not important" to "absolutely essential."

In February 2015, participants were recruited from the Research Now Healthcare physician panel. Research Now is a company that manages a panel of physicians who have opted to become members of the Research Now Healthcare panel. Email invitations for participation in this study were sent from Research Now to their physician panelists, who remained anonymous to the investigators in this study. To qualify to participate in this survey, physicians had to specialize in anesthesiology, surgery, critical care medicine, or pulmonology; have been in practice for at least 2 years since residency; rotate in surgical ICU, medical ICU, or an ICU accepting a variety of patients; and treat or consult on at least 3 to 4 ICU patients per week. Physicians who worked in cardiac, neurology, or pediatric ICUs were excluded. Subquotas were set for each specialty to ensure that a minimum number of completed surveys were received from each specialty: 125 surgeons, 125 anesthesiologists, 175 critical care medicine specialists, and 75 pulmonologists. All potential respondents were recruited by email invitation which provided a general description of the survey topic and a link for interested recipients to access the online survey. Invitations were sent to 12,435 physicians. Of these, a total of 2724 physicians attempted to access the survey, making the response rate 21.9 %. Of the 2724 who attempted to access the survey, 502 (4.0 %) made up the final participant pool that accessed the survey, qualified via the screening questions, and completed the survey prior to the set quotas being reached. Each invitation contained a unique ID that prevented any one respondent from taking the survey more than once. The participants were aware that the anonymous data collected in this survey may be published.

This research project involved obtaining the opinions of physicians about their choice for the use of various fluids for resuscitation in 3 different hypothetical patient situations. No patient data was obtained, and no questions were asked of the physicians that would help in identifying them. Any physician data was de-identified. Hence, this study was exempt from requiring institutional review board review under USA Code of Federal Regulations Title 45 Part 46.101(b)(2) by Copernicus Group IRB, because any physician information within the survey dataset was de-identified.

Statistical analysis

Several questions were based on 5-point scales and provided ordinal data which, by definition, are not normally distributed. As such, descriptive statistics were performed using a Kruskal-Wallis test to evaluate differences among the physician groups on the ordinal measures. Follow-up tests were conducted to evaluate differences between ICU types and between practice settings. t tests were used to evaluate differences across ratio variables (i.e., bolus volume). Statistical significance was assessed at the alpha level of <0.05. Descriptive analyses were performed using SPSS (version 23.0). Data analysis was done by PN.

Results

Of the 502 physicians who completed the survey, 125 (24.9 %) were anesthesiologists, 125 (24.9 %) were surgeons, 104 (20.7 %) practiced critical care medicine, and 148 (29.5 %) were pulmonologists (Table 1). The majority of anesthesiologists and surgeons practiced in surgical ICUs, while the majority of critical care medicine specialists and pulmonologists were from medical ICUs. Approximately three-fourths of the physicians from each clinical specialty practiced at nonuniversity hospitals. The average hospital size was approximately 400 beds,

Table 1 Summary of participant characteristics

		Anesthesiologists[A]	Surgeon[S]	Critical care medicine[C]	Pulmonologists[P]
		($n = 125$)	($n = 125$)	($n = 104$)	($n = 148$)
ICU type	Surgical	58.4 %	74.4 %[A]	–	–
	Medical	–	–	52.9 %	61.5 %
	ICU accepting variety of patients	41.6 %[S]	25.6 %	47.1 %[S]	38.5 %[S]
Practice setting	University hospital	24.8 %	28.0 %	31.7 %	26.4 %
	Nonuniversity hospital	75.2 %	72.0 %	68.3 %	73.6 %
Hospital size	No. of beds in the hospital	343	410	410	403
	No. of ICU beds in the hospital	35	49[A]	39	41

Superscripts A, S, C, and P denote differences between specialties that are statistically significant at $P < 0.05$
ICU intensive care unit

and the average number of ICU beds in each hospital was about 40 beds. Physician age and gender were not collected.

The decision-making process for fluid management varied considerably among physicians of all clinical specialties in this study, and there was extensive heterogeneity in the diagnostic approaches used to inform decisions for fluid management (Fig. 1). Some of the results provide unexpected insights into the ways in which physicians from different backgrounds approach ICU care. Many tests were used at varying extents by all 4 physician specialties to assess the need for volume expansion, with the 3 most frequently used indicators being blood pressure, urine output, and central venous pressure. Our observations reflected published findings of a Canadian survey (McIntyre et al. 2007) which reported that urine output and blood pressure were also the 2 most commonly cited resuscitation end-points for early septic shock. To our surprise, less invasive parameters, such as pulse pressure or systolic pressure variation and plethysmographic waveform variations, were not frequently used by physicians of any specialty. Of those who chose pulse pressure or systolic pressure variation, anesthesiologists (40 %), critical care medicine specialists (30 %), and pulmonologists (26 %) were more than 2-fold as likely to use these indicators as surgeons (14 %).

Overall, crystalloid fluid was the primary choice for fluid resuscitation (Figs. 2, 3, and 4). The second most

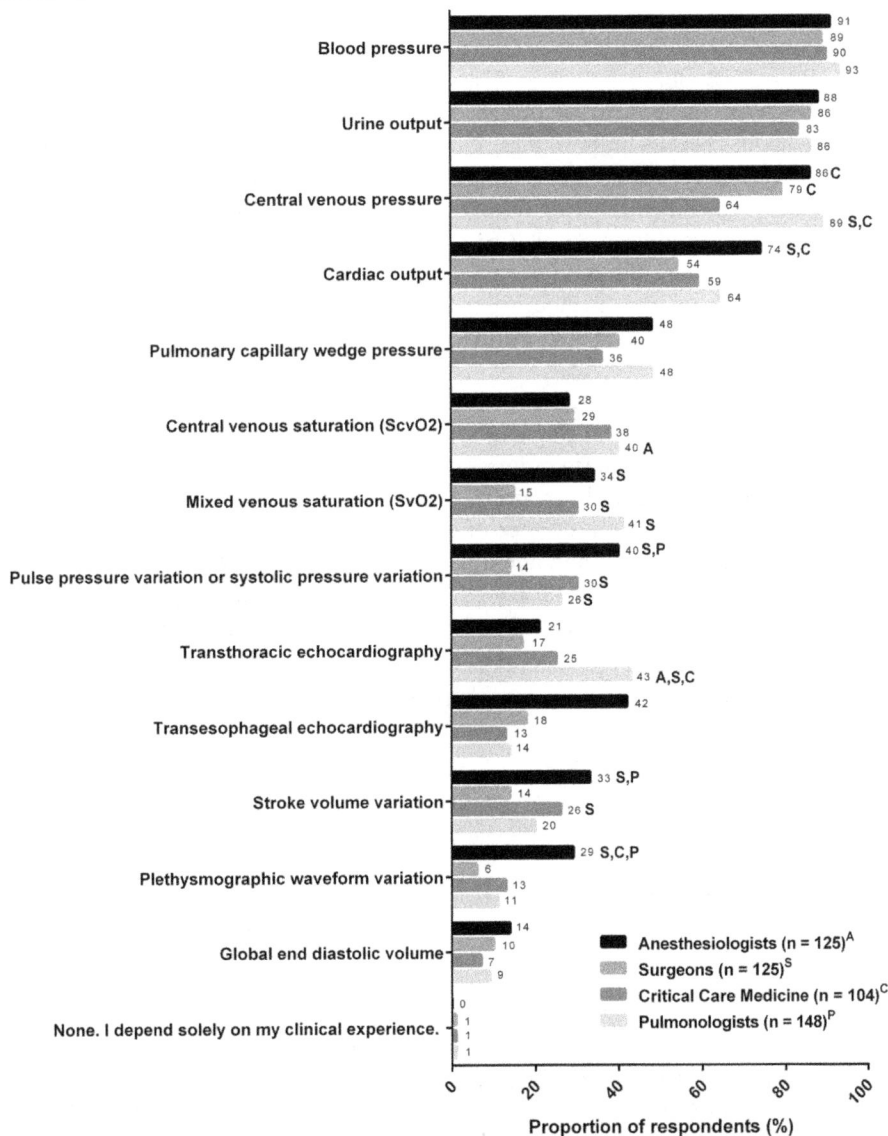

Fig. 1 Volume status indicators and diagnostic tools used in assessing fluid needs. *Superscripts A, S, C,* and *P* denote differences between specialties that are statistically significant at $P < 0.05$

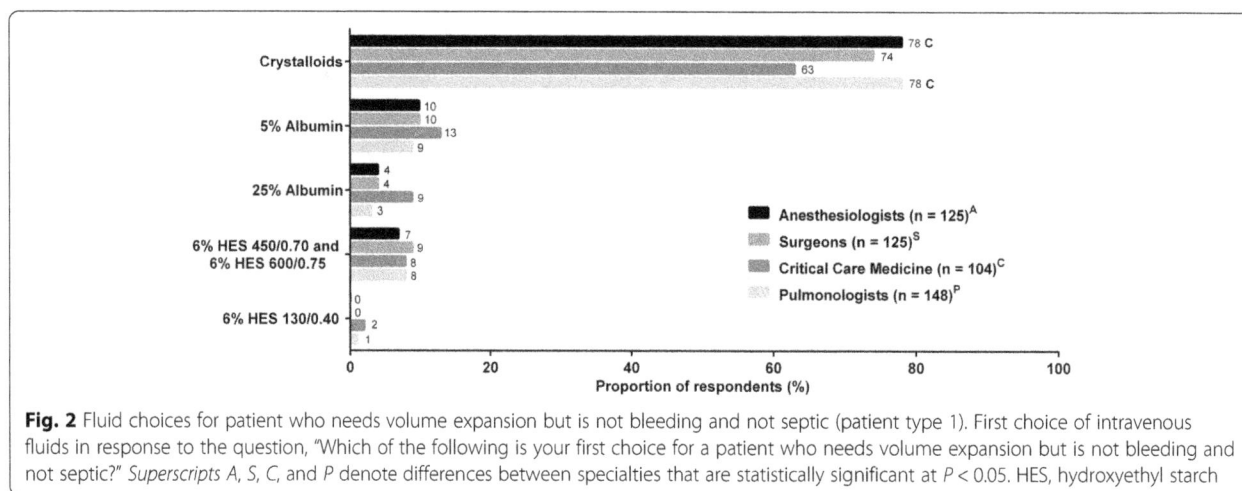

Fig. 2 Fluid choices for patient who needs volume expansion but is not bleeding and not septic (patient type 1). First choice of intravenous fluids in response to the question, "Which of the following is your first choice for a patient who needs volume expansion but is not bleeding and not septic?" *Superscripts A, S, C, and P denote differences between specialties that are statistically significant at P < 0.05. HES, hydroxyethyl starch*

commonly chosen fluid was 5 % albumin. Only a small fraction of physicians chose 25 % albumin as their first choice, and, therefore, we have elected not to present data on utilization frequency of 25 % albumin in Figs. 2, 3, and 4. Among the 4 clinical specialties of treating physicians, there were subtle, but statistically significant, differences in how fluids were being utilized for all 3 patient types. Data on the frequencies of utilization of various fluids are shown in Additional file 2: Figure S1, Additional file 3: Figure S2, and Additional file 4: Figure S3 for the 3 patient types.

For patient type 1 who needs volume expansion in the *absence of blood loss and sepsis* (Fig. 2), most physicians (63–78 %) chose crystalloids as their first choice of intravenous (IV) fluids regardless of clinical specialty, followed by 5 % albumin (9–13 %). About a quarter of all physicians reported "often" using 5 % albumin and up to 49 % "sometimes" use 5 % albumin (Additional file 2: Figure S1B). HES 450/600 were chosen by 7–9 % of

physicians, while only <2 % of physicians chose HES 130. Critical care medicine specialists seemed to prefer less crystalloids and slightly more albumin for this patient type than physicians from other specialties. In contrast to critical care medicine specialists, anesthesiologists most frequently reported "often" choosing crystalloids (Additional file 2: Figure S1A), "sometimes" choosing 5 % albumin (Additional file 2: Figure S1B) and HES 450/600 (Additional file 2: Figure S1C), but "rarely" or "never" HES 130 (Additional file 2: Figure S1D). Interestingly, the highest proportions of those who "rarely" or "never" choose HES 450/600 or HES 130 were pulmonologists.

For patient type 2 who needs volume expansion in *the presence of blood loss but is not septic* (Fig. 3), crystalloid was the first choice of IV fluids (47–65 %), followed by 5 % albumin (11–24 %) and HES 450/600 (7–20 %). Less than 5 % of physicians preferred HES 130. Although anesthesiologists made up the smallest proportion of those

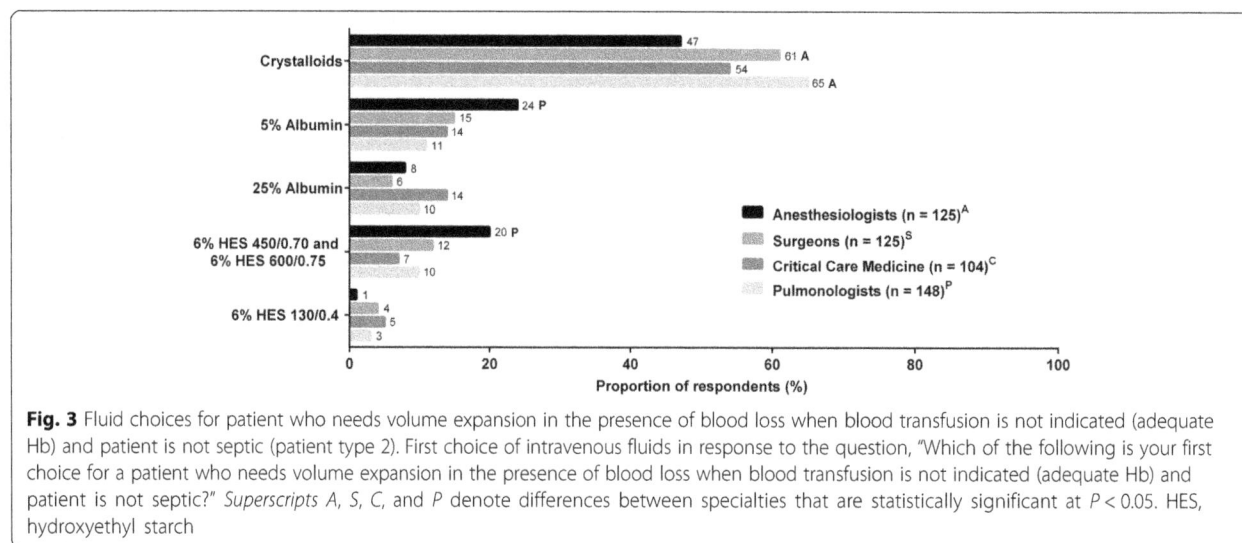

Fig. 3 Fluid choices for patient who needs volume expansion in the presence of blood loss when blood transfusion is not indicated (adequate Hb) and patient is not septic (patient type 2). First choice of intravenous fluids in response to the question, "Which of the following is your first choice for a patient who needs volume expansion in the presence of blood loss when blood transfusion is not indicated (adequate Hb) and patient is not septic?" *Superscripts A, S, C, and P denote differences between specialties that are statistically significant at P < 0.05. HES, hydroxyethyl starch*

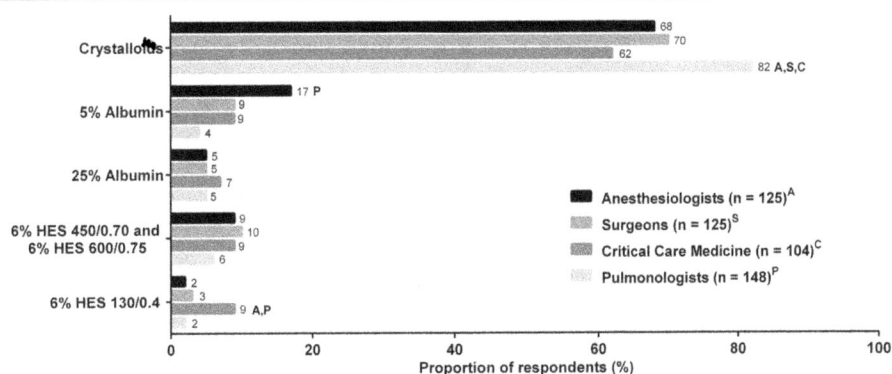

Fig. 4 Fluid choices for patient who needs volume expansion for resuscitation in sepsis (patient type 3). First choice of intravenous fluids in response to the question, "Which of the following is your first choice for a patient who needs volume expansion for resuscitation in sepsis?" *Superscripts A, S, C, and P denote differences between specialties that are statistically significant at P < 0.05. HES, hydroxyethyl starch*

who chose crystalloids (47 %) as first choice of fluid in this patient type, they were more likely to choose 5 % albumin (24 %) than pulmonologists (11 %), and they made up the highest proportion (41 %) of those who "often" chose 5 % albumin compared to any other specialties (22–25 %) (Additional file 3: Figure S2B). Surgeons (61 %) and pulmonologists (65 %) were more likely to prefer crystalloids than anesthesiologists (47 %). Moreover, pulmonologists made up the highest proportion of those who reported "always" choosing crystalloid (32 %, Additional file 3: Figure S2A) but "never" HES 450/600 (43 %, Additional file 3: Figure S2C) compared to physicians of any other specialties.

For patient type 3 who needs volume expansion *for resuscitation in sepsis* (Fig. 4), crystalloid was, again, the first-choice of fluids (62–82 %), followed by 5 % albumin (4–17 %). Pulmonologists (82 %) made up the highest proportion of physicians who chose crystalloids as the first choice of fluid. Similar to the patterns observed for patient type 2 (Fig. 3), anesthesiologists (17 %) were more likely to choose 5 % albumin as their first choice than pulmonologists (4 %), and they also made up the highest proportion of those who "often" and "sometimes" choose 5 % albumin (Additional file 4: Figure S3B). Surprisingly, up to 10 % of physicians across all specialties chose HES as first-choice fluids for this patient type despite the 2013 Food and Drug Administration boxed warning against HES use for sepsis due to increased mortality and severe renal injury (U.S. Food and Drug Administration 2013). Furthermore, we did not expect to see more physicians prefer HES 450/600 (6–10 %) over 25 % albumin (5–7 %), as the use of HES for patients with sepsis goes against the Surviving Sepsis Campaign (SSC) recommendations (Dellinger et al. 2013). Among those who chose HES 130 as their first choice, critical care medicine specialists made up the highest proportion (9 %) compared to the 2–3 % of physicians from other specialties.

When colloids were chosen as the preferred fluid for resuscitation, the 3 reasons most frequently cited for these decisions were the following: (1) more sustained volume expansion (Fig. 5a); (2) faster volume expansion (Fig. 5b); and (3) less interstitial edema (Fig. 5c). "Better respiratory function" appeared to be of less importance (Fig. 5d), and "less weight gain" (Fig. 5e) was the least important factor.

Another factor affecting the decision-making process was the practice setting from which the physicians came (Fig. 6). Subanalysis results suggest that practice patterns varied depending on whether a physician worked in university vs nonuniversity hospitals. Within the dataset for each patient type, *t* tests were used to assess for the significance of the differences between proportion of physicians from university and nonuniversity hospitals. To simplify the data, we combined 5 % and 25 % albumin into a single category named "albumin." The same was done for the 3 HES subtypes. Overall, most physicians chose crystalloids as the first choice of fluid regardless of practice setting. However, more physicians from nonuniversity hospitals compared to university hospitals chose crystalloid as their first choice for volume expansion in patient types 2 (bleeding but not septic, Fig. 6b) and 3 (septic, Fig. 6c) but not for patient type 1 (Fig. 6a). For patient type 3, physicians from university hospitals (21 %) preferred albumin more frequently relative to those from nonuniversity hospitals (12 %) (Fig. 6c). This is intriguing, as we wonder how ICU protocols at university hospitals may have played a role in distinguishing the behavior of this group toward treating patients with sepsis.

When we further analyzed data of the physicians who indicated crystalloids as the first-choice fluid based on their clinical specialties (Table 2), we found intriguing differences between how university and nonuniversity hospitals would handle the 3 different types of patients.

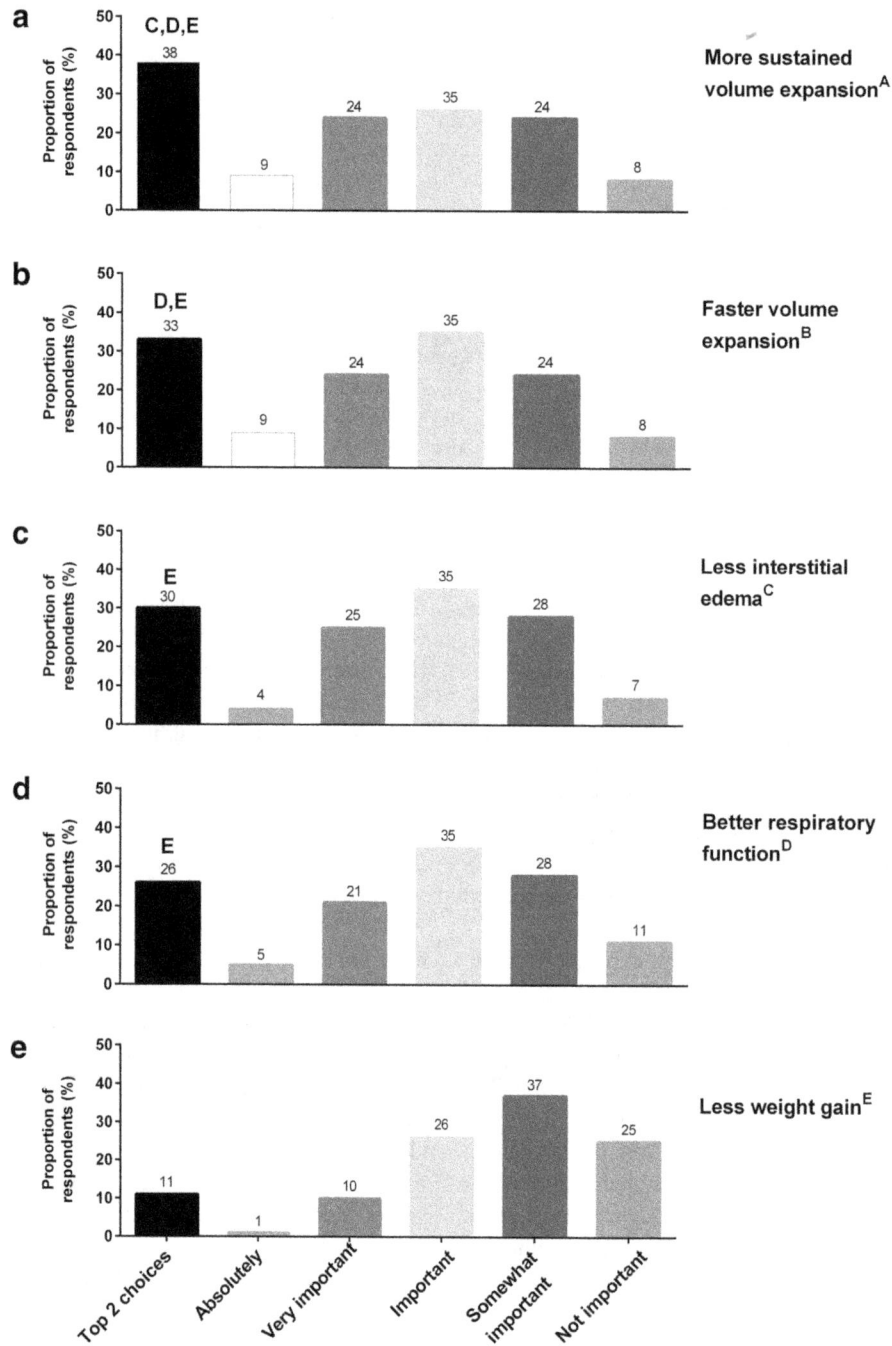

Fig. 5 Rankings of the importance of certain colloid traits when colloids are used for volume expansion. Colloid traits assessed are as follows: (**a**) more sustained volume expansion; (**b**) faster volume expansion; (**c**) less interstitial edema; (**d**) better respiratory function; (**e**) less weight gain

When the data for all clinical specialties were analyzed together, a higher proportion of physicians from nonuniversity hospitals (61.5 %) chose crystalloids for patient type 2 than those from university hospitals (45.7 %); while no difference in practice setting was found for patient types 1 and 3. When the data were analyzed based on the 4 individual clinical specialties, statistically

significant differences were detected for only anesthesiologists and surgeons; while no differences were observed among critical care medicine specialists and pulmonologists based on their practice settings. More anesthesiologists from nonuniversity hospitals than university hospitals preferred crystalloids as their first choice of fluid for patient type 2 (52.1 % vs 32.3 %,

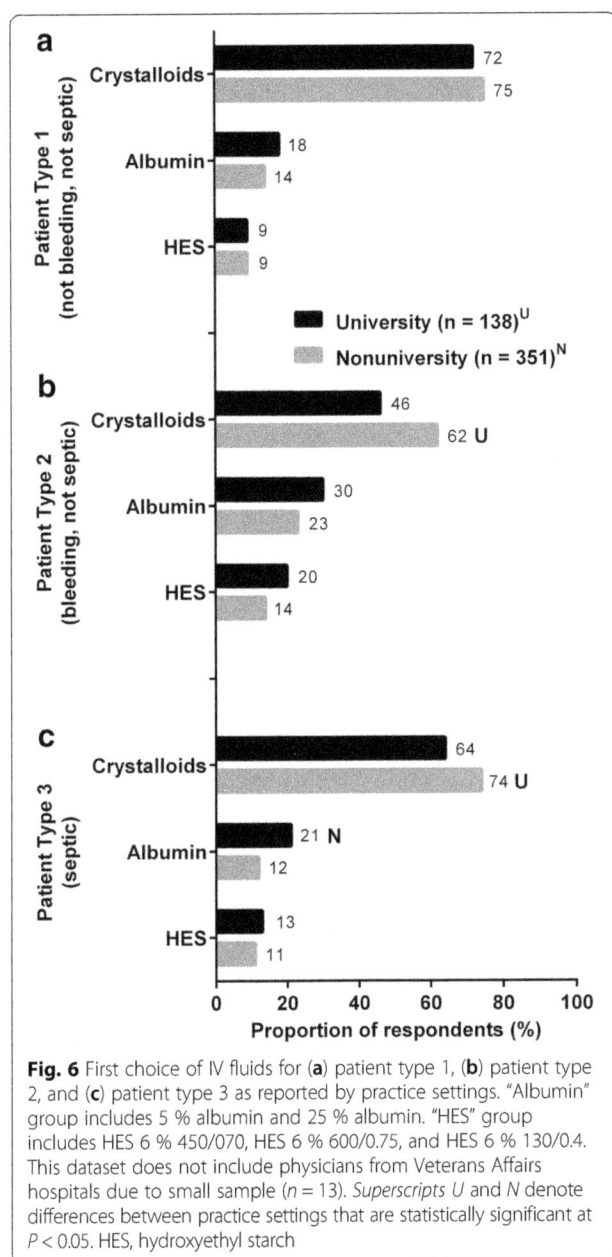

Fig. 6 First choice of IV fluids for (**a**) patient type 1, (**b**) patient type 2, and (**c**) patient type 3 as reported by practice settings. "Albumin" group includes 5 % albumin and 25 % albumin. "HES" group includes HES 6 % 450/070, HES 6 % 600/0.75, and HES 6 % 130/0.4. This dataset does not include physicians from Veterans Affairs hospitals due to small sample ($n = 13$). *Superscripts U and N denote differences between practice settings that are statistically significant at $P < 0.05$.* HES, hydroxyethyl starch

respectively) and for patient type 3 (73.4 % vs 51.6 %) but not for patient type 1. Surgeons from university hospitals (45.7 %) chose crystalloid as their first choice less frequently than those from nonuniversity hospitals (66.7 %) for patient type 2.

Interesting observations were also made regarding the preferences for bolus volume. In general, all physicians reported typical volume of colloid bolus (464.4 mL) as smaller than their typical volume of crystalloid bolus (797.4 mL). The estimated ratio of 1:1.7 for albumin to crystalloid volume in our study resembled previously published estimates from the SAFE study (1:1.4) (Finfer et al. 2004) and a systematic review/meta-

regression study across 24 reports (1:1.5) (Orbegozo Cortes et al. 2015). When bolus volume was evaluated as a function of clinical practice settings (Table 3), results from a one-sample t test indicated that physicians in nonuniversity hospitals appeared to prefer a slightly larger volume of crystalloid bolus (821.7 mL) than do physicians in university hospitals (716.5 mL), although this difference in volume was small and may not have clinical significance in most situations. Data from VA physicians were not included in this particular analysis due to small sample size ($n = 13$). To the best of our knowledge, these results are novel and have not been reported previously.

Discussion

This survey of 502 physicians from 4 clinical specialties of various ICU practice settings revealed that practice patterns in fluid resuscitation vary broadly with respect to preferences of volume status parameters and preferences for fluid types that would be used to treat patients who need volume expansion but are not bleeding and not septic (patient type 1), patients who need volume expansion due to bleeding but are not septic (patient type 2), and those who need resuscitation due to sepsis (patient type 3). For volume status parameters, the 3 most frequently preferred indicators were blood pressure, urine output, and central venous pressure; whereas, cardiac output, pulse pressure variation, and stroke volume may be considered to be better predictors of hemodynamic response to fluid loading (McDermid et al. 2014). For volume expansion, the most preferred fluid type was crystalloid, followed by 5 % albumin, regardless of the patient type considered. Surprisingly, up to 10 % of physicians still chose HES as a first choice of fluid for resuscitation in sepsis. The clinical specialties and practice settings of the treating physicians also influenced fluid choices. Among the different physician specialties, anesthesiologists appeared to prefer more colloids, particularly 5 % albumin, for patient types 2 and 3 than the other physician subgroups (Figs. 3 and 4). The data suggests that a greater proportion of university physicians than nonuniversity physicians preferred colloid as a first choice of fluids (Fig. 6).

Our finding that crystalloid was the first choice of fluid for most physicians in the USA aligned with published data from an international, cross-sectional survey (391 ICUs) in 2007 (Finfer et al. 2010), which found that the USA and New Zealand were more likely to use crystalloids than colloids; whereas, countries like Australia, China, Great Britain, Switzerland, and Sweden used more colloids than crystalloids. Furthermore, the strongest determinant of fluid choice was location of country, not measures of illness severity in their patients. Although we did not measure variations among geographic regions of the USA, we did observe differences in fluid

Table 2 Percent of physicians indicating crystalloids as first choice for volume expansion based on patient types

| | | Practice settings | |
		University hospital (*n* = 138)	Nonuniversity hospital (*n* = 351)
All clinical specialties	*n*	138	364
	Patient type 1	71.7 %	74.7 %
	Patient type 2	45.7 %	61.5 %*
	Patient type 3	64.5 %	73.6 %
Anesthesiologists only	*n*	31	94
	Patient type 1	74.2 %	79.8 %
	Patient type 2	32.3 %	52.1 %*
	Patient type 3	51.6 %	73.4 %*
Surgeons only	*n*	35	90
	Patient type 1	65.7 %	76.7 %
	Patient type 2	45.7 %	66.7 %*
	Patient type 3	60.0 %	73.3 %
Critical care medicine only	*n*	33	71
	Patient type 1	60.6 %	64.8 %
	Patient type 2	42.4 %	59.2 %
	Patient type 3	54.5 %	64.8 %
Pulmonologists only	*n*	39	109
	Patient type 1	84.6 %	75.2 %
	Patient type 2	59.0 %	67.0 %
	Patient type 3	87.2 %	79.8 %

Patient type 1: patient who needs volume expansion but is not bleeding and not septic. Patient type 2: patient who needs volume expansion in the presence of blood loss when blood transfusion is not indicated (adequate Hb) and patient is not septic. Patient type 3: patient who needs volume expansion for resuscitation in sepsis
*Statistically significant differences of $P < 0.05$ between practice settings within physician specialty

choice based on clinical practice settings. Physicians from the nonuniversity hospitals preferred crystalloids more than those from university hospitals for all 3 patient types (Fig. 6).

Specifically for patients with sepsis (patient type 3), physicians from university hospitals were the more likely to prefer albumin compared to physicians from nonuniversity hospitals. Of interest for septic patients, HES was chosen by 11 %–13 % of physicians (Fig. 6c); this was unexpected because the use of HES in septic patients does not align with SSC recommendations (Dellinger et al. 2013). Based on results from the VISEP (Brunkhorst et al. 2008), 6S (Perner et al.

2012), and CHEST (Myburgh et al. 2012) trials, the SSC recommended against the use of HES. Instead, fluid resuscitation in sepsis as defined by the SSC includes initial fluid challenge with crystalloids as the first choice of fluid (grade 1B), followed by albumin as the second choice if patients are unresponsive to large amounts of crystalloids. When compared to other fluid types, HES solutions, regardless of molecular weight, may be associated with increased mortality and acute kidney injury in patients with sepsis as well as in the general population (Myburgh et al. 2012; Brunkhorst et al. 2008; Guidet et al. 2012; Schortgen et al. 2001; Zarychanski et al. 2013).

Table 3 Bolus volumes (mL) of fluid resuscitation with colloids vs crystalloids, by practice settings

		University hospitals (*n* = 138)	Nonuniversity hospitals[a] (*n* = 351)
Colloids (mL)	Mean (SD)	411.8 (362.3)	485.5 (504.7)
Crystalloids (mL)	Mean (SD)	716.5 (539.0)	821.7 (612.8)*

SD standard deviation
*Statistically significant differences of $P < 0.05$ between practice settings as analyzed by independent-sample *t* test
[a]Excludes physicians in Veterans Affairs hospital setting (*n* = 13)

More physicians across all specialties chose colloid for patients with blood loss (patient type 2) than for the other 2 patient examples. Anesthesiologists preferred more colloid, both 5 % albumin and HES, than physicians from other specialties. This may be because anesthesiologists, relative to other specialists, are more familiar with managing blood loss, when the faster speed of shock reversal with colloid with less fluid volume required may be particularly advantageous (Rehm et al. 2000; Roger et al. 2014).

When asked about the importance of certain colloid traits when colloids are used for volume expansion, 60 % of physicians thought that the more sustained volume expansion, faster volume expansion, and less interstitial edema with colloids were either important or very important (Fig. 5), suggesting that physicians are generally aware of the potential physiological advantages of colloids. Only 8 % of respondents thought that these properties were not important. With respect to the use of albumin solutions as a specific type of colloid fluid, our data aligns with previously published data from another cross-sectional survey of 61 ICUs in Australia and New Zealand between 2007 and 2013 (Hammond et al. 2015), which found that hypo-oncotic albumin (31.6 %) was used more frequently than hyper-oncotic albumin (11.6 %). When comparing the fluid preference for resuscitation in sepsis, our data showed that physicians in the USA preferred more crystalloids over colloids (Fig. 4).

Recent publications are calling for IV fluids to be considered as drugs and for physicians to approach fluid infusions with the same considerations one would give for the pharmacokinetic and pharmacodynamic characteristics of any other treatment (Rewa and Bagshaw 2015; McDermid et al. 2014; Santi et al. 2015; Severs et al. 2015). Furthermore, Bellomo and colleagues (Bellomo et al. 2006) reported that fluid volume may be an independent predictor of changes in pH, chloride, ionized calcium, bicarbonate, base excess, and effective strong ion difference within the first 24 h of resuscitation.

Our study revealed that physicians reported using a wide range of fluid volumes for fluid boluses regardless of clinical practice settings. Published evidence indicates that initial high-volume fluid resuscitation is associated with increased overall mortality in patients with trauma-related bleeding (Wang et al. 2014) and that hyper-oncotic albumin fluids are suitable for small-volume resuscitation with no evidence of deleterious effects (Jacob et al. 2008). Evidence from well-designed network meta-analyses and clinical trials suggests that crystalloid fluids, particularly balanced solutions, seem to be the most advisable first choice, and albumin is equivalent or superior to other available fluids in severe sepsis and septic shock (Jacob et al. 2008; Rochwerg et al. 2015; Rochwerg et al. 2014; Delaney et al. 2011; SAFE Study

Investigators et al. 2011). Altogether, the data from this survey suggest that the participating physicians may prefer albumin when a smaller bolus volume is desired to achieve a more rapid and sustained volume expansion. Thus in the context of sepsis, we believe it makes sense that using small-volume fluid resuscitation, particularly with colloids (e.g., albumin) early in the course of the disease before significant EGL damage ensues, may be better at limiting fluid loss into the interstitium, leading to better intravascular volume expansion. Unfortunately, our data do not explain how physicians would approach the decision on bolus size based on the disease context.

The strength of this study is that it provides an up-to-date picture of how fluid management is practiced in the USA. Although a few international surveys on fluid resuscitation (McIntyre et al. 2007; Finfer et al. 2010; Schortgen et al. 2004) have been conducted in the past, major changes in fluid management have occurred in recent years (Hammond et al. 2015), and past data may no longer be relevant. For instance, we note that an older survey conducted by the CRYCO Study Group in 2002 showed that colloids, not crystalloids, were widely chosen as the first choice of fluid in Europe (Schortgen et al. 2004), and starches were the most frequently used colloids during that time. A limitation of this study is that it describes current practices in only the USA. We acknowledge that our study results cannot be generalized to other countries in the rest of the world. As our study is based on a survey of physician preferences, we did not report on clinical outcomes. We also recognize that the decision-making processes of physicians are complex and may vary from the situations we put forth in the survey. While our study design cannot provide details for all of the reasons underlying treatment decisions, the results allow physicians to compare their own practice patterns to other colleagues, which could be helpful given the lack of expert consensus on fluid resuscitation in critically ill patients. It is also important to provide basic background information for the design of future trials that address complicated issues, such as fluid resuscitation strategies. Although appropriate timing of fluid administration is an important topic, our survey was not designed to delineate this matter; thus, we cannot comment on how fluid resuscitation is influenced by the temporal cadence of ICUs in the USA. Based on the published literature, one could hypothesize that early fluid therapy with colloids followed by a restricted volume strategy may be associated with better outcomes (van Haren and Zacharowski 2014), especially in the context of sepsis (Lee et al. 2014).

Conclusions

This survey of physicians from different specialties caring for patients in ICUs of the USA highlights several important issues in fluid resuscitation and fluid management, which should be based on the underlying pathophysiology of the disease context of the patient. Fluid resuscitation is one component of a complex resuscitation process with changing requirements over the duration of acute illness. However, estimating the extent of hypovolemia or evaluating the response to a fluid challenge is difficult, as there is no single clinical or biochemical parameter that reflects the complexity of the circulation, particularly under rapidly changing pathological conditions. With the lack of consensus, the physicians in our study approached fluid resuscitation in a wide variety of ways, depending on their clinical specialties and practice settings. It is important for physicians to keep in mind the variability in fluid requirements of each patient necessitates a targeted and integrated assessment of volume status and on-going fluid needs (Rewa and Bagshaw 2015). Crystalloid solution is the primary fluid of choice for nonseptic and septic patients. If physicians wish to use colloids in septic patients, then according to the FDA and SSC recommendations albumin would be the logical second choice, not HES, due to recent concerns about HES safety (U.S. Food and Drug Administration 2013; Dellinger et al. 2013; Perner et al. 2012). In our survey, colloids were used more frequently in the bleeding patient type, because physicians felt that colloids provide more rapid and sustained volume expansion (Perner et al. 2012). We encourage physicians to prescribe fluids as one would any other drug, carefully considering the fluid amount, the fluid type, and the disease context specific to the patient being treated.

Additional files

Additional file 1: ICU Fluid Utilization Survey. (DOCX 308 kb)

Additional file 2: Figure S1. Fluid choices for patient who needs volume expansion but is not bleeding and not septic (patient type 1). As follow-up questions (for "Which of the following is your first choice for a patient who needs volume expansion but is not bleeding and not septic?"), the utilization frequency of (A) crystalloid, (B) 5 % albumin, (C) 6 % HES 450/0.70 AND 6 % HES 600/0.75, and (D) 6 % HES 130/0.40 was assessed by asking the question, "How often do you use each of the following in a patient when volume expansion is indicated in the absence of blood loss and sepsis?" N values for panels A–D are as follows: anesthesiologists ($n = 125$), surgeons ($n = 121$), critical care medicine ($n = 98$), pulmonologists ($n = 146$). Superscripts A, S, C, and P denote differences between specialties that are statistically significant at $P < 0.05$. HES, hydroxyethyl starch. (JPG 1674 kb)

Additional file 3: Figure S2. Fluid choices for patient who needs volume expansion in the presence of blood loss when blood transfusion is not indicated (adequate Hb) and patient is not septic (patient type 2). As follow-up questions (for "Which of the following is your first choice for a patient who needs volume expansion in the presence of blood loss when blood transfusion is not indicated (adequate Hb) and patient is not septic?"), the utilization frequency of (A) crystalloid, (B) 5 % albumin, (C) 6 % HES 450/0.70 AND 6 % HES 600/0.75, and (D) 6 % HES 130/0.40 was assessed by asking the question, "How often do you use each of the following in a patient for volume expansion in the presence of blood loss when blood transfusion is not indicated (adequate Hb) and patient is

not septic?" N values for panels A–D are as follows: anesthesiologists ($n = 125$), surgeons ($n = 121$), critical care medicine ($n = 98$), pulmonologists ($n = 146$). Superscripts A, S, C, and P denote differences between specialties that are statistically significant at $P < 0.05$. HES, hydroxyethyl starch. (JPG 1692 kb)

Additional file 4: Figure S3. Fluid choices for patient who needs volume expansion for resuscitation in sepsis (patient type 3). As follow-up questions (for "Which of the following is your first choice for a patient who needs volume expansion for resuscitation in sepsis?" As follow-up questions, the utilization frequency of (A) crystalloid, (B) 5 % albumin, (C) 6 % HES 450/0.70 AND 6 % HES 600/0.75, and (D) 6 % HES 130/0.40 was assessed by asking the question, "How often do you use each of the following or a patient who needs volume expansion for resuscitation in sepsis?" N values for panels A–D are as follows: anesthesiologists ($n = 125$), surgeons ($n = 120$), critical care medicine ($n = 98$), pulmonologists ($n = 146$). Superscripts A, S, C, and P denote differences between specialties that are statistically significant at $P < 0.05$. HES, hydroxyethyl starch. (JPG 1701 kb)

Abbreviations

6S: Scandinavian Start for Severe Sepsis/Septic Shock Study; ALBIOS: Albumin Italian Outcome Sepsis Study; CHEST: Crystalloid Versus Hydroxyethyl Starch Trial; CRISTAL: Colloids Versus Crystalloids for the Resuscitation of the Critically Ill Trial; EGL: endothelial glycocalyx layer; FIRST: Fluids in Resuscitation of Severe Trauma Trial; Hb: hemoglobin; HES: hydroxyethyl starches; ICU: intensive care unit; IV: intravenous; SAFE: Saline and Albumin Fluid Evaluation Trial; SSC: Surviving Sepsis Campaign; VISEP: Efficacy of Volume Substitution and Insulin Therapy in Severe Sepsis Study.

Acknowledgements

Tam Nguyen-Cao, PhD of Grifols provided literature searches and medical writing assistance under the direction of the authors. This study was funded by Grifols (Research Triangle Park, NC), a manufacturer of albumin.

Authors' contributions

TEM and CSB designed the study and generated the questionnaire. MB edited the questionnaire and provided a critical review of the manuscript. PN refined the questionnaire along with TEM and CSB and performed all data analyses. All authors reviewed the manuscript thoroughly and approved the final draft.

Competing interests

TEM has research funded by Edwards Lifesciences and is a speaker for Edwards Lifesciences, Grifols, and Cheetah Medical. CSB is a speaker and member of advisory boards for Grifols, Hospira/Pfizer, and Orion; he is also a speaker for NWAS. MB is an employee of Grifols. PN has no competing interests.

Author details

[1]Department of Anesthesiology, Duke University Medical Center, Durham, NC 27710, USA. [2]Department of Medical Affairs, Grifols, 79 TW Alexander Dr. Bldg. 4101, Research Triangle Park, NC 27709, USA. [3]One Research, LLC, 1150 Hungry Neck Blvd., Suite C-303, Charleston, SC 29464, USA.

References

Aditianingsih D, George YW. Guiding principles of fluid and volume therapy. Best Pract Res Clin Anaesthesiol. 2014;28(3):249–60. doi:10.1016/j.bpa.2014.07.002.
Ait-Oufella H, Maury E, Lehoux S, Guidet B, Offenstadt G. The endothelium: physiological functions and role in microcirculatory failure during severe sepsis. Intensive Care Med. 2010;36(8):1286–98. doi:10.1007/s00134-010-1893-6.
Annane D, Siami S, Jaber S, Martin C, Elatrous S, Declere AD, et al. Effects of fluid resuscitation with colloids vs crystalloids on mortality in critically ill patients presenting with hypovolemic shock: the CRISTAL randomized trial. JAMA. 2013;310(17):1809–17. doi:10.1001/jama.2013.280502.
Becker BF, Chappell D, Jacob M. Endothelial glycocalyx and coronary vascular permeability: the fringe benefit. Basic Res Cardiol. 2010;105(6):687–701. doi: 10.1007/s00395-010-0118-z.

Bellomo R, Morimatsu H, French C, Cole L, Story D, Uchino S, et al. The effects of saline or albumin resuscitation on acid-base status and serum electrolytes. Crit Care Med. 2006;34(12):2891–7. doi:10.1097/01.CCM.0000242159.32764.86.

Brunkhorst FM, Engel C, Bloos F, Meier-Hellmann A, Ragaller M, Weiler N, et al. Intensive insulin therapy and pentastarch resuscitation in severe sepsis. N Engl J Med. 2008;358(2):125–39. doi:10.1056/NEJMoa070716.

Caironi P, Tognoni G, Masson S, Fumagalli R, Pesenti A, Romero M, et al. Albumin replacement in patients with severe sepsis or septic shock. N Engl J Med. 2014;370(15):1412–21. doi:10.1056/NEJMoa1305727.

Cherpanath TG, Aarts LP, Groeneveld JA, Geerts BF. Defining fluid responsiveness: a guide to patient-tailored volume titration. J Cardiothorac Vasc Anesth. 2014;28(3):745–54. doi:10.1053/j.jvca.2013.12.025.

Delaney AP, Dan A, McCaffrey J, Finfer S. The role of albumin as a resuscitation fluid for patients with sepsis: a systematic review and meta-analysis. Crit Care Med. 2011;39(2):386–91. doi:10.1097/CCM.0b013e3181ffe217.

Dellinger RP, Levy MM, Rhodes A, Annane D, Gerlach H, Opal SM, et al. Surviving Sepsis Campaign: international guidelines for management of severe sepsis and septic shock, 2012. Intensive Care Med. 2013;39(2):165–228. doi:10.1007/s00134-012-2769-8.

Elixhauser A, Friedman B, Stranges E. Septicemia in U.S. Hospitals, 2009: Statistical Brief #122. Rockville (MD): Healthcare Cost and Utilization Project (HCUP) Statistical Briefs; 2006.

Finfer S, Bellomo R, Boyce N, French J, Myburgh J, Norton R, et al. A comparison of albumin and saline for fluid resuscitation in the intensive care unit. N Engl J Med. 2004;350(22):2247–56. doi:10.1056/NEJMoa040232.

Finfer S, Liu B, Taylor C, Bellomo R, Billot L, Cook D, et al. Resuscitation fluid use in critically ill adults: an international cross-sectional study in 391 intensive care units. Crit Care. 2010;14(5):R185. doi:10.1186/cc9293.

Guidet B, Martinet O, Boulain T, Philippart F, Poussel JF, Maizel J, et al. Assessment of hemodynamic efficacy and safety of 6 % hydroxyethyl starch 130/0.4 vs. 0.9 % NaCl fluid replacement in patients with severe sepsis: the CRYSTMAS study. Crit Care. 2012;16(3):R94. doi:10.1186/cc11358.

Hammond NE, Taylor C, Saxena M, Liu B, Finfer S, Glass P, et al. Resuscitation fluid use in Australian and New Zealand Intensive Care Units between 2007 and 2013. Intensive Care Med. 2015;41(9):1611–9. doi:10.1007/s00134-015-3878-y.

Hoste EA, Maitland K, Brudney CS, Mehta R, Vincent JL, Yates D, et al. Four phases of intravenous fluid therapy: a conceptual model. Br J Anaesth. 2014;113(5):740–7. doi:10.1093/bja/aeu300.

Jacob M, Chappell D. Reappraising Starling: the physiology of the microcirculation. Curr Opin Crit Care. 2013;19(4):282–9. doi:10.1097/MCC.0b013e3283632d5e.

Jacob M, Chappell D, Conzen P, Wilkes MM, Becker BF, Rehm M. Small-volume resuscitation with hyperoncotic albumin: a systematic review of randomized clinical trials. Crit Care. 2008;12(2):R34. doi:10.1186/cc6812.

James MF, Michell WL, Joubert IA, Nicol AJ, Navsaria PH, Gillespie RS. Resuscitation with hydroxyethyl starch improves renal function and lactate clearance in penetrating trauma in a randomized controlled study: the FIRST trial (Fluids in Resuscitation of Severe Trauma). Br J Anaesth. 2011;107(5):693–702. doi:10.1093/bja/aer229.

Johansson PI, Stensballe J, Rasmussen LS, Ostrowski SR. A high admission syndecan-1 level, a marker of endothelial glycocalyx degradation, is associated with inflammation, protein C depletion, fibrinolysis, and increased mortality in trauma patients. Ann Surg. 2011;254(2):194–200. doi:10.1097/SLA.0b013e318226113d.

Lee SJ, Ramar K, Park JG, Gajic O, Li G, Kashyap R. Increased fluid administration in the first three hours of sepsis resuscitation is associated with reduced mortality: a retrospective cohort study. Chest. 2014;146(4):908–15. doi:10.1378/chest.13-2702.

McDermid RC, Raghunathan K, Romanovsky A, Shaw AD, Bagshaw SM. Controversies in fluid therapy: type, dose and toxicity. World J Crit Care Med. 2014;3(1):24–33. doi:10.5492/wjccm.v3.i1.24.

McIntyre LA, Hebert PC, Fergusson D, Cook DJ, Aziz A, Canadian Critical Care Trials Group. A survey of Canadian intensivists' resuscitation practices in early septic shock. Crit Care. 2007;11(4):R74. doi:10.1186/cc5962.

Myburgh JA. Fluid resuscitation in acute medicine: what is the current situation? J Intern Med. 2015;277(1):58–68. doi:10.1111/joim.12326.

Myburgh JA, Mythen MG. Resuscitation fluids. N Engl J Med. 2013;369(13):1243–51. doi:10.1056/NEJMra1208627.

Myburgh JA, Finfer S, Bellomo R, Billot L, Cass A, Gattas D, et al. Hydroxyethyl starch or saline for fluid resuscitation in intensive care. N Engl J Med. 2012;367(20):1901–11. doi:10.1056/NEJMoa1209759.

Navarro LH, Bloomstone JA, Auler Jr JO, Cannesson M, Rocca GD, Gan TJ, et al. Perioperative fluid therapy: a statement from the international Fluid Optimization Group. Perioper Med (Lond). 2015;4:3. doi:10.1186/s13741-015-0014-z.

Opperer M, Poeran J, Rasul R, Mazumdar M, Memtsoudis SG. Use of perioperative hydroxyethyl starch 6 % and albumin 5 % in elective joint arthroplasty and association with adverse outcomes: a retrospective population based analysis. BMJ. 2015;350:h1567. doi:10.1136/bmj.h1567.

Orbegozo Cortes D, Gamarano Barros T, Njimi H, Vincent JL. Crystalloids versus colloids: exploring differences in fluid requirements by systematic review and meta-regression. Anesth Analg. 2015;120(2):389–402. doi:10.1213/ANE.0000000000000564.

Perner A, Haase N, Guttormsen AB, Tenhunen J, Klemenzson G, Aneman A, et al. Hydroxyethyl starch 130/0.42 versus Ringer's acetate in severe sepsis. N Engl J Med. 2012;367(2):124–34. doi:10.1056/NEJMoa1204242.

Polderman KH, Varon J. Do not drown the patient: appropriate fluid management in critical illness. Am J Emerg Med. 2015;33(3):448–50. doi:10.1016/j.ajem.2015.01.051.

Rehm M, Orth V, Kreimeier U, Thiel M, Haller M, Brechtelsbauer H, et al. Changes in intravascular volume during acute normovolemic hemodilution and intraoperative retransfusion in patients with radical hysterectomy. Anesthesiology. 2000;92(3):657–64.

Rewa O, Bagshaw SM. Principles of fluid management. Crit Care Clin. 2015;31(4):785–801. doi:10.1016/j.ccc.2015.06.012.

Rochwerg B, Alhazzani W, Sindi A, Heels-Ansdell D, Thabane L, Fox-Robichaud A, et al. Fluid resuscitation in sepsis: a systematic review and network meta-analysis. Ann Intern Med. 2014;161(5):347–55. doi:10.7326/M14-0178.

Rochwerg B, Alhazzani W, Gibson A, Ribic CM, Sindi A, Heels-Ansdell D, et al. Fluid type and the use of renal replacement therapy in sepsis: a systematic review and network meta-analysis. Intensive Care Med. 2015;41(9):1561–71. doi:10.1007/s00134-015-3794-1.

Roger C, Muller L, Deras P, Louart G, Nouvellon E, Molinari N, et al. Does the type of fluid affect rapidity of shock reversal in an anaesthetized-piglet model of near-fatal controlled haemorrhage? A randomized study. Br J Anaesth. 2014;112(6):1015–23. doi:10.1093/bja/aet375.

SAFE Study Investigators, Finfer S, McEvoy S, Bellomo R, McArthur C, Myburgh J, et al. Impact of albumin compared to saline on organ function and mortality of patients with severe sepsis. Intensive Care Med. 2011;37(1):86–96. doi:10.1007/s00134-010-2039-6.

Santi M, Lava SA, Camozzi P, Giannini O, Milani GP, Simonetti GD, et al. The great fluid debate: saline or so-called "balanced" salt solutions? Ital J Pediatr. 2015;41:47. doi:10.1186/s13052-015-0154-2.

Schortgen F, Lacherade JC, Bruneel F, Cattaneo I, Hemery F, Lemaire F, et al. Effects of hydroxyethyl starch and gelatin on renal function in severe sepsis: a multicentre randomised study. Lancet. 2001;357(9260):911–6. doi:10.1016/S0140-6736(00)04211-2.

Schortgen F, Deye N, Brochard L, CRYCO Study Group. Preferred plasma volume expanders for critically ill patients: results of an international survey. Intensive Care Med. 2004;30(12):2222–9. doi:10.1007/s00134-004-2415-1.

Severs D, Rookmaaker MB, Hoorn EJ. Intravenous solutions in the care of patients with volume depletion and electrolyte abnormalities. Am J Kidney Dis. 2015;66(1):147–53. doi:10.1053/j.ajkd.2015.01.031.

Steppan J, Hofer S, Funke B, Brenner T, Henrich M, Martin E, et al. Sepsis and major abdominal surgery lead to flaking of the endothelial glycocalix. J Surg Res. 2011;165(1):136–41. doi:10.1016/j.jss.2009.04.034.

U.S. Food and Drug Administration. FDA Safety Communication: boxed warning on increased mortality and severe renal injury, and additional warning on risk of bleeding, for use of hydroxyethyl starch solutions in some settings. 2013. http://www.fda.gov/biologicsbloodvaccines/safetyavailability/ucm358271.htm. Accessed 18 September 2015

van Haren F, Zacharowski K. What's new in volume therapy in the intensive care unit? Best Pract Res Clin Anaesthesiol. 2014;28(3):275–83. doi:10.1016/j.bpa.2014.06.004.

Vincent JL, De Backer D. Circulatory shock. N Engl J Med. 2013;369(18):1726–34. doi:10.1056/NEJMra1208943.

Wang CH, Hsieh WH, Chou HC, Huang YS, Shen JH, Yeo YH, et al. Liberal versus restricted fluid resuscitation strategies in trauma patients: a systematic review and meta-analysis of randomized controlled trials and observational studies*. Crit Care Med. 2014;42(4):954–61. doi:10.1097/CCM.0000000000000050.

Weinbaum S, Tarbell JM, Damiano ER. The structure and function of the
    endothelial glycocalyx layer. Annu Rev Biomed Eng. 2007;9:121–67. doi:10.
    1146/annurev.bioeng.9.060906.151959.

Zarychanski R, Abou-Setta AM, Turgeon AF, Houston BL, McIntyre L, Marshall JC,
    et al. Association of hydroxyethyl starch administration with mortality and
    acute kidney injury in critically ill patients requiring volume resuscitation: a
    systematic review and meta-analysis. JAMA. 2013;309(7):678–88. doi:10.1001/
    jama.2013.430.

6

Care of elderly patients: a prospective audit of the prevalence of hypotension and the use of BIS intraoperatively in 25 hospitals

Alex Wickham[1], David Highton[2], Daniel Martin[3,4*] and The Pan London Perioperative Audit and Research Network (PLAN)[5]

Abstract

Background: Anaesthesia is frequently complicated by intraoperative hypotension (IOH) in the elderly, and this is associated with adverse outcome. The definition of IOH is controversial, and although management guidelines for IOH in the elderly exist, the frequency of IOH and typical clinically applied treatment thresholds are largely unknown in the UK.

Methods: We audited frequency of intraoperative blood pressure against national guidelines in elderly patients undergoing surgery. Depth of anaesthesia (DOA) monitoring was also audited due to the association between low DOA values and IOH with increased mortality (as part of "double" and "triple low" phenomena) and because it is a suggested management strategy to reduce IOH.

Results: Twenty-five hospitals submitted data on 481 patients. Hypotension varied depending on the definition, but affected 400 patients (83.3 %) using the AAGBI standard. Furthermore, 2.9, 13.5, and 24.6 % had mean arterial blood pressures <50, <60, and <70 mmHg for 20 min, respectively, and 136 (28.4 %) had systolic blood pressure decrease by 20 % for 20 min. DOA monitors were used for 45 (9.4 %) patients.

Conclusions: IOH is common and use of DOA monitors is less than implied by guidelines. Improved management of IOH may be a simple intervention with real potential to reduce morbidity in this vulnerable group.

Keywords: Elderly, Intraoperative hypotension, Depth of anaesthesia

Background

Older patients are vulnerable to perioperative complications due to a combination of physiological frailty and comorbid disease and now constitute an increasing proportion of the surgical population (Griffiths et al. 2014). Changes in intraoperative haemodynamics and oxygen delivery have been a focus of interest in the mechanism of perioperative organ dysfunction (Lobo and de Oliveira 2013) and therefore may be of increased relevance in older patients. Blood pressure and depth of anaesthesia

influence organ (particularly cerebral) perfusion and oxygenation and are routinely manipulated intraoperatively. Recently, this has been a focus of interest in the Anaesthesia Sprint Audit of Practice (ASAP) (ASAP collaboration team 2014) highlighting a high prevalence of intraoperative hypotension (IOH) in patients who sustained fractured necks of femur.

Hypotension occurs frequently during anaesthesia and is associated with adverse outcomes in the elderly. These include stroke, compromised postoperative neurological performance, acute kidney injury, myocardial infarction, and increased 30-day and 1-year mortality (Bijker et al 2009; Bijker et al 2012; Yocum et al. 2009; Sun et al. 2015; Walsh et al. 2013; Monk et al 2005; Mascha et al 2015). Thus, the Association of Anaesthetists of Great

* Correspondence: daniel.martin@ucl.ac.uk
[3]Division of Surgery and Interventional Science, Royal Free Hospital, University College London, Pond Street, London NW3 2QG, UK
[4]Royal Free Perioperative Research, Department of Anaesthesia, Royal Free Hospital, Pond Street, London NW3 2QG, UK
Full list of author information is available at the end of the article

Britain and Ireland (AAGBI) guidelines recommend IOH should be avoided in older patients (Griffiths et al. 2014), although the specific thresholds that constitute hypotension remain a topic of considerable debate (Bijker et al. 2007; Warner and Monk 2007; Brady and Hogue 2013). Both the prevalence of hypotension and associated complications vary widely in the literature, in part due to the range of threshold values used to define hypotension. The AAGBI recommend avoiding >20 % drop in systolic blood pressure (Griffiths et al. 2014), whilst drops of >30 % mean arterial pressure (MAP) and MAP <55 mmHg have been associated with stroke, myocardial ischaemia, and kidney injury (Bijker et al. 2009; Walsh et al. 2013). The treatment threshold applied in clinical anaesthetic practice in the UK is largely unreported, and this is key to addressing improvement.

Excessive anaesthetic depth is implicated in the mechanism of haemodynamic compromise, has been associated with myocardial infarction and stroke, postoperative delirium and, when combined with hypotension and low inspired anaesthetic concentration, increased mortality (Leslie et al. 2010; Radtke et al 2013; Sessler et al. 2012; Willingham et al. 2014; Willingham et al. 2015), a phenomenon referred to as the 'triple-low'. Patients exhibiting the triple low for 60 min or longer are a particularly high risk group, with a quadrupled risk of 30-day mortality. The National Institute for Health and Care Excellence (NICE) recommends using electroencephalogram (EEG) based DOA monitors for patients at 'higher risk of adverse outcomes', specifically citing 'older patients' (National Institute for Health and Clinical Excellence 2012), and this might be a means to reduce the risk of haemodynamic compromise.

Maintaining intraoperative blood pressure and depth of anaesthesia within broadly normal limits are thus generally accepted standards, supported by recent evidence and national guidelines, and might influence outcomes for elderly patients. It is known that established standards are not met in the hip fracture population (ASAP collaboration team 2014), yet the frequency of such deviations is unknown in other older surgical populations in the UK. The aim of this audit was to characterise the incidence of IOH and the use of DOA monitoring in older surgical patients against current standards. A secondary goal was to assess the feasibility of the newly formed trainee-led Pan London Perioperative Audit and Research Network (www.uk-plan.net). The latter methodology is part of a national programme of network-based, trainee-led collaborations that aim to deliver audit, research and quality improvement projects.

Methods

A prospective snapshot audit was conducted across 25 hospitals in London within the PLAN network. The project was confirmed to be a clinical audit by Imperial College Healthcare NHS Trust Clinical Governance department; they confirmed that research ethics committee approval and individual patient consent were not required because it is an audit and not research. Appropriate approval for the audit was obtained from clinical governance departments locally at each participating hospital.

Patients aged 65 years or older having a surgical procedure under general anaesthesia were included. Patients receiving sedation or regional anaesthesia as the sole method of anaesthesia, intracranial neurosurgery, cardio-pulmonary bypass (non-pulsatile hypotension implicit) or jet ventilation were excluded. Audit standards and definitions were identified from consensus statements, research and national guidance. The AAGBI standard, 'a fall in systolic blood pressure of more than 20 % from pre-induction baseline... is a suitable limit' (Griffiths et al. 2014), was used for IOH. The standard for DOA monitoring, 'the use of EEG based depth of anaesthesia monitors is recommended... in patients at risk of adverse outcomes', was taken from NICE guidelines (National Institute for Health and Clinical Excellence 2012).

Data was collected from the anaesthetic record by anaesthetic trainees who were independent of the clinical care of the patients over two locally determined weekdays in July and August 2014. To ensure no cases were missed, trainees collected data on 'non-clinical' days or used study leave and worked closely with nursing staff in each recovery area of their hospital. All patients passing through recovery were assessed for inclusion. Data were collected using a paper case report form.

Blood pressure values were recorded from the anaesthetic chart (either handwritten paper forms, or an electronic print out or log), which are typically documented every 5 min. The values were taken at 5-min intervals for both non-invasive and invasive monitoring. Preoperative blood pressure was determined using a reading from pre-assessment clinic, the theatre care plan or ward observation chart (last recorded value). Pre-induction blood pressure documented was the blood pressure taken immediately prior to the induction of anaesthesia. Where multiple hypotensive episodes occurred, total cumulative hypotensive time was calculated. If different degrees of hypotension occurred at separate time points, the lowest value was taken to calculate the degree of drop from the pre-induction pressure. The frequency of recording DOA values varies, but is typically every 15 min. Types of DOA monitoring and cumulative duration of scores less than 40 were documented.

Statistics were calculated using R version 3.2.0 (© 2015 The R Foundation for Statistical Computing). Data were examined for normality using the Shapiro-Wilk test. Paired data was compared using the Wilcoxon matched pairs test. Categorical data analyses were made using chi square test with Fisher's correction. All tests were two tailed, and significance was taken as $p < 0.05$. Continuous data is presented as median (IQR [range]), categorical data as number (proportion).

Results

Twenty-five hospitals submitted data for 481 patients. The median number of patients per hospital was 19 (IQR 16–23, range 7–60). Results were received from 11 (44.0 %) district general hospitals, 11 (44.0 %) teaching hospitals and 3 (12.0 %) single specialty hospitals. One case was not completed beyond detail on gender and was therefore excluded from analysis. Paper-based anaesthetic records were used in 411 (85.6 %) cases whilst printed computerised records were available in 6 (24.0 %) hospitals and therefore used for 69 (14.4 %) cases. Incomplete recording of blood pressure was present in 12 cases on paper notes (2.5 %) compared with 0 cases with an electronic record. The patient and surgery characteristics, frequency of systolic hypotension and prolonged IOH are shown in Table 1.

The method for measuring intraoperative blood pressure was recorded in 478 cases (99.4 %), and 89 (18.6 %) patients in this group had invasive monitoring. Preoperative blood pressure values were not documented in 47 cases (9.8 %). Stage 1 hypertension (BP >140/90 mmHg (National Institute for Health and Clinical Excellence 2011) was present in 38 (7.9 %) patients preoperatively.

Although the systolic blood pressure was significantly higher pre-induction ($p = 0.02$), the effect size was small, median preoperative blood pressure 140/77 mmHg, and pre-induction 140/78 mmHg (Table 2).

Figure 1 illustrates the frequency of hypotension as a function of the definition used, and it can be seen that this causes considerable variation in the reported IOH. Table 3 details the prevalence of IOH using different thresholds: 0–20.0, 20.1–40.0 and ≥40.1 % drop from pre-induction baseline systolic blood pressure. Hypotension of more than 20.0 % drop occurred in 400 patients (83.3 %), and in 188 (39.2 %), the drop was ≥40.1 %. In 141 (29.4 %), this lasted for longer than 20 min. Systolic hypotension (>20 % drop) occurred across all patient age groups (65–74, 75–84, ≥85 years old), in all surgical specialities and in both elective and unscheduled surgery (see Table 1). Lowest reported intraoperative systolic (87 versus 80 mmHg) and mean (61 versus 57 mmHg) blood pressure values were significantly lower in patients whose blood pressure was recorded electronically compared with those whose blood pressure was handwritten ($p < 0.001$ and $p = 0.005$, respectively); 129 (26.8 %) patients had mean arterial pressures less than 55 mmHg at some point during their surgery; this persisted for over 20 min in 45 (9.6 %) patients.

Regional anaesthesia was used in combination with general anaesthesia in 95 (19.9 %) cases, most commonly in orthopaedic surgery (39, 41.5 % of orthopaedic cases) and colorectal surgery (16, 35.6 % of colorectal cases). There were no significant differences IOH (>20 % of

Table 1 Patient characteristics, frequency of intraoperative systolic hypotension (≥20 % from pre induction value) and prolonged hypotension. Values are number (percentage)

Variable		Patient characteristics	Frequency of systolic hypotension	Frequency of systolic hypotension lasting >20 min
Gender	Female	234 (48.9)	201 (85.9)	67 (27.4)
	Male	245 (51.2)	197 (80.4)	74 (31.6)
Age	65–74	286 (59.5)	244 (85.3)	100 (35.0)
	75–84	152 (31.6)	119 (78.3)	35 (23.0)
	>85	43 (8.9)	35 (81.4)	6 (14.0)
Surgical speciality	General, breast and endocrine	188 (9.1)	158 (84.0)	48 (25.5)
	Orthopaedics, trauma, plastic and spinal	145 (30.2)	115 (79.3)	37 (25.5)
	Other	36 (7.5)	29 (80.6)	11 (30.6)
	Gynaecology	35 (7.3)	29 (82.9)	15 (42.9)
	Vascular	25 (5.2)	23 (92.0)	12 (48.0)
	ENT	22 (4.6)	20 (90.9)	8 (36.6)
	Thoracic	18 (3.7)	13 (72.2)	7 (38.9)
	Ophthalmology	12 (2.5)	12 (100.0)	3 (25.0)
NCEPOD classification	Immediate	5 (1.0)	4 (80.0)	1 (20.0)
	Urgent	64 (13.3)	57 (89.1)	15 (23.4)
	Expedited	32 (6.7)	24 (75.0)	13 (40.6)
	Elective	379 (79.0)	314 (82.9)	113 (29.8)

Table 2 Preoperative, pre-induction and intraoperative blood pressure. Values are median (IQR [range])

	Preoperative (mmHg)	Pre-induction (mmHg)	Lowest intraoperative (mmHg)	Difference between preoperative and pre-induction value (Wilcoxon matched pairs)
Systolic	140 [125–151 (90–209)]	140 [125–155 (80–215)]	90 [80–100 (46–157)]	$p = 0.02$
Diastolic	77 [69–85 (23–114)]	78 [68–85 (38–178)]	50 [42–58 (25–94)]	$p = 1.00$

pre-induction systolic baseline) incidence in patients who received combined regional and general anaesthesia techniques in comparison with those who received general anaesthesia alone ($\chi^2 = 0.3634$). Additionally, there were no significant differences in the occurrence of intraoperative systolic hypotension between the different types of regional anaesthesia ($\chi^2 = 0.5774$).

Depth of anaesthesia monitoring was used in 46 (9.6 %) patients in 11 (44.0 %) hospitals, although 24 (52.2 %) patients' data came from 2 hospitals. Twenty-nine (63.0 %) patients had intraoperative total intravenous anaesthesia (TIVA) and 17 (37.0 %) had inhalational anaesthesia. In those patients where DOA monitors were used, 37 (80.4 %) used BIS and 9 (19.6 %) used Entropy. Thirty-seven (80.4 %) of these patients had a DOA scores <40. In 33 (89.2 %) patients, this was combined with a systolic blood pressure reduction greater than 20 %. Twenty-seven (73.0 %) patients had a DOA score <40 for longer than 20 min.

Discussion

We have demonstrated that IOH, as described by current definitions, is extremely common in the centres studied. Although this did vary dependant on definition, a large proportion (39 %) experienced a drop ≥40.1 %, a degree of IOH that has previously been associated with excess stroke, myocardial ischaemia and kidney injury. DOA monitoring was not used as often as suggested by NICE guidelines (National Institute for Health and Clinical Excellence 2012). However, when it was used, DOA scores less than 40 were common and this was frequently accompanied by hypotension. The formation of a trainee network to complete this project permitted the rapid completion of an audit project across a large number of hospitals within a defined geographical area.

Our results are consistent with those from ASAP in patients having proximal femoral fracture repair (ASAP collaboration team 2014), which reported IOH affected 56–89 % of patients dependant on which definition was used. IOH prevalence depends on the threshold used

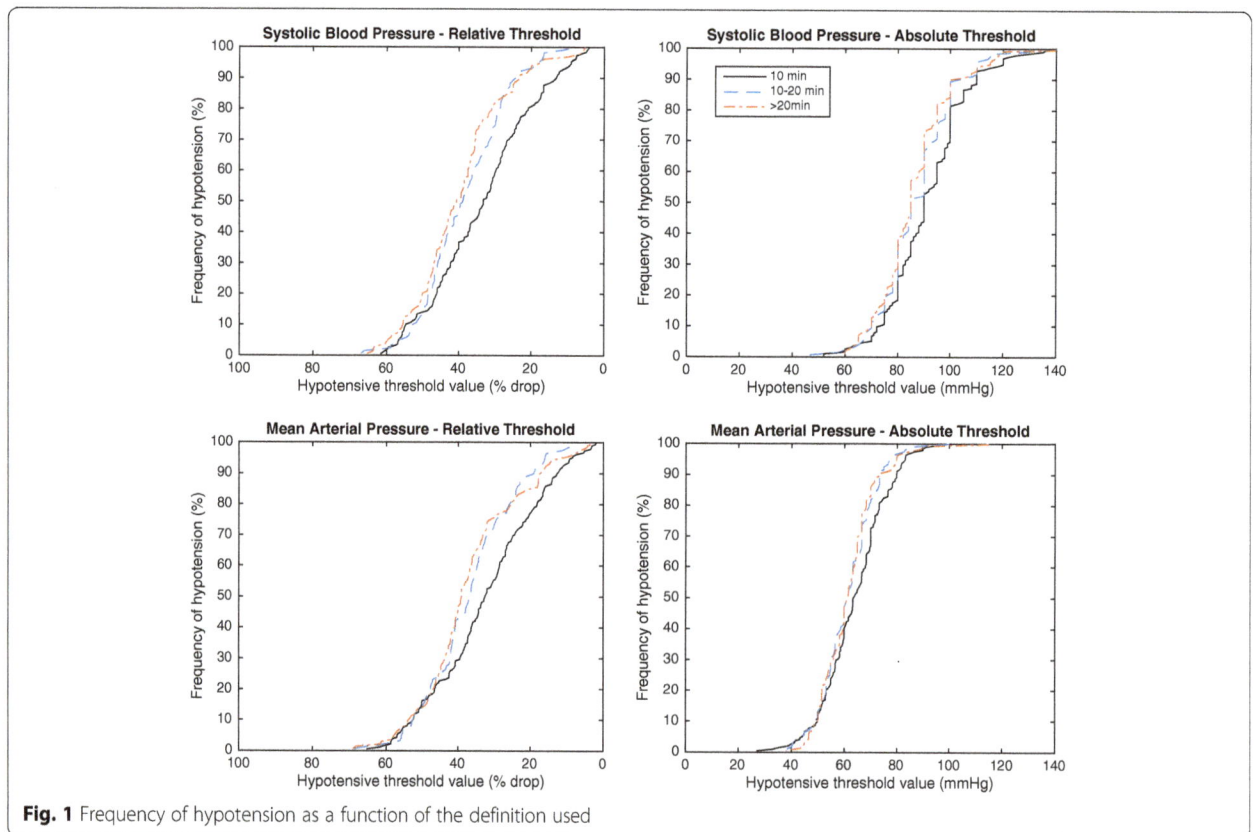

Fig. 1 Frequency of hypotension as a function of the definition used

Table 3 Duration of intraoperative systolic hypotension. Data was available for 461 cases. Values are number (proportion). Drop defined from pre-induction systolic blood pressure

Drop in systolic blood pressure	<10 min	10–20 min	>20 min	Total
0–20.0 %	54 (11.37 %)	7 (1.5 %)	5 (1.0 %)	66 (13.8 %)
20.1–40.0 %	82 (17.1 %)	57 (11.9 %)	68 (14.2 %)	207 (43.1 %)
>40.1 %	60 (12.5 %)	60 (12.5 %)	68 (14.2 %)	188 (39.2 %)
Total	196 (40.8 %)	124 (25.8 %)	141 (29.4 %)	461

(Bijker et al. 2007) (relative reduction or absolute value) and component (systolic, diastolic or mean pressure), there being no universally agreed definition. We used the AAGBI definition of hypotension (Griffiths et al. 2014), a 20 % reduction in systolic blood pressure from preoperative baseline. This is a broad definition and therefore may generate high rates of IOH, but it is a suitably cautious physiological value for the older patient set by a national organisation that produces robust guidance. One might expect a large difference between our findings and those from ASAP, as the frailty of the hip fracture population may predispose to hypotensive episodes. However, we demonstrate that IOH in excess of present recommendations is a wider feature commonly affecting older surgical patients. This is also consistent with large international studies (Bijker et al. 2009) indicating it is not an issue isolated to this investigation.

The risk of harm from IOH relates to both degree and total duration, with elderly patients less able to tolerate any period of hypotension (Bijker et al. 2009). Mean arterial blood pressure less than 55 mmHg have been linked to increased morbidity in several large studies (Sun et al 2015; Walsh et al. 2013), and we found that this affected a quarter of our population. Our audit adds to these studies by demonstrating that despite national standards, both greater degrees of hypotension and duration of hypotension are common in elderly patients. Invasive arterial monitoring was used in approximately one in five patients, in keeping with AAGBI recommendations (Griffiths et al. 2014), perhaps suggesting anaesthetists recognise frailty in older patients and more readily choose invasive monitoring. However, many other practical strategies might also be employed to reduce IOH: cautious induction (Griffiths et al. 2014; Pandit et al. 2014), minimisation of anaesthesia dose guided by DOA monitoring (Willingham et al. 2015; Pandit et al. 2014, Ballard et al 2012), guided intraoperative fluid resuscitation (Pearse et al. 2014) and individualised alarm settings. Whether treatment for IOH can be effective at reducing morbidity remains to be examined in prospective studies, but the high prevalence of IOH below thresholds associated with complications (>40 % drop, MAP <55 mmHg) strongly suggests that additional treatment has the potential to improve outcome in a considerable number of patients.

Several studies have reported that combined low DOA scores (<40) and hypotension are associated with harm (Sessler et al. 2012; Willingham et al. 2014), although this remains a topic of debate and the 'triple low' phenomenon has been recently both questioned (Kertai et al. 2014) and supported (Willingham et al. 2015). Almost three quarters of patients whose DOA was monitored in our study had a combined 'double low' (concomitant BIS <40 and hypotension). Whilst we acknowledge that this was a small number of patients (33), it suggests that the technology is not being applied in an effort to minimise anaesthetic dose or lack of confidence to reduce dose below certain thresholds based on this technique. Whilst NICE guidelines on DOA monitoring have provoked some criticisms (Smith et al. 2013), particularly around who constitutes the 'higher risk' category, older people are well recognised to have an increased risk of perioperative complications. Subsequent to this, both the AAGBI (Griffiths et al. 2014) and Fifth National Audit Project of the Royal College of Anaesthetists (NAP5) report (Pandit et al. 2014) endorsed DOA monitoring to avoid excessively deep anaesthetic states and associated hypotension, suggesting a rationale for more widespread use in the elderly.

PLAN is a trainee-led collaborative research and audit network supported by the London Academy of Anaesthesia. The structure is similar to other trainee networks (South West Anaesthetic Research Matrix 2014); projects are proposed and voted for by members and then coordinated by the proposer supported by a core committee. Our sample of 481 patients is sufficient to assess the common intraoperative targets measured and the feasibility of delivering this investigation at a larger scale, when outcomes data could also be collected. International studies have typically used retrospective analysis of electronic records; however, this is unavailable in the majority of UK departments. Trainees collected data based in recovery ensuring capture of all cases. Our aim was to assess adherence to targets rather than outcomes (which have been established by other investigators); therefore, we did not collect comprehensive patient and treatment details or postoperative outcomes, all of which potentially limit the scope of our findings. The high rate of paper anaesthetic charts in our study may cause some hypotensive episodes to be missed due to 'smoothing' and inaccuracies in handwritten records (Van Schalkwyk et al. 2011), meaning the true rate may actually be higher than reported. However, the written record is likely to still reflect the thresholds the anaesthetist considers important even if it deviates from electronic notes, and this is the key information of interest when informing an improvement strategy. There was variety in the quantity of data submitted from the different hospitals, and we did not assess the number or seniority of anaesthetists delivering care; therefore, our results might possibly disproportionately reflect the practice of a smaller sample of practitioners.

Conclusions

We have demonstrated that IOH is widely prevalent in elective and unscheduled surgery in older patients in a UK setting. DOA monitoring, which might be used to minimise excessively deep anaesthesia and associated hypotension, is infrequently used. Our results suggest the need for a larger national UK investigation of practice to further clarify the clinical threshold employed for treatment of IOH in the context of patient factors and outcome. Although prospective interventional studies are required to establish an effect of tighter blood pressure control, it is unlikely that a drop of >40 % should be tolerated. Greater awareness of this issue may enable local quality improvement and improved outcomes. National studies using trainee networks have the potential to deliver these goals.

Abbreviations

AAGBI: Association of Anaesthetists of Great Britain and Ireland; IOH: intraoperative hypotension; NAP5: Fifth National Audit Project of the Royal College of Anasthetists; NCEPOD: National Confidential Enquiry into Patient Outcome and Death; NICE: National Institute for Health and Clinical Excellence.

Acknowledgements

We thank all members contributing to data collection (www.uk-plan.net/QUINCE) and commenting on the drafts, the departments of anaesthesia for granting study leave and the London Academy of Anaesthesia for their support. All collaborators and their roles are listed below.
The project leads are Alex Wickham and David Highton.
The members of the PLAN Committee are Sibtain Anwar, Sohail Bampoe, Carsten Bantel, Mevan Gooneratne, David Highton, Philip Hopkins, Annie Hunningher, Carolyn Johnston, Helen Laycock, Daniel Martin, James O'Carroll, Peter Odor, Sioned Philips, Anil Visram and Harriet Wordsworth.
The local trust project contributors are Lena Al-Shammari, Glenn Arnold, Farrah Ayob, Steven Barrett, Linden Baxter, James Bland, Oliver Blightman, Nadia Blunt, Sara Bowman, Toni Boyce, Edward Burdett, Maria Chereshneva, Stuart Cleland, Vanessa Cowie, Jugdeep Dhesi, Matthew Dickinson, Wei Du, Amy Dukoff-Gordon, Lliam Edger, Zara Edwards, Kerry Elliot, James Gill, Sophia Grobler, Paul Halford, Sarah Hodge, Brian Hogan, Omar Hussain, Shaman Jhanji, Rob John, Craig Johnstone, Roshmi Kumar, Alice Loughnan, Val Luoma, Samson Ma, Anna Markiewicz, Jon Mathers, Stuart McCorkell, Joanna Moore, Clare Morkane, Ahmer Mosharaf, Ramy Mottaleb, Kenneth Murray, Finn Nesbit, Lisa Nicholls, Alice O'Neil, Cheng Ong, Simon Parrington, George Perrett, Vivekanandan Ponnampolam, Junia Rahman, Kausi Rao, Sonia Renwick, Jan Schumacher, Akshay Shah, Vinnie Sodhi, Rebecca Szekely, Drinka Uzeirbegovic, Duncan Wagstaff, Ximena Watson, Tim Wigmore, Jo Wilson, and Trudi Young.

Authors' contributions

AW prepared, revised and edited the draft. DH and DM revised and edited the drafts. All members of PLAN listed at www.uk-plan.net/QUINCE were able to comment on and suggest amendments to the article. All authors read and approved the final manuscript.

Authors' information

AW is an anaesthetic registrar in London and a member of PLAN.
DH is an anaesthetic and intensive care speciality registrar in London. He co-founded PLAN.
DM is a consultant in anaesthesia and intensive care.

Competing interests

The authors declare that they have no competing interests.

Author details

[1]Department of Anaesthetics, Imperial College Healthcare NHS Trust, London, UK. [2]Neurocritical Care, the National Hospital for Neurology and Neurosurgery, University College London Hospitals, Queen Square, London, UK. [3]Division of Surgery and Interventional Science, Royal Free Hospital, University College London, Pond Street, London NW3 2QG, UK. [4]Royal Free Perioperative Research, Department of Anaesthesia, Royal Free Hospital, Pond Street, London NW3 2QG, UK. [5]The London Academy of Anaesthesia, London, UK.

References

ASAP collaboration team. Falls and Fragility Fracture Audit Programme of the National Hip Fracture Database: Anaesthesia Sprint Audit of Practice 2014. London: Royal College of Physicians; 2014.

Ballard C, Jones E, Gauge N, Aarsland D, Nilsen OB, Saxby BK, Lowery D, Corbett A, Wesnes K, Katsaiti E, Arden J, Amaoko D, Prophet N, Purushothaman B, Green D. Optimised anaesthesia to reduce post operative cognitive decline (POCD) in older patients undergoing elective surgery, a randomised controlled trial. PLoS One. 2012;7(6):e37410. doi:10.1371/journal.pone.0037410.

Bijker BJ, van Klei W, Kappen TH, van Wolfswinkel L, Moons KGM, Kalkman CJ. Incidence of intraoperative hypotension as a function of the chosen definition. Anesthesiology. 2007;107:213–20.

Bijker JB, van Klei WA, Vergouwe Y, Eleveld DJ, van Wolfswinkel L, Moons KG, Kalkman CJ. Intraoperative hypotension and 1-year mortality after noncardiac surgery. Anesthesiology. 2009;111:1217–26.

Bijker JB, Persoon S, Peelen LM, Moons KG, Kalkman CJ, Kappelle LJ, van Klei WA. Intraoperative hypotension and perioperative ischemic stroke after general surgery: a nested case-control study. Anesthesiology. 2012;116:658–64.

Brady K, Hogue CW. Intraoperative hypotension and patient outcome. Does one size fit all? Anesthesiology. 2013;119:495–7.

Griffiths R, Beech F, Brown A, Dhesi J, Foo I, Goodall J, Harrop-Griffiths W, Jameson J, Love N, Pappenheim K, White S. AAGBI working party: perioperative care of the elderly 2014. Anaesthesia. 2014;69 Suppl 1:81–98.

Kertai MD, White WD, Gan TJ. Cumulative duration of "triple low" state of low blood pressure, low bispectral index, and low minimum alveolar concentration of volatile anesthesia is not associated with increased mortality. Anesthesiology. 2014;121:18–28.

Leslie K, Myles PS, Forbes A, Chan MTV. The effect of bispectral index monitoring on long-term survival in the B-aware trial. Anesth Analg. 2010;110:816–22.

Lobo SM, de Oliveira NE. Clinical review: what are the best hemodynamic targets for noncardiac surgical patients? Crit Care. 2013;17:210.

Mascha EJ, Dongsheng Y, Weiss S, Sessler DI. Intraoperative mean arterial pressure variability and 30-day mortality in patients having noncardiac surgery. Anesthesiology. 2015;123:79–91.

Monk TG, Saini V, Weldon BC, Sigl JC. Anesthetic management and one-year mortality after noncardiac surgery. Anesth Analg. 2005;100:4–10.

National Institute for Health and Clinical Excellence. NICE clinical guideline 127: clinical management of primary hypertension in adults. London: NICE; 2011.

National Institute for Health and Clinical Excellence. NICE diagnostics guidance 6. Depth of Anaesthesia monitors – Bispectral Index (BIS), E-Entropy and Narcotrend-Compact M. London: NICE; 2012.

Care of elderly patients: a prospective audit of the prevalence of hypotension and the use of BIS...

51

Pandit JJ, Cook TM, et al. 5th National Audit Project of The Royal College of Anaesthetists and the Association of Anaesthetists of Great Britain and Ireland: Accidental Awareness during General Anaesthesia in the United Kingdom and Ireland. London: The Royal College of Anaesthetists and the Association of Anaesthetists of Great Britain and Ireland; 2014.

Pearse RM, Harrison DA, MacDonald N, Gillies MA, Blunt M, Ackland G, Grocott MP, Ahern A, Griggs K, Scott R, Hinds C, Rowan K, OPTIMISE Study Group. Effect of a perioperative, cardiac output-guided hemodynamic therapy algorithm on outcomes following major gastrointestinal surgery: a randomized clinical trial and systematic review. J Am Med Assoc. 2014; 311(21):2181–90.

Radtke FM, Franck M, Lendner J, Kruger S, Wernecke KD, Spies CD. Monitoring depth of anaesthesia in a randomized trial decreases the rate of postoperative delirium but not postoperative cognitive dysfunction. Br J Anaesth. 2013;110 Suppl 1:98–105.

Sessler DI, Sigl JC, Kelley SD, Chamoun NG, Manberg PJ, Saager L, Kurz A, Greenwald S. Hospital stay and mortality are increased in patients having a "triple low" of low blood pressure, low bispectral index, and low minimum alveolar concentration of volatile anesthesia. Anesthesiology. 2012;116:1195–203.

Smith D, Andrzejowski J, Smith A. Certainty and uncertainty: NICE guidance on 'depth of anaesthesia' monitoring. Anaesthesia. 2013;68:1000–5.

South West Anaesthetic Research Matrix. Sedation practice in six acute hospitals—a snapshot survey. Anaesthesia. 2014;70(4):407–15.

Sun LY, Wijeysundera DN, Tait GA, Beattie WS. Association of intraoperative hypotension with acute kidney injury after elective noncardiac surgery. Anesthesiology. 2015;123:00–00.

Van Schalkwyk JM, Lowes D, Frampton C, Merry AF. Does manual anaesthetic record capture remove clinically important data? Br J Anaesth. 2011;107(4):546–52.

Walsh M, Devereaux PJ, Garg AX, Kurz A, Turan A, Rodseth RN, Cywinski J, Thabane L, Sessler DI. Relationship between intraoperative mean arterial pressure and clinical outcomes after noncardiac surgery: toward an empirical definition of hypotension. Anesthesiology. 2013;119:507–15.

Warner MA, Monk TG. The impact of lack of standardised definitions on the speciality. Anesthesiology. 2007;107:198–9.

Willingham M, Ben Abdallah A, Gradwohl S, Helsten D, Lin N, Villafranca A, Jacobsohn E, Avidan M, Kaiser H. Association between intraoperative electroencephalographic suppression and postoperative mortality. Br J Anaesth. 2014;113(6):1001–8.

Willingham MD, Karren E, Shanks AM, O'Connor MF, Jacobsohn E, Kheterpal S, Avidan MS. Minimum alveolar concentration, and low bispectral index is associated with postoperative death. Anesthesiology. 2015;123:775–85.

Yocum GT, Gaudet JG, Teverbaugh LA, Quest DO, McCormick PC, Sander Connelly Jr S, Heyer EJ. Neurocognitive performance in hypertensive patients after spine surgery. Anesthesiology. 2009;110(2):254–61.

7

Postoperative pulmonary complications following major elective abdominal surgery

Kamlesh Patel[1], Fatemeh Hadian[1], Aysha Ali[1], Graham Broadley[1], Kate Evans[1], Claire Horder[1], Marianne Johnstone[1], Fiona Langlands[1], Jake Matthews[1], Prithish Narayan[1], Priya Rallon[1], Charlotte Roberts[1], Sonali Shah[1] and Ravinder Vohra[1,2]*

Abstract

Background: Postoperative pulmonary complications (PPC) are an under-reported but major cause of perioperative morbidity and mortality. The aim of this prospective, contemporary, multicentre cohort study of unselected patients undergoing major elective abdominal surgery was to determine the incidence and effects of PPC.

Methods: Data on all major elective abdominal operations performed over a 2-week period in December 2014 were collected in six hospitals. The primary outcome measure of PPC at 7 days was used. Univariate and multivariate analyses were performed to investigate how different factors were associated with PPC and the effects of such complications.

Results: Two hundred sixty-eight major elective abdominal operations were performed, and the internal validation showed that the data set was 99 % accurate. Thirty-two (11.9 %) PPC were reported at 7 days. PPC was more common in patients with a history of chronic obstructive pulmonary disease compared to those with no history (26.7 vs. 10.2 %, $p < 0.001$). PPC was not associated with other patient factors (e.g. age, gender, body mass index or other comorbidities), type/method of operation or postoperative analgesia. The risk of PPC appeared to increase with every additional minute of operating time independent of other factors (odds ratio 1.01 (95 % confidence intervals 1.00–1.02), $p = 0.007$). PPC significantly increase the length of hospital stay (10 vs. 3 days). Attendance to the emergency department within 30 days (27.3 vs. 10.6 %), 30-day readmission (21.7 vs. 9.9 %) and 30-day mortality (12.5 vs. 0.0 %) was higher in those with PPC.

Conclusions: PPC are common and have profound effects on outcomes. Strategies need to be considered to reduce PPC.

Keywords: Pulmonary complications, Morbidity, Surgery, Postoperative

Background

An estimated 234 million patients undergo major surgery worldwide every year (Weiser et al. 2008). Approximately 16 % will suffer a complication within 30 days (Kazaure et al. 2012). These include well-defined complications e.g. thromboembolic complications (NICE 2010) and surgical site infections (NICE 2013) and others which are likely to be under-reported as they do not form part of the current hospital quality measures.

One set of under-reported complications are postoperative pulmonary complications (PPC). These include a spectre of clinical conditions. PPC includes postoperative hypoxia, atelectasis, bronchospasm, pulmonary infection, pulmonary infiltrate, aspiration pneumonitis, acute respiratory distress syndrome, pleural effusions and pulmonary oedema (Arozullah et al. 2000). Depending on the severity, these can be self-limiting, require ward-based interventions e.g. antibiotics or physiotherapy, or readmission to critical care, reintubation and even death.

* Correspondence: ravsvohra@hotmail.com
[1]West Midlands Research Collaborative, Academic Department of Surgery, School of Cancer Sciences, University of Birmingham, Birmingham B15 2TH, UK
[2]Nottingham Oesophago-Gastric Unit, Nottingham University Hospitals, Nottingham, UK

Some estimates suggest that the incidence of PPC is anywhere between 5 and 40 % of patients following surgeries involving the abdomen (Seiler et al. 2009; Hemmes et al. 2014; Niggebrugge et al. 1999; Treschan et al. 2012). PPC is associated with a 30-day mortality of 18 % compared with 2.5 % for those without PPC (Khuri et al. 2005). Even after risk adjustment, at 5 years post surgery, PPC is associated with a 66 % lower survival (Khuri et al. 2005). In those who do survive, the limited available evidence suggests a detrimental effect of PPC on early and late health-related quality of life (Thompson et al. 2006). Following major elective abdominal surgery, PPC results in six to nine extra hospital days and costs the healthcare system an additional $30,000 per patient (Dimick et al. 2004).

This data relates to studies conducted over 10 years ago. The incidence and effects of PPC may have changed with the advances in perioperative anaesthetic techniques e.g. non-invasive positive pressure ventilation, pain control adjuncts and enhanced recovery protocols (Hemmes et al. 2014; Kehlet and Wilmore 2008). The aim of this prospective multicentre cohort study of unselected patients undergoing major elective abdominal surgery was to determine the incidence and effects of PPC.

Methods

Over the past 8 years, trainee-led networks in the UK have adopted a collaborative approach to deliver prospective population-level data collections and measure patient, disease, surgical and hospital variables with short-term endpoints such as readmissions and complications (Bhangu et al. 2013). Using these networks, a prospective, multicentre cohort study across six hospitals in the UK was conducted over a 2-week period in December 2014.

Inclusion and exclusion criteria

All patients over the age of 18 years undergoing major (defined as a postoperative hospital stay of > 1 day) elective surgery (patients admitted either the day of surgery or the night before) in the study period were included. Consecutive patients undergoing benign and cancer resections on the stomach, liver, pancreas, biliary tree, small bowel, colon, rectum, bladder, kidneys and abdominal aorta were included here. Organ transplantation and emergency operations were excluded. Cholecystectomy was also excluded as the majority are performed as a day case procedure.

Primary outcome

The primary outcome measure of PPC at 7 days was used (Additional file 1: Table S1). Demographic,

intraoperative and postoperative data at day 30 were collected (Additional file 1: Table S2). The definitions for all data were derived from two recent randomised controlled trials (The PROVE Network Investigators 2014; Futier et al. 2013). Patients were investigated and diagnosed with respiratory complications as per 'routine care' at each institution.

Explanatory variables

Demographic and intraoperative data were collected here as potential explanatory variables for PPC at day 7 (Additional file 1: Table S2). Further, postoperative data at day 30 were also collected (Additional file 1: Table S2).

Data validation

To standardise data quality, a quality assurance programme has been developed for previous studies (Vohra et al. 2015). This included a detailed study protocol, a pilot phase, and a requirement for a minimum of 95 % data completeness at submission. Case ascertainment and data accuracy were further validated by independent investigators at selected hospitals, who checked data correctness from 10 % of patients against original medical records. These independent investigators were not involved in the original data collection.

Ethical approval

The protocol did not require research registration or consent from patients as only anonymous observational data were collected. Data collection was entirely independent of patient management, and therefore, patient management was not altered as a result of the study. This was confirmed by the online National Research Ethics Service (NRES) decision tool (http://www.hra-decisiontool-s.org.uk/research/) used to determine whether a study requires review from a research ethics committee in the UK National Health Service (NHS). This decision was further supported by the Research and Development Director at University Hospitals Birmingham NHS Foundation Trust, UK. The study was registered as a 'clinical audit' or 'service evaluation' at each participating hospital under the supervision of a named senior investigator (consultant or attending surgeon).

Statistical analysis

Data were collected and analysed in clinically relevant categories. Univariate and multivariate analyses, including factors with a $p < 0.05$ on univariate analysis, were performed to investigate how different factors were associated with PPC and the sequelae of such complications. Missing data for predictor values were replaced using the multiple imputation method to create five imputed datasets; all predictor and outcome variables will be entered into the predictive models for imputation.

Statistical analyses were conducted using SPSS v21 (IBM, Armonk, NY, USA). Statistical significance was set at $p < 0.050$. The report of this study was prepared in accordance to the guidelines set by the Strengthening the Reporting of Observational Studies in Epidemiology (STROBE) statement for observational studies (Von Elm et al. 2007).

Results
Demographics
Over the 2-week period, a total of 268 consecutive major elective abdominal operations were performed in the six hospitals. Case ascertainment and accuracy of collected data were above 99 and 98 %, respectively, when compared with a 20 % sample checked independently against the original medical records. Missing data were 0.8 % within the entire dataset. General demographic data is shown in Table 1. Median age of the cohort was 66 years, 61.9 % were male, 53.7 % were ASA grade 1 or 2 and 31 % were having a cancer operation. In addition, it is notable that 84.3 % were administered perioperative antibiotics, 63.1 % had open operations and despite all operations being classed as major operations, elective critical care use was 19.4 %. Endotracheal tubes were mainly used reflecting the duration and grade of the operations performed.

Outcomes at day 7 and 30 (Table 2)
A total of 32 (11.9 %) PPC were reported at 7 days, and suspected pulmonary infection was the most common ($n = 24$, 9 %). The median length of hospital stay for the cohort was 4 days, and 30-day mortality was 1.5 % ($n = 4$). Readmissions at 30 days were 17 % which reflects the grade of operations performed.

Effect of pre and perioperative factors (Tables 3 and 4)
Risk factors for PPC by day 7 were a history of chronic obstructive pulmonary disease, undergoing an operation for a malignancy and a postoperative nasogastric tube. In addition, the duration of surgery associated with PPC at day 7 as was the intraoperative analgesia strategy and a change to this strategy in the first 24 h. PPC was not associated with age, gender, body mass index, other co-morbidities, smoking or type or method of operation (open vs. laparoscopic).

When these significant factors were included in a multivariate model, chronic obstructive pulmonary disease was independently associated with development of a PPC (Table 4). Further, the risk of PPC appeared to increase with every additional minute of operating time independent of other factors (odds ratio 1.01 (95 % confidence intervals 1.00–1.02), $p = 0.007$).

Table 1 General demographics

n	268
Age (years, IQR)	66 (53–75)
Male	166 (61.9)
Body mass index (kilograms/metres^2, IQR)	27.3 (24.0–31.2)
American Society of Anesthesiologists physical status classification system	
1	32 (11.9)
2	112 (41.8)
3	71 (26.5)
4	7 (2.6)
Unknown	46 (17.2)
Current smoker	42 (15.7)
Chronic obstructive pulmonary disease	30 (11.2)
Previous cerebrovascular accident	23 (8.6)
Urea (milligrams per decilitre, IQR)	5.4 (4.5–7.0)
Proton pump inhibitor	89 (33.2)
Steroids	16 (6.0)
Cancer operation	83 (31.0)
Type of operation	
Gastric	28 (10.4)
Hepatobiliary/pancreatic	19 (7.1)
Small bowel	13 (4.9)
Colorectal	76 (28.4)
Urological	57 (21.3)
Vascular	62 (23.1)
Other	13 (4.9)
Perioperative antibiotics	226 (84.3)
Type of intubation	
Laryngeal mask airway	60 (22.4)
Cuffed/uncuffed endotracheal tube	207 (77.2)
Unknown	1 (0.4)
Method of operation	
Laparoscopic	77 (28.7)
Laparoscopic-assisted	6 (2.2)
Laparoscopic converted to open	8 (3.0)
Open	169 (63.1)
Endovascular	8 (3.0)
Bowel resection	74 (27.6)
Nasogastric tube	9 (3.4)
Duration of surgery (minutes, IQR)	145 (87–210)
Elective critical care admission	52 (19.4)
Analgesia use in the first 24 h	
Epidural	40 (14.9)
Patient controlled analgesia	50 (18.7)
Wound catheter	2 (0.7)
Oral analgesia only	173 (64.6)
Unknown	3 (1.1)
Change in analgesia strategy in the first 24 h	171 (63.8)
Incentive spirometer	3 (1.1)

Table 2 Selected outcomes within seven and thirty days

At 7 days	
Severe hypoxia	6 (2.2)
Bronchospasm	1 (0.4)
Suspected pulmonary infection	24 (9.0)
Pulmonary infiltrate	11 (4.1)
Aspiration pneumonitis	2 (0.7)
Acute respiratory distress syndrome	2 (0.7)
Atelectasis	13 (4.9)
Pleural effusion	10 (3.7)
Pulmonary oedema	6 (2.2)
Any postoperative pulmonary complication	32 (11.9)
Readmission to critical care	7 (2.6)
Reintubation	5 (1.9)
Length of hospital stay (days, IQR)	4 (1–7)
At 30 days	
Accident and emergency attendance	22 (8.2)
Readmission	46 (17.2)
All complications	59 (22.0)
Non-pulmonary complications	37 (13.8)
Mortality	4 (1.5)

Impact of PPC at day 30

The four postoperative deaths occurred exclusively in patients who developed PPC. PPC increased the median length of hospital stay by 7 days, attendance to the emergency department by 38.8 % and readmissions by 45.6 % compared to if no PPC occurred (Table 5).

Discussion

This prospective multicentre cohort study investigated pulmonary complications in an unselected cohort following major elective abdominal surgery. The data set was internally and independently validated. The incidence of PPC was 11.9 %. PPC were associated with pre-operative and intraoperative risk factors. Despite the small cohort, the development of PPC had a significant impact on length of hospital stay and 30-day outcomes. The mortalities within our cohort were exclusively in patients with a PPC. Cause of death was not examined as part of the study, and thus, we were unable to infer causality; however, length of stay and outcomes data support the morbidity secondary to PPC.

PPC have been estimated by both retrospective cohort studies and in randomised controlled trials (Seiler et al. 2009; Hemmes et al. 2014; Niggebrugge et al. 1999; Treschan et al. 2012; Holte et al. 2007; Squadrone et al. 2005; Pöpping et al. 2008). This has produced a wide disparity in the reported incidence of PPC. The definitions of PPC used in this cohort study were derived from two recent randomised controlled trials investigating differences in tidal volume settings in patients undergoing major elective abdominal surgery performed by an open procedure (Hemmes et al. 2014; Futier et al. 2013). These two studies estimated the incidence of PPC between 20 and 40 %. The incidence estimated in the data presented here was lower than previously described despite high internal study validity. This may be explained by differences in patients' risk factors (e.g. smoking status) and surgical procedures between the unselected cohort studied here and those randomised in previous studies (Hemmes et al. 2014; Futier et al. 2013). Another explanation may be the high numbers of laparoscopic and laparoscopic-assisted procedures performed in this series. However, these approaches are linked with longer operating times, which in this study and previous studies are associated with a higher incidence of PPC (Canet et al. 2010).

PPC was associated with worse 30-day outcomes in this study. The most striking impact of PPC was the effect on hospital length of stay. Median hospital length of stay was extended from 3 to 10 days if a PPC occurred. This is similar to data from 2001 to 2002 from the National Surgical Quality Improvement Project (NSQIP) in the USA (Dimick et al. 2004) which demonstrated that a PPC resulted in an additional six hospital days. Other infectious, cardiovascular and thromboembolic complications resulted in an additional three, two and three hospital days, respectively. In addition, PPC were associated with three times higher healthcare costs compared to other complications.

Other studies have shown continued demonstrable effects of a PPC 5 years following the index event (Khuri et al. 2005). PPCs have a multifactorial aetiology including ventilation-perfusion mismatch and hypoxemia which is a consequence of general anaesthesia, postoperative pain, diaphragmatic dysfunction, decreased chest wall compliance and depressed airway reflexes (Canet et al. 2010; Gazarian 2006; Ebell 2007). This is confounded by bacterial entry into the lower respiratory tract by aspiration of oral and pharyngeal pathogens at the time of intubation and continued leakage of secretions containing bacteria around the endotracheal tube cuff when patients are ventilated for prolonged periods (days to weeks) (du Moulin et al. 1982; Cook et al. 1998; American Thoracic Society, Infectious Diseases Society of America 2005). Colonisation of the lower respiratory tract can overwhelm the patients' mechanical, humoral, and cellular defences to establish infection following surgery (Craven and Steger 1996). Chronic airway inflammation, copious airway secretions and use of preoperative steroids causing immunosuppression may be to blame for increased PPC in patients with COPD (Banerjee et al. 2004).

Table 3 Effect of perioperative variables on PPC

	PPC No. (%)	Yes (%)	
n	236	32	
Age (years, IQR)	67 (53–76)	60 (57–67)	0.404
Gender			0.647
Male	145 (61.4)	21 (65.6)	
Female	91 (38.6)	11 (34.4)	
Body mass index (kilograms/metres^2, IQR)	27.3 (23.8–30.5)	27.1 (25.6–29.9)	0.742
American Society of Anesthesiologists physical status classification system			0.244
1	50 (21.2)	3 (9.4)	
2	119 (50.4)	13 (40.6)	
3	58 (24.7)	12 (37.6)	
4	6 (2.5)	2 (6.2)	
Unknown	3 (1.2)	2 (6.2)	
Current smoker	36 (15.3)	6 (18.8)	0.662
Chronic obstructive pulmonary disease	22 (9.3)	8 (25.0)	0.009
Previous cerebrovascular accident	21 (8.9)	2 (6.3)	0.603
Urea (milligrams per decilitre, IQR)	5.6 (4.5–7.3)	5.4 (4.0–9.4)	0.886
Proton pump inhibitor	80 (33.9)	9 (28.1)	0.515
Steroids	13 (5.5)	3 (9.4)	0.390
Cancer operation	67 (28.4)	15 (46.9)	0.035
Type of operation			0.270
Gastric	24 (10.2)	4 (12.5)	
Hepatobiliary/pancreatic	17 (7.2)	2 (6.3)	
Small bowel	12 (5.1)	1 (3.1)	
Colorectal	66 (28.0)	10 (31.3)	
Urological	55 (23.3)	2 (6.3)	
Vascular	52 (22.0)	10 (31.3)	
Other	10 (4.2)	3 (9.2)	
Perioperative antibiotics	200 (84.7)	26 (81.3)	0.860
Type of intubation			0.946
Laryngeal mask airway	54 (22.9)	6 (18.8)	
Cuffed/uncuffed endotracheal tube	181 (76.7)	26 (81.2)	
Unknown	1 (0.4)	0 (0.0)	
Method of operation			0.722
Laparoscopic	72 (30.5)	5 (15.6)	
Laparoscopic-assisted	5 (2.1)	1 (3.1)	
Laparoscopic converted to open	6 (2.5)	2 (6.3)	
Open	145 (61.4)	24 (75.0)	
Endovascular	8 (3.5)	0 (0.0)	
Bowel resection	61 (25.8)	13 (17.6)	0.079

Table 3 Effect of perioperative variables on PPC *(Continued)*

Nasogastric tube	6 (2.5)	3 (9.4)	0.011
Duration of surgery (minutes, IQR)	100 (55–170)	212 (182–294)	<0.001
Elective critical care admission	33 (14.0)	19 (59.4)	<0.001
Analgesia use in the first 24 h			<0.001
Epidural	26 (11.0)	14 (43.8)	
Patient controlled analgesia	40 (16.9)	10 (31.3)	
Wound catheter	2 (0.1)	0 (0.0)	
Oral analgesia only	166 (70.3)	7 (21.8)	
Unknown	2 (0.1)	1 (3.1)	
Change in analgesia strategy in the first 24 h	148 (62.7)	23 (71.9)	0.014
Incentive spirometer	1 (0.4)	2 (6.3)	<0.001

A patient safety summit statement recently recommended that PPC should be a measure of healthcare quality as it is likely to require a multifaceted and multidisciplinary approach to reduce the incidence (Shander et al. 2011). The definitions used here were monitored successfully by junior surgeons with high internal study validity using prospective cross-sectional methodology described previously (Vohra et al. 2015). These data fields could be used to provide ongoing monitoring of PPC incidence. High incidences of PPC, following patient stratification and risk adjustment, may be used to indicate deficiencies in the perioperative care of patients undergoing major surgery.

Table 4 Selected factors and adjusted odds ratios for postoperative pulmonary complications

	OR (95 % CI)	p value
Chronic obstructive pulmonary disease	16.77 (2.56–109.88)	0.003
Cancer operation	5.13 (0.41–62.5)	0.205
Nasogastric tube	2.15 (0.33–4.01)	0.411
Duration of surgery	1.01 (1.00–1.02)	0.007
Elective critical care admission	4.45 (0.45–43.75)	0.200
Analgesia use in the first 24 h		
Epidural	Reference	
Patient controlled analgesia	0.83 (0.05–15.26)	0.898
Wound catheter	3.05 (0.40–22.98)	0.279
Oral analgesia only	2.56 (0.23–10.54)	0.636
Change in analgesia strategy in the first 24 h	0.24 (0.02–2.70)	0.247
Incentive spirometer	2.93 (0.12–23.83)	0.782

Table 5 Outcomes and postoperative pulmonary complications (PPC)

	PPC		
	No (%)	Yes (%)	
Length of hospital stay (days, IQR)	3 (1–6)	10 (7–16)	< 0.001
At 30 days			
Accident and Emergency attendance	26 (11.0)	6 (27.3)	0.014
Readmission	22 (9.3)	10 (21.7)	0.014
Mortality	0 (0.0)	4 (12.5)	< 0.001

Conclusions

This study highlights the frequency at which PPC occur and their subsequent effects on short-term outcomes. Other studies have shown further implications for long-term patient morbidity.

The development of any PPC is associated with significant morbidity reflected in worse 7- and 30-day outcomes as demonstrated here. Standardised care bundles and other novel strategies need to be considered to reduce PPC across all surgical patients.

Abbreviations

COPD: chronic obstructive pulmonary disease; PPC: postoperative pulmonary complications.

Acknowledgements

West Midlands Research Collaborative. The study was self-funded by members of the West Midlands Research Collaborative. No external funding was sought.

Authors' contributions

RV was responsible for the study design. FH, AA, GB, KE, CH, MJ, FL, JM, PN, PR, CR and SS collected the data. RV was responsible for the input of the data and its analysis. KP, FH, AA, GB, KE, CH, MJ, FL, JM, PN, PR, CR, SS and RV contributed to the compilation of the manuscript. KP and RV were responsible for the review and refinement of the final manuscript. All authors have read and approved the final manuscript.

Competing interests

The authors declare that they have no competing interests.

References

American Thoracic Society, Infectious Diseases Society of America. Guidelines for the management of adults with hospital-acquired, ventilator-associated, and healthcare-associated pneumonia. Am J Respir Crit Care Med. 2005;171(4): 388–416.

Arozullah AM, Daley J, Henderson WG, Khuri SF. Multifactorial risk index for predicting postoperative respiratory failure in men after major noncardiac surgery. The National Veterans Administration Surgical Quality Improvement Program. Ann Surg. 2000;232:242–53.

Banerjee D, Khair OA, Honeybourne D. Impact of sputum bacteria on airway inflammation and health status in clinical stable COPD. Eur Respir J. 2004;23: 685–91.

Bhangu A, Kolias AG, Pinkney T, Hall NJ, Fitzgerald JE. Surgical research collaboratives in the UK. Lancet. 2013;382(9898):1091–2.

Canet J, Gallart L, Gomar C, Paluzie G, Vallès J, Castillo J. Prediction of postoperative pulmonary complications in a population-based surgical cohort. Anesthesiology. 2010;113:1338–50.

Cook D, De Jonghe B, Brochard L, Brun-Buisson C. Influence of airway management on ventilator-associated pneumonia: evidence from randomized trials. JAMA. 1998;279:781–7.

Craven DE, Steger KA. Nosocomial pneumonia in mechanically ventilated adult patients: epidemiology and prevention in 1996. Semin Respir Infect. 1996;11: 32–53.

Dimick JB, Chen SL, Taheri PA, Henderson WG, Khuri SF, Campbell Jr DA. Hospital costs associated with surgical complications: a report from the private-sector National Surgical Quality Improvement Program. J Am Coll Surg. 2004a;199:531–7.

du Moulin GC, Paterson DG, Hedley-Whyte J, Lisbon A. Aspiration of gastric bacteria in antacid-treated patients: a frequent cause of postoperative colonisation of the airway. Lancet. 1982;1:242–5.

Ebell MH. Predicting postoperative pulmonary complications. Am Fam Physician. 2007;75:1837–8.

Futier E, Constantin JM, Paugam-Burtz C, Pascal J, Eurin M, et al. A trial of intraoperative low-tidal-volume ventilation in abdominal surgery. N Engl J Med. 2013a;369(5):428–37.

Gazarian PK. Identifying risk factors for postoperative pulmonary complications. AORN J. 2006;84:616–25. quiz 627–630.

Hemmes SN, Gama de Abreu M, Pelosi P, Schultz MJ, PROVE Network Investigators for the Clinical Trial Network of the European Society of Anaesthesiology. High versus low positive end-expiratory pressure during general anaesthesia for open abdominal surgery (PROVHILO trial): a multicentre randomised controlled trial. Lancet. 2014;384(9942):495–503.

Holte K, Foss NB, Andersen J, Valentiner L, Lund C, Bie P, et al. Liberal or restrictive fluid administration in fast-track colonic surgery: a randomized, double-blind study. Br J Anaesth. 2007;99(4):500–8.

Kazaure HS, Roman SA, Sosa JA. Association of postdischarge complications with reoperation and mortality in general surgery. Arch Surg. 2012;147:1000–7.

Kehlet H, Wilmore DW. Evidence-based surgical care and the evolution of fast-track surgery. Ann Surg. 2008;248(2):89–98.

Khuri SF, Henderson WG, DePalma RG, Mosca C, Healey NA, Kumbhani DJ, et al. Determinants of long-term survival after major surgery and the adverse effect of postoperative complications. Ann Surg. 2005;242(3):326–41 [discussion 341-343].

NICE. Surgical site infection. NICE quality standard 49. 2013. Available online at http://www.nice.org.uk/guidance/qs49/resources/guidance-surgical-site-infection-pdf. Accessed 12 jan 2015.

NICE. Venous thromboembolism prevention quality standard. NICE quality standard 3. 2010. Available online at http://www.nice.org.uk/guidance/qs3/resources/guidance-venous-thromboembolism-prevention-quality-standard-pdf. Accessed 12 jan 2015.

Niggebrugge AH, Trimbos JB, Hermans J, Steup WH, Van De Velde CJ. Influence of abdominal-wound closure technique on complications after surgery: a randomised study. Lancet. 1999;353(9164):1563–7.

Pöpping DM, Elia N, Marret E, Remy C, Tramèr MR. Protective effects of epidural analgesia on pulmonary complications after abdominal and thoracic surgery: a meta-analysis. Arch Surg. 2008;143(10):990–9.

Seiler CM, Deckert A, Diener MK, Knaebel HP, Weigand MA, Victor N, et al. Midline versus transverse incision in major abdominal surgery: a randomized, double-blind equivalence trial (POVATI: ISRCTN60734227). Ann Surg. 2009; 249(6):913–20.

Shander A, Fleisher LA, Barie PS, Bigatello LM, Sladen RN, Watson CB. Clinical and economic burden of postoperative pulmonary complications: patient safety summit on definition, risk reducing interventions, and preventive strategies. Crit Care Med. 2011;39:2163–72.

Squadrone V, Coha M, Cerutti E, Schellino MM, Biolino P, Occella P, et al. Continuous positive airway pressure for treatment of postoperative hypoxemia: a randomized controlled trial. JAMA. 2005;293(5):589–95.

The PROVE Network Investigators. High versus low positive end-expiratory pressure during general anaesthesia for open abdominal surgery (PROVHILO trial): a multicentre randomised controlled trial. Lancet. 2014;384(9942):495–503.

Thompson DA, Makary MA, Dorman T, Pronovost PJ. Clinical and economic outcomes of hospital acquired pneumonia in intra-abdominal surgery patients. Ann Surg. 2006;243(4):547–52.

Treschan TA, Kaisers W, Schaefer MS, Bastin B, Schmalz U, Wania V, et al. Ventilation with low tidal volumes during upper abdominal surgery does not improve postoperative lung function. Br J Anaesth. 2012a;109(2):263–71.

Vohra RS, Spreadborough P, Johnstone M, Marriott P, Bhangu A, Alderson D, et al. West Midlands Research Collaborative. Protocol for a multicentre, prospective, population-based cohort study of variation in practice of cholecystectomy and surgical outcomes (The CholeS study). BMJ Open. 2015;5:1.

Von Elm E, Altman DG, Egger M, Pocock SJ, Gøtzsche PC, Vandenbroucke JP. Strengthening the reporting of observational studies in epidemiology (STROBE) statement: guidelines for reporting observational studies. BMJ. 2007;335(7624):806–8.

Weiser TG, Regenbogen SE, Thompson KD, Haynes AB, Lipsitz SR, Berry WR, et al. An estimation of the global volume of surgery: a modelling strategy based on available data. Lancet. 2008;372(9633):139–44.

8

Physical activity levels in locally advanced rectal cancer patients following neoadjuvant chemoradiotherapy and an exercise training programme before surgery

Lisa Loughney[1,2,3*], Malcolm A. West[1,2,4], Borislav D. Dimitrov[5], Graham J. Kemp[2,6], Michael PW. Grocott[1,2] and Sandy Jack[1,2]

Abstract

Background: The aim of this pilot study was to measure changes in physical activity level (PAL) variables, as well as sleep duration and efficiency in people with locally advanced rectal cancer (1) before and after neoadjuvant chemoradiotherapy (CRT) and (2) after participating in a pre-operative 6-week in-hospital exercise training programme, following neoadjuvant CRT prior to major surgery, compared to a usual care control group.

Methods: We prospectively studied 39 consecutive participants (27 males). All participants completed standardised neoadjuvant CRT: 23 undertook a 6-week in-hospital exercise training programme following neoadjuvant CRT. These were compared to 16 contemporaneous non-randomised participants (usual care control group). All participants underwent a continuous 72-h period of PA monitoring by SenseWear biaxial accelerometer at baseline, immediately following neoadjuvant CRT (week 0), and at week 6 (following the exercise training programme).

Results: Of 39 recruited participants, 23 out of 23 (exercise) and 10 out of 16 (usual care control) completed the study. In all participants ($n = 33$), there was a significant reduction from baseline (pre-CRT) to week 0 (post-CRT) in daily step count: median (IQR) 4966 (4435) vs. 3044 (3265); $p < 0.0001$, active energy expenditure (EE) (kcal): 264 (471) vs. 154 (164); $p = 0.003$, and metabolic equivalent (MET) (1.3 (0.6) vs. 1.2 (0.3); $p = 0.010$). There was a significant improvement in sleep efficiency (%) between week 0 and week 6 in the exercise group compared to the usual care control group (80 (13) vs. 78 (15) compared to (69 ((24) vs. 76 (20); $p = 0.022$), as well as in sleep duration and lying down time ($p < 0.05$) while those in active EE (kcal) (152 (154) vs. 434 (658) compared to (244 (198) vs. 392 (701) or in MET (1.3 (0.4) vs. 1.5 (0.5) compared to (1.1 (0.2) vs. 1.5 (0.5) were also of importance but did not reach statistical significance ($p > 0.05$). An apparent improvement in daily step count and overall PAL in the exercise group was not statistically significant.

(Continued on next page)

* Correspondence: ll2y12@soton.ac.uk
[1]Anaesthesia and Critical Care Research Area, NIHR Respiratory Biomedical Research Unit, University Hospital Southampton NHS Foundation Trust, CE93, MP24, Tremona Road, Southampton SO16 6YD, UK
[2]Integrative Physiology and Critical Illness Group, Clinical and Experimental Sciences, Faculty of Medicine, University of Southampton, CE93, MP24, Tremona Road, Southampton SO16 6YD, UK
Full list of author information is available at the end of the article

(Continued from previous page)

Conclusions: PAL variables, daily step count, EE and MET significantly reduced following neoadjuvant CRT in all participants. A 6-week pre-operative in-hospital exercise training programme improved sleep efficiency, sleep duration and lying down time when compared to participants receiving usual care.

Trial registration: Clinicaltrials.gov NCT01325909

Keywords: Rectal cancer, Neoadjuvant cancer treatment, Physical activity, Exercise, Prehabilitation, Surgery

Background

Cancer treatment reduces physical fitness, which appears to be worse in those receiving surgery and radiotherapy in combination with chemotherapy than in those receiving radiotherapy or surgery alone (Moros et al. 2010). Changes in fitness are clinically important: neoadjuvant chemo- and chemoradiotherapy (CRT) reduce physical fitness, objectively measured using cardiopulmonary exercise testing (CPET), which is associated with increased in-hospital morbidity following advanced rectal cancer resection (West et al. 2014) and decreased 1-year overall survival following upper gastrointestinal cancer resection (Jack et al. 2014).

Physical fitness is closely connected with physical activity (PA), although relationships of cause and effect are complex. Remaining physically active during and after cancer treatment improves cancer-related fatigue, psychological distress, quality of life, as well as overall survival and reduces the probability of cancer recurrence (Thomas et al. 2014). Increasing PA following cancer diagnosis may reduce the risk of cancer-specific death in people with breast and non-metastatic colorectal cancer (Holmes et al. 2005; Meyerhardt et al. 2006) or death from any cause in non-metastatic colorectal cancer (Meyerhardt et al. 2006). Exercise training during chemotherapy has a significant beneficial effect on tumour progression and chemotherapy efficacy in solid tumours (Jones and Alfano 2013).

For people diagnosed with locally advanced rectal cancer [tumour, node, metastasis (TNM) stage >T3N+ magnetic resonance imaging (MRI) identified circumferential resection margin threatened cancer], the standard treatment is neoadjuvant CRT followed by surgery (Pucciarelli et al. 2009; Wasserberg 2014). The aim of this pilot study was to measure changes in daily PAL in people with locally advanced rectal cancer scheduled to undergo neoadjuvant CRT followed by surgical resection with a curative intent. We aimed to evaluate changes in daily step count (numbers of steps taken) and overall PAL pre- and post- neoadjuvant CRT in all participants in an attempt to quantify the impact of neoadjuvant CRT on PAL. We also aimed to evaluate changes in daily step count and overall PAL at the start and end of a pre-operative 6-week in-hospital exercise training programme, commenced after completion of neoadjuvant CRT, comparing changes with those observed in a usual care control group (no formal exercise intervention). Exploratory aims included observing changes in other PAL variables such as: total energy expenditure (EE) (daily living EE) and active EE (PA-induced EE) PA duration; lying down time; sleep duration and efficiency; and metabolic equivalent (MET) (intensity of PA) in all participants following neoadjuvant CRT and compare changes in the exercise group compared to the usual care control group.

Methods
Participants and study design

This prospective pilot, non-randomised, parallel group, interventional controlled trial was a nested study of a clinical trial (West et al. 2015). This pilot study was approved by the North West Liverpool East Research and Ethics Committee (11/H1002/12) and registered with clinicaltrials.gov (NCT01325909). Written informed consent was obtained from all participants. We recruited consecutive participants between March 2011 and February 2014 referred to the Colorectal Multi-Disciplinary Team, aged ≥18 years, with locally advanced (MRI-defined) circumferential resection margin threatened, operable rectal cancer, undergoing standardised neoadjuvant CRT with no distant metastasis and with WHO performance status <2 (Oken et al. 1982) (categorised between 0 (fully active) to 4 (completely disabled, cannot carry out self-care: totally confined to bed or chair). Exclusion criteria were as follows: inability to give informed consent, non-resectable disease, inability to perform CPET or bicycle exercise due to lower limb dysfunction, and participants who declined surgery or neoadjuvant CRT or who received non-standard neoadjuvant CRT. After completing neoadjuvant CRT, participants were allocated to the exercise training group by default. If unable to commit to the exercise schedule (or living >15 miles from the hospital), they were asked to act as contemporaneously recruited controls (no formal exercise intervention) with the same PA monitoring follow-up. Participant characteristics such as age, gender, past medical history, ASA score (the ASA score is a subjective assessment of patients overall health, categorised into five classes: I (healthy fit patient) to V (patient who is not expected to live 24 h without surgery); and WHO status were collected at the baseline visit.

All participants underwent a continuous 72-h period of PA monitoring using SenseWear biaxial accelerometer (Fig. 1). PAL was measured during weekdays at baseline (2 weeks before neoadjuvant CRT), immediately following neoadjuvant CRT (week 0) and at week 3 and week 6. Participants in the exercise training group undertook a 6-week supervised in-hospital exercise training programme (3 sessions per week). The exercise training intensities were responsive to each individual CPET at week 0 and week 3 (informed and altered according to measured work rates at oxygen uptake at lactate threshold and at peak exercise). Exercise training consisted of 40 min (including 5 min warm-up and 5 min cooldown) of interval training on an electromagnetically braked cycle ergometer (Optibike Ergoline GmbH, Germany). The interval training programme consisted of alternating moderate (80% of work rate at oxygen uptake

at lactate threshold—4 by 3-min intervals) to severe (50% of the difference in work rates between oxygen uptake at peak and lactate threshold—4 by 2-min intervals) intensities (total 20 min) for the first two sessions. This was then increased to 40 min (6×3-min intervals at moderate intensity and 6×2-min intervals at severe intensity). The exercise training protocol and procedures are described elsewhere (West et al. 2015).

TNM staging involved flexible sigmoidoscopy for histological diagnosis, colonoscopy, chest, abdomen, and pelvis computer-aided tomography (CT), and 1.5 T pelvic magnetic resonance imaging (MRI). All participants underwent 5 weeks neoadjuvant CRT. Standardised radiotherapy consisted of 45 Gy in 25 fractions on weekdays using a 3D conformal technique with CT guidance. Oral capecitabine (825 mg m^{-2}) was given twice daily on radiotherapy days. No participants received brachytherapy.

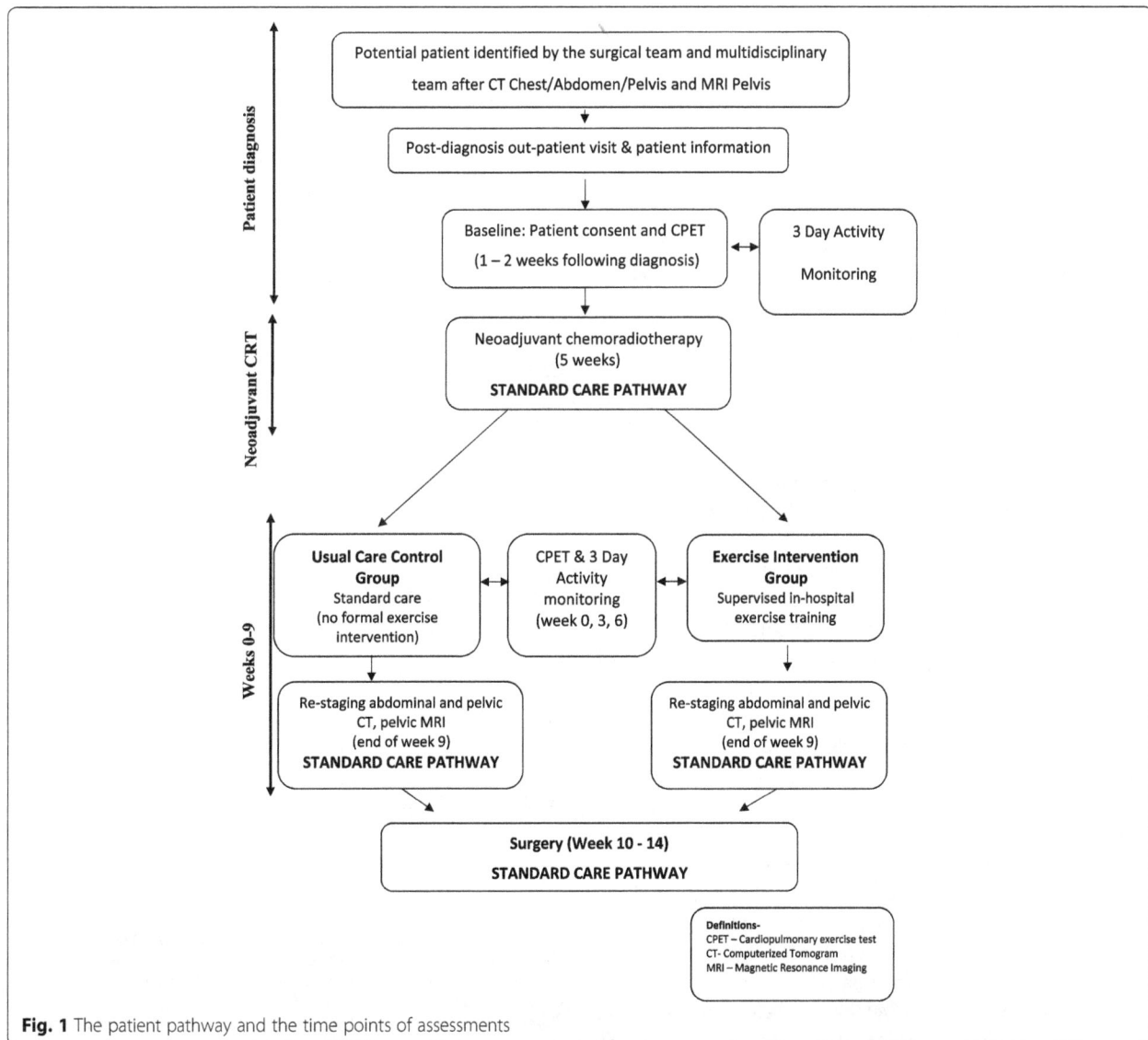

Fig. 1 The patient pathway and the time points of assessments

At 9 weeks post-neoadjuvant CRT, participants were restaged using chest, abdomen, and pelvic CT and pelvic MRI. The colorectal Multi-Disciplinary Team was blind to PAL results and participant allocation.

Measurements

Daily PAL was measured in all participants using a multi-sensor accelerometer (SenseWear Pro® armband; BodyMedia, Inc., Pittsburgh, PADL, USA). The Sense-Wear Amrband Pro is a reliable estimation of resting EE and provides useful information on daily EE when compared to indirect calorimetry (cancer patients) (Cereda et al. 2007) and reasonable agreement on daily EE when compared with doubly labelled water (free living-adults) (St-Onge et al. 2007). The PA accelerometer was worn on the upper right arm continuously for three consecutive weekdays (except when bathing). Participants in the exercise training group removed the PA monitor during in-hospital exercise training sessions.

The armband estimates EE using measurements from a biaxial accelerometer and sensors that quantify galvanic skin response, heat flux, and skin temperature The device records and reports daily movement: total and active EE, PA duration, number of steps, lying down time, average MET, sleep duration and efficiency (number of minutes of sleep divided by number of minutes in bed). The SenseWear Pro can distinguish between lying down and sleep time by using algorithms that detect the characteristics combination of orientation, motion, temperature and skin conductivity with each state.

Statistical methods

This was a nested study of a clinical trial, which was powered to detect changes in objectively measured physical fitness (West et al. 2015). Therefore, no a priori formal power calculation was undertaken for such a PA pilot study.

Continuous variables are reported as mean (range), mean (SD) or median and inter-quartile range (IQR), depending on distribution, and categorical variables as frequency (%). The Shapiro-Wilk test for normality of distributions was applied. Descriptive statistics and univariate statistical comparisons of patient characteristics between the groups were undertaken: for continuous variables, a two-sample t test when relevant distributional assumptions were met and the Mann–Whitney U-test otherwise; for categorical variables, $\chi2$ tests or, when cell counts were insufficient, Fisher's exact test.

Generalised linear mixed models, with a repeated effect for the comparison between the consecutive visits, were used to obtain restricted maximum likelihood (REML) solutions with an unstructured type of the covariance matrix for all or selected measurements in the two groups. Least square means with 95% CIs were

obtained. $p < 0.05$ was taken as statistically significant. All analyses were performed with the statistical software IBM SPSS Statistics Ver.22 (IBM Corporation, Armonk, NY, USA).

Results

A total of 39 participants were recruited of whom 23 (exercise group) and 10 (usual care control group) completed the study (6 participants withdrew consent (dropped out) in the usual care control group: 4 before baseline measurements and 2 during the study). There were significant baseline differences between groups in age, ASA and WHO performance status: the usual care control group were older with poorer subjective performance (Table 1). Further details of participant characteristics are reported elsewhere (West et al. 2015).

There was a significant reduction in daily step count between pre-neoadjuvant CRT (baseline) and post-neoadjuvant CRT (week 0) in all participants (4966 (4435) vs. 3044 (3265); $p < 0.0001$), active EE (kcal) (264 (471) vs. 154 (164); $p < 0.005$), and MET (1.3 (0.6) vs. 1.2 (0.3) $p < 0.05$; table 2) (Additional file 1: Table S1 shows overall PAL as mean (SD) and median and inter-quartile range (IQR). Following the 6-week exercise intervention, the exercise group compared to the usual care control group showed significant improvements in sleep efficiency (%) (78 (13) vs. 80 (15) compared to (69 (24) vs. 76 (20); $p = 0.022$), sleep duration (min) (190 (269) vs.

Table 1 Characteristics of patients scheduled for neoadjuvant cancer treatment and surgery

	Exercise ($n = 23$)	Control ($n = 10$)	p value
Age (year)*	64 (45–82)	72 (62–84)	0.015
Gender M:F (%)	15 (65): 8 (35)	8 (80): 2 (20)	0.710
Past medical history[a]	10 (44)	5 (50)	0.617
Heart failure	3 (13)	1 (10)	
Diabetes	2 (9)	1 (10)	
Ischaemic heart disease	5 (22)	3 (30)	
Cerebrovascular disease	0	0	
ASA[b]			0.003
I	11 (48)	0	
II	10 (44)	9 (90)	
III	2 (9)	1 (10)	
WHO performance status[b]			0.035
0	18 (78)	0	
1	5 (22)	9 (90)	
2	0	1 (10)	

Values presented as mean (range). Participants who dropped out of the study are not included in participant characteristics
[a]Frequencies with percentages in parentheses, smoking status assessed as currently smoking: yes (1) vs no (0)
[b]Number of patients (%) WHO performance status and ASA physical status
*$p < 0.05$ was taken as statistically significant

Table 2 Pre- and post-neoadjuvant CRT physical activity variables

Physical activity variables	Group	Pre-neoadjuvant CRT	Post-neoadjuvant CRT	Change, % change	p value
Step count* (steps/day)	Exercise (n = 23)	5705.3 (3746)	3723 (2867)	−2755 (4152), −44 (20)	<0.0001
	Usual care control (n = 10)	3701.5 (3569)	2274 (3690)	−4 (2600), −0.1 (78)	
	Overall (n = 33)	4966 (4435)	3044.2 (3265)		
MET*	Exercise (n = 23)	1.4 (0.5)	1.3 (0.4)	−0.03 (0.3), −2.3 (15)	0.010
	Usual care control (n = 10)	1.3 (0.9)	1.1 (0.2)	−0.1 (0.3), −8 (14)	
	Overall (n = 33)	1.3 (0.6)	1.2 (0.3)		
Active EE (kcal/day)*	Exercise (n = 23)	229 (482.3)	152 (153.7)	−115 (499), −30 (93)	0.003
	Usual care control (n = 10)	354 (443.5)	244.3 (198.3)	−223 (861), −47 (70)	
	Overall (n = 33)	264.3 (471.3)	154 (163.9)		
PA duration (min/day)	Exercise (n = 23)	61 (97.3)	38 (68)	31 (105), 8 (140)	0.45
	Usual care control (n = 10)	69 (83)	50 (4)	−34 (151), −41 (52)	
	Overall (n = 33)	64 (80.3)	39 (46)		
Lying down (min/day)	Exercise (n = 23)	250 (367.3)	360 (351.7)	6 (211), 2 (40)	0.443
	Usual care control (n = 10)	351.4 (432.4)	541.3 (360.4)	119 (263), 28 (71)	
	Overall (n = 33)	363 (423.9)	483.5 (416.5)		
Sleep efficiency (%)	Exercise (n = 7)	78 (9.1)	78 (13)	0.2 (15), 0.3 (21)	0.917
	Usual care control (n = 7)	69 (20)	69 (24)	−4 (23), −5 (30)	
	Overall (n = 14)	75 (11)	73 (22)		
Sleep duration (min/day)	Exercise (n = 23)	220 (330)	190 (269)	0 (141), 0 (35)	0.847
	Usual care control (n = 10)	264.5 (284)	265 (315)	143 (235), 56 (85)	
	Overall (n = 33)	260 (285)	44 (318)		
Total EE (kcal/day)	Exercise (n = 23)	1668 (932)	1701 (921)	−234 (1013), −0.1 (63)	0.33
	Usual care control (n = 10)	1867 (833)	1741 (416)	−241 (1019), 7 (147)	
	Overall (n = 33)	1668 (846)	1707 (722)		

Values are presented as median (IQR). Absolute change (no brackets) and relative (percentage) change (in brackets) are based on the difference between post-neoadjuvant CRT (week 0) and pre-neoadjuvant CRT (baseline) within each group. All data is averaged over the 72-h period of PA monitoring. Note: due to an upgrade in software during data collection, sleep efficiency is reported in 7/23 (exercise) and 7/10 (usual care control)

EE energy expenditure, *PA* physical activity

*$p < 0.05$ is taken as statistically significant

369 (81) compared to (265 (315) vs. 299 (39); $p = 0.028$) and lying down time (min) (360 (352) vs. 47 (476) compared to (541 (360) vs. 341 (372); $p = 0.029$, Table 3) (Additional file 1: Table S2 shows overall PAL data as mean (SD) and median and inter-quartile range (IQR). Note: (1) the exercise training group took the PA monitors off for the duration of each in-hospital exercise session (120 min/week × 6 weeks): (2) sleep efficiency data is presented in only seven participants in the exercise intervention and usual care control group: this is due to an upgrade in software during data collection.

Discussion

This pilot study shows that neoadjuvant CRT significantly reduced daily step count, active EE and MET in people with newly diagnosed locally advanced rectal cancer. Furthermore, neoadjuvant CRT had a generally negative effect on the other exploratory PA variables, although findings were not statistically significant. People

who participated in the 6-week in-hospital exercise training programme, in the time interval following neoadjuvant CRT and prior to surgery, showed significant improvements in sleep efficiency, sleep duration and lying down time compared to the usual care control group. Furthermore, the exercise group showed an improvement in daily step count and active EE, although these findings did not reach statistical significance.

It has been previously been reported that neoadjuvant chemo- and chemoradiotherapy significantly reduce physical fitness and this change is associated with postoperative complications and reduced 1-year survival in locally advanced rectal and upper gastrointestinal cancer (West et al. 2014; Jack et al. 2014). However, little is known about its effect on PAL and to our knowledge, we are the first to report daily PAL in people with locally advanced rectal cancer scheduled for neoadjuvant cancer treatment and surgery. PAL is commonly quantified by using MET which is scored as follows: ≥1.70 (active

Table 3 Changes in physical activity variables (week 0–week 6)

Physical activity variables	Group	Week 0	Week 3	Week 6	Change, % change	p value
Step count (steps/day)	Exercise (n = 23)	3723 (2867)	6333 (5291)	5401 (3869)	−1544 (5800), 22 (52)	0.728
	Usual care control (n = 10)	2274 (3690)	6422 (7158)	4792 (4370)	1580 (1732), 57 (70)	
MET	Exercise (n = 23)	1.3 (0.4)	1.5 (0.4)	1.5 (0.5)	−0.1 (0.6), 7 (38)	0.440
	Usual care control (n = 10)	1.1 (0.2)	1.2 (0.3)	1.5 (0.5)	0.2 (2), 17 (174)	
Active EE (kcal/day)	Exercise (n = 23)	152 (154)	355 (486)	434 (658)	181 (1228), 46 (92)	0.743
	Usual care control (n = 10)	244 (198)	322 (517)	392 (701)	320 (1368), 110 (284)	
PA duration (min/day)	Exercise (n = 23)	38 (68)	76 (70)	84 (110)	35 (185), 41 (105)	0.992
	Usual care control (n = 10)	39 (46)	66 (89)	89 (132)	85 (243), 100 (276)	
Lying down (min/day)*	Exercise (n = 23)	360 (352)	95 (438)	47 (476)	18 (332), 4 (82)	0.029
	Usual care control (n = 10)	541 (360)	321 (352)	341 (372)	10 (292), 2 (82)	
Sleep efficiency (%)*	Exercise (n = 7)	78 (13)	78 (14)	80 (15)	6 (28), 6 (39)	0.022
	Usual care control (n = 7)	69 (24)	66 (14)	76 (20)	6 (11), 7 (17)	
Sleep duration (min/day)*	Exercise (n = 23)	190 (265)	405 (70)	369 (81)	0 (141), 1 (52)	0.028
	Usual care control (n = 10)	265 (315)	197 (244)	299 (39)	143 (235), 3 (112)	
Total EE (kcal/day)	Exercise (n = 23)	1707 (921)	1949 (769)	1869 (924)	−2 (1177), −0.1 (63)	0.701
	Usual care control (n = 10)	1741 (416)	1962 (730)	1673 (1169)	147 (2705), 7 (147)	

Values presented as median (IQR). Absolute change (no brackets) and relative (percentage) change (in brackets) at week 6 from baseline (pre-neoadjuvant CRT presented in Table 2) within the groups. All data is averaged over the 72-h period of PA monitoring. Note: due to an upgrade in software at the time of data collection, sleep efficiency is reported in 7/23 (exercise) and 7/10 (usual care control)

*p < 0.05 is taken as statistically significant

person); 1.40–1.69 (predominantly sedentary); <1.40 (very inactive); and 1.2 (chair- or bed-bound) (Black et al. 1996). We reported a MET score at cancer diagnosis 1.3 (0.6) which significantly reduced to 1.2 (0.3) following neoadjuvant CRT. This MET score suggests that people in our study were predominantly sedentary following neoadjuvant CRT. Although findings were not statistically significant, we reported lying down time at cancer diagnosis 363 (424) min compared to 484 (417) following completing neoadjuvant CRT. We also reported that, at cancer diagnosis prior to commencing cancer treatment, people in our study had a lower than recommended daily step count (7000–10,000) of 4966 steps (4435) which further reduced to 3044 steps (3265) following neoadjuvant CRT. Daily step count reported following CRT in our study is comparable to daily step count reported in people living with Chronic Obstructive Pulmonary Disease (COPD) (Tudor-Locke et al. 2009). Although little is known about low levels of PA in people with cancer, low levels of PA in people with COPD is associated with development of systemic consequences such as skeletal muscle weakness, osteoporosis, cardiovascular disease (Booth et al. 2000) and with hospital admission and mortality (Garcia-Aymerich et al. 2006).

Participation in the exercise programme had a positive influence on PAL outside the programme similar to findings reported in other studies in people with breast cancer who participated in an exercise programme during adjuvant cancer treatment (Campbell et al. 2005; Adamsen et al. 2009). Although findings were not significant, we reported an improvement in active EE and MET following participation in the exercise programme initiated following neoadjuvant CRT and before surgery. We also showed that daily step count 3 weeks following completion of neoadjuvant CRT (week 0) almost doubled in both groups compared to week 0 but further reduced at week 6, more so in the usual care control group (it must be noted, there were no statistical changes in daily step count following participation in the exercise programme therefore caution is required while interpreting our findings). Additionally, following participation in the exercise programme, there was a significant improvement in sleep efficiency (as well as sleep duration and lying down time) which may be clinically important: sleep disturbance in people with cancer is the second most common reported symptom (Cleeland et al. 2013). Sixty-one percent of people with breast cancer undergoing chemotherapy and radiotherapy report having significant sleep problems (measured using Pittsburgh Sleep Quality Index) which is related to poor health-related quality of life (HRQoL) (Fortner et al. 2002). To our knowledge, only one other study in people with breast cancer scheduled for multimodal treatment (surgery and adjuvant cancer treatment) has assessed sleep disturbance in the context of exercise training during cancer treatment (measured using General Sleep Disturbance response scale) (Naraphong et al. 2015). Although findings from this study did not reach statistical significance, there was a decline in sleep disturbance following a 12-week exercise programme.

To date, measures assessing PAL in people with cancer mainly include subjective self-reported measures such as: Short Form Health Survey (SF-36) (Campbell et al. 2005; Mock et al. 2005; Hoffman et al. 2014); Physical Activity Questionnaire (PAQ) (Mock et al. 2005); Scottish Physical Activity Questionnaire (SPAQ) (Campbell et al. 2005); and leisure time physical activity (Adamsen et al. 2009), all of which provide a patient's personal perception of their daily activities. Such questionnaires have been found to be of limited validity and reliability (Shepard 2003). Patients' estimations of time spent on activities have been shown to be inconsistent when compared to values recorded using PA monitors (Hoffman et al. 2014). PA monitors have been validated as a measure of PAL in several patient cohorts such as in people with physical disabilities, COPD (Pitta et al. 2005; Rabinovich et al. 2013) and spinal cord injury (Hiremath et al. 2013). PA monitors provide direct measures of specific behaviours such as steps per day (Matthews et al. 2012) as well as the time spent being active (intensity of activity), standing, sitting and lying (Pitta et al. 2005). One recent study reported that cancer patients participating in a lifestyle intervention during chemotherapy reported 366% higher moderate-to-vigorous intensity PA (MPVA) using the International PA Questionnaire compared to measures collected using SenseWear accelerometers (Vassbakk-Brovold et al. 2016). Our study highlights that objective measures of PAL throughout the cancer care journey are worthy of attention: they are relatively simple to undertake and to date have not been used in the perioperative setting.

Strengths of this study include its prospective design, the homogenous study population (only operable locally advanced rectal cancer patients), the clearly defined exercise intervention and the standardised neoadjuvant CRT regime. PA was averaged over a 72-h period, measured in an objective manner using validated SenseWear activity monitors. Furthermore, participants in the exercise group did not wear the PA monitors during exercise sessions. Potential weaknesses of this study include its design as a relatively small pilot study, which was powered to detect changes in objectively measured physical fitness (West et al. 2015), and the limitation of recruitment to one single centre, which may limit generalisability of results. This was a non-randomised design study (i.e. participants in the usual care control group were people who were living >15 miles from the hospital) and there was significant baseline differences between groups

in age, ASA and WHO performance status: the usual care control group were older with poorer subjective performance. Furthermore, differences exist in group sample size, 23/23 (exercise) and 10/16 (usual care control) completed the study. Sleep efficiency data were only available for 7 in each group: this was due to an upgrade in software during data collection.

Conclusions
Our study shows that neoadjuvant CRT significantly reduces MET score, active EE and daily step count in people with locally advanced rectal. People who participated in a 6-week in-hospital exercise training programme following neoadjuvant CRT showed a significant improvement in sleep efficiency, sleep duration and lying down time and an apparent improvement in daily step count and overall PAL compared to the usual care control group.

Abbreviations
COPD: Chronic obstructive pulmonary disease; CPET: Cardiopulmonary exercise test; CRT: Chemo-radiotherapy; CT: Computer-aided tomography; EE: Energy expenditure; HRQoL: Health-related quality of life; IQR: Inter-quartile range; MET: Metabolic equivalent threshold; MRI: Magnetic resonance imaging; PA: Physical activity; PAL: Physical activity levels; PAQ: Physical activity questionnaire; REML: Restricted maximum likelihood; SD: Standard deviation; SF-36: Short form health survey; SPAQ: Scottish physical activity questionnaire; TNM: Tumour, nodes, metastasis

Acknowledgements
Not applicable.

Funding
Not applicable.

Authors' contributions
MAW, GJK, MPWG and SJ conceived the study. LL, MAW, GJK, MPWG and SJ contributed to study design. BDD undertook the statistical analysis. LL drafted the manuscript which underwent revision by all other authors. All authors read and approved the final manuscript.

Competing interests
The authors declare that they have no competing interests.

Author details
[1]Anaesthesia and Critical Care Research Area, NIHR Respiratory Biomedical Research Unit, University Hospital Southampton NHS Foundation Trust, CE93, MP24, Tremona Road, Southampton SO16 6YD, UK. [2]Integrative Physiology and Critical Illness Group, Clinical and Experimental Sciences, Faculty of Medicine, University of Southampton, CE93, MP24, Tremona Road,

Southampton SO16 6YD, UK. [3]MedEx Research Cluster, School of Health and Human Performance, Dublin City University, Dublin, Ireland. [4]Academic Unit of Cancer Sciences, Faculty of Medicine, University of Southampton, Southampton, UK. [5]Academic Unit of Primary Care and Population Sciences, Faculty of Medicine, University of Southampton, Southampton, UK. [6]Department of Musculoskeletal Biology and MRC – Arthritis Research UK Centre for Integrated research into Musculoskeletal Ageing (CIMA), Faculty of Health and Life Sciences, University of Liverpool, Liverpool, UK.

References

Adamsen L, Quist M, Andersen C, Moller T, Herrstedt J, Kronborg D, et al. Effect of a multimodal high intensity exercise intervention in cancer patients undergoing chemotherapy: randomised controlled trial. BMJ. 2009;339:3410.

Black AE, Coward WA, Cole TJ, Prentice AM. Human energy expenditure in affluent societies: an analysis of 574 doubly-labelled water measurements. Eur J Clin Nutr. 1996;50:72–92.

Booth FW, Gordon SE, Carlson CJ, Hamilton MT. Waging war on modern chronic diseases: primary prevention through exercise biology. J Appl Physiol. 2000;88(2):774–87.

Campbell A, Mutrie N, White F, McGuire F, Kearney N. A pilot study of a supervised group exercise programme as a rehabilitation treatment for women with breast cancer receiving adjuvant treatment. Eur J Oncol Nurs. 2005;9(1):56–63.

Cereda E, Turrini M, Ciapanna D, Marbello L, Pietrobelli A, Corradi E. Assessing energy expenditure in cancer patients: a pilot validation of a new wearable device. JPEN J Parenter Enteral Nutr. 2007;31(6):502–7.

Cleeland CS, Zhao F, Chang VT, Sloan JA, O'Mara AM, Gilman PB, et al. The symptom burden of cancer: Evidence for a core set of cancer-related and treatment-related symptoms from the Eastern Cooperative Oncology Group Symptom Outcomes and Practice Patterns study. Cancer. 2013;119(24):4333–40.

Fortner BV, Stepanski EJ, Wang SC, Kasprowicz S, Durrence HH. Sleep and Quality of Life in Breast Cancer Patients. J Pain Symptom Manage. 2002;24:5.

Garcia-Aymerich J, Lange P, Benet M, Schnohr P, Anto JM. Regular physical activity reduces hospital admission and mortality in chronic obstructive pulmonary disease: a population based cohort study. Thorax. 2006;61(9):772–8.

Hiremath SV, Ding D, Farringdon J, Vyas N, Cooper RA. Physical activity classification utilizing SenseWear activity monitor in manual wheelchair users with spinal cord injury. Spinal Cord. 2013;51(9):705–9.

Hoffman AJ, Brintnall RA, von Eye A, Jones LW, Alderink G, Patzelt LH, et al. Home-based exercise: promising rehabilitation for symptom relief, improved functional status and quality of life for post-surgical lung cancer patients. J Thorac Dis. 2014;6(6):632–40.

Holmes MD, Chen WY, Feskanich D, Kroenke CH, Colditz GA. Physical Activity and Survival After Breast Cancer Diagnosis. JAMA. 2005;11(5):106.

Jack S, West MA, Raw D, Marwood S, Ambler G, Cope TM, et al. The effect of neoadjuvant chemotherapy on physical fitness and survival in patients undergoing oesophagogastric cancer surgery. Eur J Surg Oncol. 2014;40(10):1313–20.

Jones LW, Alfano CM. Exercise-oncology research: past, present, and future. Acta Oncol. 2013;52(2):195–215.

Matthews CE, Hagstromer M, Pober DM, Bowles HR. Best practices for using physical activity monitors in population-based research. Med Sci Sports Exerc. 2012;44(1):68–76.

Meyerhardt JA, Giovannucci EL, Holmes MD, Chan AT, Chan JA, Colditz GA, et al. Physical activity and survival after colorectal cancer diagnosis. J Clin Oncol. 2006;24(22):3527–34.

Mock V, Frangakis C, Davidson NE, Ropka ME, Pickett M, Poniatowski B, et al. Exercise manages fatigue during breast cancer treatment: a randomized controlled trial. Psychooncology. 2005;14(6):464–77.

Moros MT, Ruidiaz M, Caballero A, Serrano E, Martinez V, Tres A. Effects of an exercise training program on the quality of life of women with breast cancer on chemotherapy. Rev Med Chil. 2010;138(6):715–22.

Naraphong W, Lane A, Schafer J, Whitmer K, Wilson BR. Exercise intervention for fatigue-related symptoms in Thai women with breast cancer: A pilot study. Nurs Health Sci. 2015;17(1):33–41.

Oken MM, Creech RH, Tormey DC, Horton J, Davis TE, McFadden ET, et al. Toxicity and response criteria of the Eastern Cooperative Oncology Group. J Clin Oncol. 1982;5(6):649–55.

Pitta F, Troosters T, Spruit MA, Decramer M, Gosselink R. Activity monitoring for assessment of physical activities in daily life in patients with chronic obstructive pulmonary disease. Phys Med Rehab. 2005;86(10):1979–85.

Pucciarelli S, Gagliardi G, Maretto I, Lonardi S, Friso ML, Uros E, et al. Long-Term Oncologic Results and Complications After Preoperative Chemoradiotherpay for Rectal Cancer: A Single-Institution Experience After a Median Follow-Up of 95 Months. Ann Surg Oncol. 2009;16:893–9.

Rabinovich RA, Louvaris Z, Raste Y, Langer D, Van Remoortel H, Giavedoni S, et al. Validity of physical activity monitors during daily life in patients with COPD. Eur Respir J. 2013;42(5):1205–15.

Shepard RJ. Limits to the measurement of habitual physical activity by questionnaires. BRJ Sports Med. 2003;37(3):197–206.

St-Onge M, Mignault D, Allison D, Rabasa-Lhoret R. Evaluation of a portable device to measure daily energy expenditure in free-living adults. Am J Clin Nutr. 2007;85(3):742–9.

Thomas RJ, Holm M, Al-Adhami A. Physical activity after cancer: An evidence review of the international literature. Br J Med Pract. 2014;7(1):708.

Tudor-Locke C, Washington TL, Hart TL. Expected values for steps/day in special populations. Prev Med. 2009;49(1):3–11.

Vassbakk-Brovold K, Kersten C, Fegran L, Mjåland O, Mjåland S, Seiler S, et al. Cancer patients participating in a lifestyle intervention during chemotherapy greatly over-report their physical activity level: a validation study. BMC Sports Sci Med Rehabil. 2016;8:10.

Wasserberg N. Interval to surgery after neoadjuvant treatment for colorectal cancer. World J Gastroenterol. 2014;20(15):4256–62.

West MA, Loughney L, Barben CP, Sripadam R, Kemp GJ, Grocott MP, et al. The effects of neoadjuvant chemoradiotherapy on physical fitness and morbidity in rectal cancer surgery patients. Eur J Surg Oncol. 2014;40(11):1421–8.

West MA, Loughney L, Lythgoe D, Barben CP, Sripadam R, Kemp GK, et al. Effect of prehabilitation on objectively measured physical fitness after neoadjuvant treatment in preoperative rectal cancer patients: a blinded interventional pilot study. Br J Anaesth. 2015;114(2):244–51.

9

Enhanced recovery protocols for colorectal surgery and postoperative renal function

Charles R. Horres[1], Mohamed A. Adam[2], Zhifei Sun[2], Julie K. Thacker[2], Richard E. Moon[1], Timothy E. Miller[1] and Stuart A. Grant[1]*

Abstract

Background: While enhanced recovery protocols (ERPs) reduce physiologic stress and improve outcomes in general, their effects on postoperative renal function have not been directly studied.

Methods: Patients undergoing major colorectal surgery under ERP (February 2010 to March 2013) were compared with a traditional care control group (October 2004 October 2007) at a single institution. Multivariable regression models examined the association of ERP with postoperative creatinine changes and incidence of postoperative acute kidney dysfunction (based on the Risk, Injury, Failure, Loss, and End-stage renal disease criteria).

Results: Included were 1054 patients: 590 patients underwent surgery with ERP and 464 patients without ERP. Patient demographics were not significantly different. Higher rates of neoplastic and inflammatory bowel disease surgical indications were found in the ERP group (81 vs. 74%, $p = 0.045$). Patients in the ERP group had more comorbidities (ASA ≥ 3) (62 vs. 40%, $p < 0.001$). In unadjusted analysis, postoperative creatinine increase was slightly higher in the ERP group compared with control (median 0.1 vs. 0 mg/dL, $p < 0.001$), but levels of postoperative acute kidney injury were similar in both groups ($p = 0.998$). After adjustment with multivariable regression, postoperative changes in creatinine were similar in ERP vs. control ($p = 0.25$).

Conclusions: ERP in colorectal surgery is not associated with a clinically significant increase in postoperative creatinine or incidence of postoperative kidney injury. Our results support the safety of ERPs in colorectal surgery and may promote expanding implementation of these protocols.

Trial registration: Not applicable, prospective data collection and retrospective chart review only.

Keywords: Enhanced recovery, Goal-directed fluid therapy, Perioperative acute kidney injury, RIFLE criteria

Background

Enhanced recovery protocols (ERPs) are multimodal approaches focusing on improving patient surgical outcomes through preoperative optimization and emphasis on standardized evidence-based interventions in perioperative patient care. A growing body of evidence suggests that ERPs significantly reduce the incidence of perioperative complications, length of hospitalization, and health care costs for patients undergoing colorectal surgery (Miller et al., 2014; Zhuang et al., 2013; Lv, 2012).

Acute kidney injury (AKI) is a relatively common postoperative complication after colorectal surgery (Masoomi et al., 2012). Although the etiology of AKI following surgery is multifactorial, it has been traditionally thought that liberal fluid administration may be beneficial in the perioperative period, when patients are predisposed to reductions in renal blood flow (Fearon et al., 2005; Lyon et al., 2012).

ERPs attempt to avoid fluid overload during both the intraoperative and postoperative periods. Intraoperatively, low-dose maintenance crystalloid infusions are advocated to maintain zero fluid balance. In addition, many centers use goal-directed fluid therapy to optimize stroke volume and deliver fluids only to patients who

* Correspondence: grant021@mc.duke.edu
[1]Department of Anesthesiology, Duke University, DUMC 3094, Durham, NC 27710, USA
Full list of author information is available at the end of the article

are volume-responsive, as judged by stroke volume assessment (Miller et al., 2015). In the postoperative period, intravenous fluids are discontinued after resumption of oral fluid intake, most often in the immediate postoperative period (Miller et al., 2014). Permissive oliguria is tolerated and is not necessarily treated with fluid boluses in the absence of other indicators of hypovolemia.

Increased use of neuraxial analgesia is another component of ERPs. This has been shown to improve postoperative pain control and return of gastrointestinal motility (Steinbrook, 1998). At the same time, the sympatholysis produced by epidural analgesia causes arterial vasodilation (Clemente & Carli, 2008). An increased incidence of postoperative hypotension has been observed in patients treated with epidural analgesia under ERPs (Marret et al., 2007; Gupta & Gan, 2016).

Although there is good evidence for the benefits of avoiding fluid overload, concerns have been raised that the more restrictive fluid management approach in ERPs, permissive oliguria, and the increased use of epidural analgesia common to ERPs may increase the risk for postoperative AKI. Unfortunately, there is a scarcity of data examining the impact of ERP on postoperative kidney function after colorectal surgery. While small studies comparing ERPs to traditional care have reported similar rates of acute kidney dysfunction in their enhanced recovery and conventional therapy cohorts, these studies were underpowered to detect changes in individual complications (Huebner et al., 2014; Hübner et al., 2013; Ihedioha et al., 2015). Large studies, meta-analyses, and systematic reviews comparing ERPs to conventional care have not specifically set out to compare renal outcomes from traditional management to ERPs, so these studies are limited by a lack of granularity that precludes inference about the adjusted renal effects of ERPs (Bakker et al., 2015; Gustafsson et al., 2011; Ren et al., 2012; Varadhan et al., 2010; Aarts et al., 2012; ERAS Compliance Group, 2015; Shida et al., 2015; Dhruva Rao et al., 2015; Spanjersberg et al., 2015; Greco et al., 2014; Gillissen et al., 2013; Gravante & Elmussareh, 2012; Rawlinson et al., 2011). Therefore, we sought to examine directly the effects of an ERP on changes in postoperative creatinine levels and the incidence of postoperative AKI following colorectal surgery.

Methods
Study cohort
The study included patients undergoing major elective colorectal surgery under ERP (between February 2010 and March 2013) or without ERP (between October 2004 and October 2007) at the Duke University Medical Center. Eligible procedures for inclusion were segmental colectomy, total abdominal colectomy, total abdominal colectomy with end ileostomy, total proctocolectomy with ileoanal pouch, low anterior resection, and abdominoperineal resection. The study included both laparoscopic and open procedures. Procedures were performed by board-certified colorectal surgeons. Patients with preoperative renal dysfunction (defined as creatinine > 1.5) were excluded. The Duke Institutional Review Board approved this study (IRB#: Pro00061780).

Colorectal ERP
Specifics of the Duke ERP and data demonstrating improvements in colorectal surgery outcomes have been published previously (Miller et al., 2014; Adam et al., 2015). Briefly, this protocol was composed of three phases: preoperative, intraoperative, and postoperative. In the preoperative phase, patients received education on the program and details about their role. To minimize preoperative fasting, clear liquids were permitted until 3 h before the time of anesthesia induction. In addition, patients were given a carbohydrate-rich drink 3 h before induction. All patients received standardized preoperative antibiotics and thromboprophylaxis, as well as multimodal strategies for pain management and postoperative nausea and vomiting. Bowel preparation was not routinely employed. In the intraoperative phase, minimally invasive surgical approaches and use of epidural analgesia were encouraged. Ninety-two percent of ERP patients received thoracic epidural analgesia. Maintenance crystalloid therapy was delivered via an infusion pump at 1–3 ml/kg/h. Cardiac output monitors were used to perform goal-directed fluid therapy, with 250 ml boluses of Voluven® (Fresenius Kabi Norge AS, Halden, Norway) given to optimize cardiac output. Esophageal Doppler (EDM™ Deltex Medical, Inc., Irving, TX) was used for non-invasive cardiac output monitoring, and the LiDCORapid™ (LiDCO Ltd., Cambridge, UK) was used if invasive cardiac monitoring was established. During the intraoperative and postoperative periods, oliguria was tolerated if signs or symptoms of hypovolemia were absent. Postoperatively, diet and ambulation were initiated on the day of surgery. Intravenous fluids were most often stopped by 06:00 on postoperative day 1 and only restarted if there were clinical concerns about intolerance of oral intake. The head of the bed was kept at 30°, and epidural anesthesia was continued for up to 72 h following surgery. Figure 1 provides a summary of changes implemented under the ERP that are likely to affect patient fluid balance.

Data source
Data were extracted from two databases—a control cohort, previously identified by review of the Duke Innovian® (Draeger, Inc. Telford PA) perioperative database, and the enhanced recovery cohort, collected in a prospectively maintained database. Patient age, gender, race,

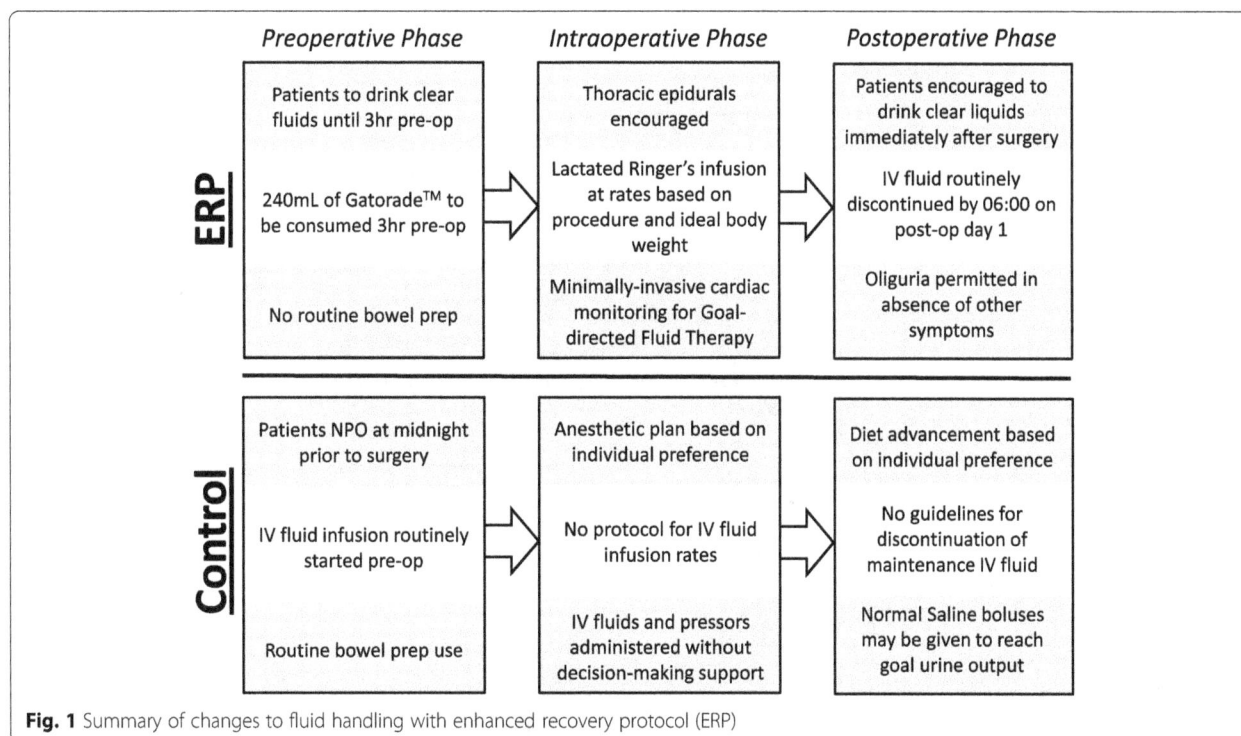

	Preoperative Phase	Intraoperative Phase	Postoperative Phase
ERP	Patients to drink clear fluids until 3hr pre-op — 240mL of Gatorade™ to be consumed 3hr pre-op — No routine bowel prep	Thoracic epidurals encouraged — Lactated Ringer's infusion at rates based on procedure and ideal body weight — Minimally-invasive cardiac monitoring for Goal-directed Fluid Therapy	Patients encouraged to drink clear liquids immediately after surgery — IV fluid routinely discontinued by 06:00 on post-op day 1 — Oliguria permitted in absence of other symptoms
Control	Patients NPO at midnight prior to surgery — IV fluid infusion routinely started pre-op — Routine bowel prep use	Anesthetic plan based on individual preference — No protocol for IV fluid infusion rates — IV fluids and pressors administered without decision-making support	Diet advancement based on individual preference — No guidelines for discontinuation of maintenance IV fluid — Normal Saline boluses may be given to reach goal urine output

Fig. 1 Summary of changes to fluid handling with enhanced recovery protocol (ERP)

American Society of Anesthesiologists (ASA) classification, surgical indication, surgical approach, and extent of surgical resection were extracted from each dataset. Serum creatinine data were collected by the study team via retrospective chart review. Preoperative serum creatinine was defined as the serum creatinine obtained in closest proximity to the date of surgery, usually within 1 week of the procedure. Peak postoperative serum creatinine was defined as the highest creatinine level obtained during the 30 days following surgery. For all patients, the 30-day period allowed for capture of creatinine levels obtained during the inpatient period, follow-up appointment, and readmissions for complications. All patients had a minimum of postoperative day 1 serum creatinine level, pre-discharge serum creatinine level, and follow-up appointment serum creatinine level. Internal auditing was performed to ensure data accuracy. A patient inclusion/exclusion flow diagram is included as Fig. 2.

Statistical analysis

The primary outcome measure of the study was the incidence of postoperative AKI. AKI was stratified into three classes: No Kidney Injury, Acute Kidney Injury ($2\times$ increase in creatinine), and Acute Kidney Failure ($3\times$ increase in creatinine). These creatinine change cutoffs correspond to the Acute Dialysis Quality Initiative's Risk, Injury, Failure, Loss, and End-stage renal disease (RIFLE) classification (Bellomo et al., 2004). Urine output definitions of renal injury were not used because urine output was not strictly tracked in the ERP group, as the

protocol calls for early discontinuation of urinary catheters. The risk category was not included, as it does not correspond to actual renal injury.

Relevant patient demographic data, perioperative creatinine, and operative characteristics were compared between the ERP and the pre-implementation (control) groups using Pearson's chi-square/Fisher's exact tests for categorical variables. The Wilcoxon rank-sum test was used to compare continuous variables.

Multivariable linear regression modeling was employed to examine the adjusted association between ERP vs. control with changes in postoperative serum creatinine levels while accounting for the effects of patient age, gender, race, ASA score, surgical indication, surgical extent, and surgical approach, and preoperative creatinine level. All statistical analyses were performed using R 3.2.1 (R Foundation for Statistical Computing; Vienna, Austria).

Results
Patient and treatment characteristics

A total of 1054 patients were included, 590 (56%) of whom were treated in the ERP group and 464 (44%) patients were in the control group. Patient demographic characteristics were not significantly different between the two groups (Table 1). ASA class tended to be higher in the ERP group (for example, ASA ≥ 3: 62 vs. 40%, $p < 0.001$). The ERP group included fewer colectomies (52 vs. 88%) and more rectal resections (48 vs. 12%) (all $p < 0.001$). Use of laparoscopy was more frequent in the ERP group (60 vs. 49%, $p < 0.001$). Although the total

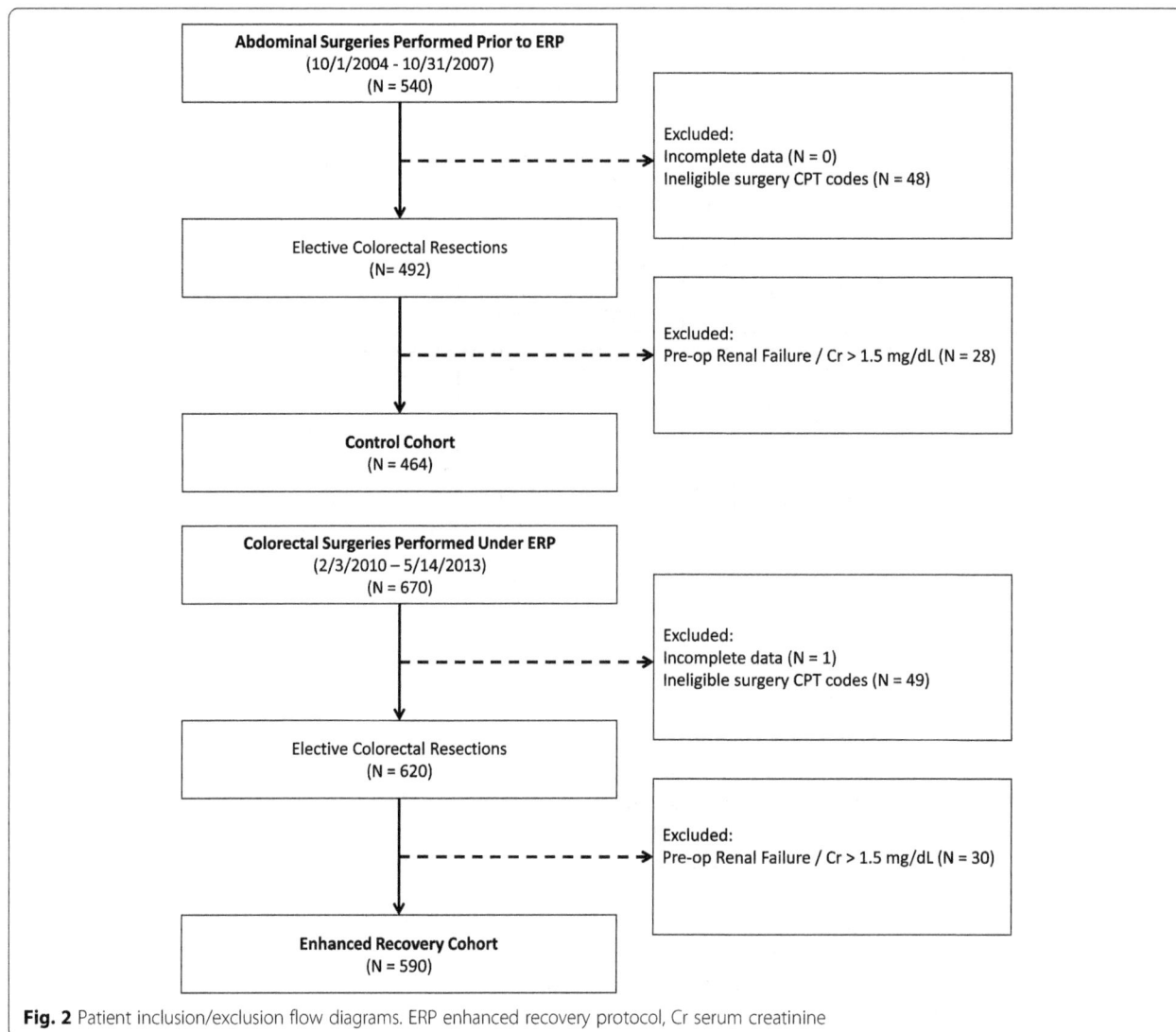

Fig. 2 Patient inclusion/exclusion flow diagrams. ERP enhanced recovery protocol, Cr serum creatinine

volume of fluid administered intraoperatively was not significantly different between the groups ($p = 0.233$), more colloid was administered in the ERP group (median 500 mL control vs. 1000 mL ERP; $p < 0.001$).

Treatment outcomes

Although statistically significant, median serum creatinine levels were not clinically different between groups preoperatively (0.9 vs. 0.9 mg/dL) or postoperatively (1.0 vs. 1.0 mg/dL). However, differences between the preoperative and postoperative serum creatinine levels were slightly higher in the ERP group than in control (median 0.1 vs. 0.0 mg/dL, respectively, $p < 0.001$) (Table 2, Fig. 3).

Compared with control, patients undergoing surgery in the ERP group had no significant differences in incidence of acute kidney injury (3.7% ERP vs. 3.7%) and acute kidney failure (0.8% ERP vs. 0.9%) ($p = 0.998$).

After adjustment for patient age, gender, race, ASA score, surgical indication, extent of surgery, and surgical approach, ERP vs. control was not associated with significant changes in postoperative serum creatinine levels ($p = 0.251$) (Table 3). Factors associated with significant increases in postoperative serum creatinine were older patient age, male gender, black race, and use of open surgical approach.

Discussion

This large single-institution study examined the impact of an optimized ERP on perioperative renal function of patients undergoing major colorectal surgery. In unadjusted analysis, patients undergoing surgery within ERP had a small statistically significant increase in postoperative serum creatinine. However, after adjustment for patient and procedure mix, implementation of an ERP was not associated with a statistically significant

Table 1 Patient demographics and treatment characteristics: ERP vs. control

	Control (N = 464)	ERP (N = 590)	p value
Age (years, median [IQR])	60 [51–71]	60 [48–68]	0.175
Sex			0.316
Male	48.9% (227)	52.0% (307)	
Female	51.1% (237)	48.0% (283)	
Race			0.749
White	72.6% (337)	74.7% (441)	
Black	23.5% (109)	21.7% (128)	
Others	3.9% (18)	3.6% (21)	
ASA classification			< 0.001
1	1.7% (8)	3.9% (23)	
2	58.4% (271)	34.4% (203)	
≥ 3	39.9% (185)	61.7% (364)	
Indication			0.045
Benign	25.8% (120)	19.3% (114)	
IBD	11.3% (52)	12.9% (76)	
Neoplastic	62.9% (292)	67.8% (400)	
Extent of surgery			< 0.001
Colectomy	88.1% (409)	52.4% (309)	
Proctectomy	11.9% (55)	47.6% (281)	
Surgical approach			< 0.001
Laparoscopic	48.7% (226)	59.9% (353)	
Open	51.3% (238)	40.1% (237)	
Intra-op total fluid (mL, median [IQR])	3760 [2460–5351]	3468 [2688–4536]	0.233
Intra-op colloid (mL, median [IQR])	500 [0–1000]	1000 [750–1500]	< 0.001
Pre-op hemoglobin (mg/dL, median [IQR])	13.4 [11.8–14.5]	13.3 [11.8–14.5]	0.401

ERP enhanced recovery protocol, *ASA* American Society of Anesthesiologists, *IQR* interquartile range, *IBD* inflammatory bowel disease

increase in the levels of postoperative serum creatinine. Further, the incidences of postoperative AKI and acute kidney failure were similar between patients treated with ERP vs. without ERP.

Overall, very few studies have tracked the incidence of renal complications within ERPs. Most individual studies present either a pooled complication rate (overall complications) or a limited subset of individual postoperative complications, which did not include acute kidney injury or failure. Similarly, meta-analyses and systematic reviews of ERPs for colorectal surgery report only classifications of "major" and "minor" complications (Huebner et al., 2014; Hübner et al., 2013; Ihedioha et al., 2015; Bakker et al., 2015; Gustafsson et al., 2011; Ren

Table 2 Unadjusted renal outcomes in patients treated with ERP vs. traditional care

	Control (N = 464)	ERP (N = 590)	All patients (N = 1054)	p value
Preoperative creatinine (mg/dL, median [IQR])	0.9 (0.8–1.1)	0.9 (0.7–1.0)	0.9 (0.8–1.1)	0.002
Max postoperative creatinine (mg/dL, median [IQR])	1.0 (0.8–1.2)	1.0 (0.8–1.2)	1.0 (0.8–1.2)	0.008
Creatinine differences (mg/dL)	0.0 (0.0–0.1)	0.1 (0.0–0.3)	0.1 (0.0–0.2)	< 0.001
Level of postoperative kidney injury				0.998
No kidney injury	95.5% (443)	95.4% (563)	95.4% (1006)	
Acute kidney injury (2× increase)	3.7% (17)	3.7% (22)	3.7% (39)	
Acute kidney failure (3× increase)	0.9% (4)	0.8% (5)	0.9% (9)	

Acute kidney injury and failure thresholds set at 2× and 3× increase in creatinine, based on RIFLE criteria cutoffs. Wilcoxon rank-sum test was used to compare creatinine ranges; Mann–Whitney U test was used to compare incidences of kidney injury and failure
ERP enhanced recovery protocol, *IQR* interquartile range

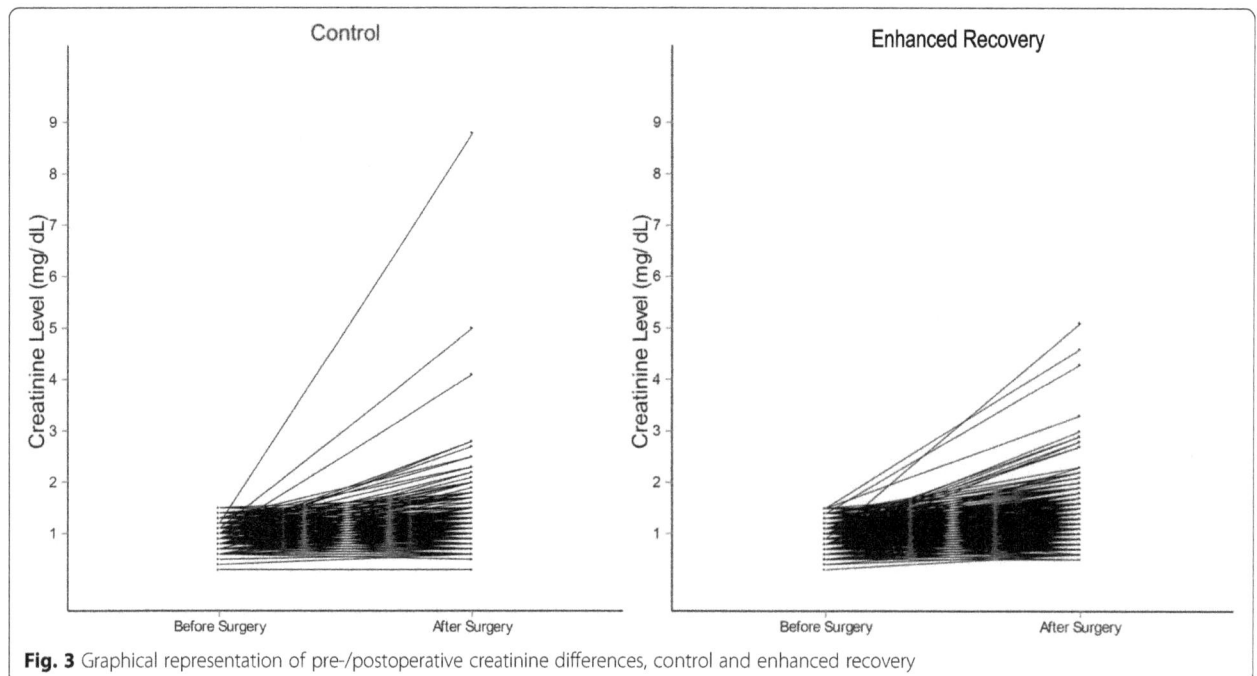

Fig. 3 Graphical representation of pre-/postoperative creatinine differences, control and enhanced recovery

et al., 2012; Varadhan et al., 2010; Aarts et al., 2012; ERAS Compliance Group, 2015; Shida et al., 2015; Dhruva Rao et al., 2015; Spanjersberg et al., 2015; Greco et al., 2014; Gillissen et al., 2013; Gravante & Elmussareh, 2012; Rawlinson et al., 2011).

In one study, 268 patients undergoing resection with established care were compared with 78 patients treated within an ERP. The rates of acute renal failure were reported as 2.2% in the established care group and 3.8% in the ERP group, which were not significantly different between the two groups (p = 0.37) (Huebner et al., 2014). While that smaller study showed equivalent renal outcomes between the ERP and traditional pathway, it was not clear how renal function and/or failure were defined. Another limitation of that study was the small size that precluded adjustment for possible confounders that have

known effects on renal function, such as patient age, comorbidities, extent of surgery, and operative technique. A small-cohort review study from the Mayo Clinic compared postoperative hemodynamics in patients who received treatment within an ERP with or without intrathecal analgesia. The study reported a 2.5% incidence of renal failure among its 163 patients (Hübner et al., 2013). That study used the Acute Kidney Injury Network criteria for renal injury and tracked creatinine and urine output, but it was still limited by small cohort size and the lack of a control group.

In our study, after adjustment for possible confounding factors, the rates of acute kidney injury or failure were similar between the ERP and traditional care groups. Our rates of acute kidney failure were lower than the rates reported in the studies discussed above

Table 3 Adjusted associations between ERP and postoperative creatinine differences

Co-variables	Estimated Δ Creatinine	Lower 95% confidence interval	Upper 95% confidence interval	p value
ERP vs. control	0.035	− 0.024	0.093	0.251
Increasing age	0.004	0.002	0.005	< 0.001
Female vs. male	− 0.282	− 0.334	− 0.231	< 0.001
Black vs. white	0.089	0.027	0.151	0.005
ASA 2 vs. ≤ 1	− 0.084	− 0.239	0.072	0.293
ASA ≥ 3 vs. ≤ 1	− 0.012	− 0.167	0.143	0.878
IBD vs. benign	0.031	− 0.065	0.127	0.529
Neoplastic vs. benign	− 0.009	− 0.073	0.055	0.784
Proctectomy vs. colectomy	0.031	− 0.032	0.094	0.333
Open vs. laparoscopic approach	0.102	0.047	0.156	< 0.001

(0.9% vs. 2–4%). This may be due to differences in definitions of acute renal failure, as well as the effect of the small sample sizes in the earlier studies. We utilized the RIFLE criteria to help define postoperative renal function. The RIFLE criteria were initially proposed as a standardized definition of kidney dysfunction to permit for better comparison of studies: these criteria have been validated as having clinical and prognostic significance (Lopes & Jorge, 2013). Basing our creatinine change cutoffs on this validated classification system improves the objectivity of our end-points, as well as the generalizability and clinical significance of our results.

Limitations of our investigation include those that are common to retrospective studies, such as the potential for selection bias. After 2010, all patients undergoing elective colorectal surgery at Duke University Hospital were treated in accordance with the hospital's enhanced recovery pathway and included in a prospectively maintained database. To improve similarity between the datasets, patients in the pre-ERP cohort who underwent multiple intra-abdominal procedures and emergency colorectal surgeries were excluded. The baseline characteristics of the patients in the control and ERP cohorts were comparable, and we performed multivariable adjustment to account for possible confounders.

An important limitation specific to this study is that the control and ERP groups are separated by time. As a result, there are several institutional variables that were not controlled in our analysis, such as changes in equipment, perioperative staff, and trainees involved in cases. There was only one lead surgeon who oversaw cases in both groups, and lead surgeon was not one of the factors included in our multivariable analysis. As a single institution study, this analysis benefited from greater standardization in fluid handling and perioperative patient care protocols, but our results may have less generalizability.

Hydroxyethyl starch (HES) was used during procedures in both groups. HES exposure was not included in the multivariable adjustment. More colloid was used intraoperatively in the ERP cohort, and all ERP patients received at least 250 mL of HES on incision as part of the goal-directed fluid therapy protocol. The maximum dose of HES in the ERP protocol was 50 mL/kg. As usage of synthetic colloid solutions has been linked to increased incidences of renal failure, it is possible that the protocolized usage of HES affected the observed incidence of renal complications in the ERP cohort (Brunkhorst et al., 2008; Schortgen et al., 2001).

In our analysis, the extent of surgery (e.g., partial colectomy vs. total abdominal colectomy) tended to be greater and the ASA scores tended to be higher in the ERP cohort, so remaining dissimilarities between the pre-ERP and ERP datasets would likely overestimate the ERP's impact on postoperative kidney injury. Additionally, it is possible that the enhanced recovery cohort captured incidences of renal dysfunction more stringently, as the introduction of this protocol also included resident education to order labs more judiciously, so that patients who appeared to be doing well clinically would be less likely to have had their serum creatinine tracked. Urine output was not as rigorously tracked for patients following ERP, so the urine output criteria for RIFLE classification were not used. The classification of surgical extent and approach was based on CPT codes, which may not accurately reflect the intraoperative techniques and decision-making.

In conclusion, this study evaluated patients undergoing colorectal surgery to assess the potential deleterious effect of enhanced recovery protocol on renal function. By tracking subclinical changes in creatinine, controlling for potential confounders in a diverse population, and employing large patient cohorts to better detect small differences in rates of perioperative AKI, our review rigorously demonstrates that the historical presumptions about the risk of kidney failure with enhanced recovery schemes in colorectal surgery are unfounded in patients without preexisting kidney disease. Given the increasing application of enhanced recovery principles to other surgical specialties, our findings also provide valuable information with regard to the safety of ERPs.

Conclusions

This study is the first and largest examining the adjusted effect of enhanced recovery principles and intentional fluid management versus traditional care on changes in postoperative creatinine and the incidence of postoperative AKI in colorectal surgery. While clinically insignificant changes in creatinine were observed in unadjusted analysis, the application of enhanced recovery protocols in our colorectal surgery population was not significantly associated with changes in creatinine after adjusting for patient and procedure characteristics. Using outcomes stratified with creatinine cutoffs from the RIFLE criteria, we showed no difference in rates of acute kidney injury or failure between traditional and enhanced recovery perioperative management. As such, intentional fluid management strategies, as part of an enhanced recovery protocol, do not appear to increase the risk of postoperative acute kidney dysfunction.

Abbreviations
AKI: Acute kidney injury; ASA: American Society of Anesthesiologists; ERP: Enhanced recovery protocol; HES: Hydroxyethyl starch; IBD: Inflammatory bowel disease; RIFLE: Risk, Injury, Failure, Loss, and End-stage renal disease

Acknowledgements
Not applicable.

Funding
There were no sources of funding for the preparation of this study.

Authors' contributions

CRH participated in the study design, extracted information from electronic medical records for inclusion in the datasets, prepared the datasets for statistical analysis and was the main contributor in writing the manuscript. MAA collected and managed the data for the ERP, participated in the study design, assisted in the statistical analysis, and participated in manuscript editing. ZS participated in the study design, was the main contributor to the statistical analysis of the datasets, and was involved in manuscript editing. JKT participated in the study design, data collection, and manuscript editing. REM oversaw the collection of data for the pre-ERP dataset and participated in manuscript editing. TEM and SAG participated in the study design and manuscript editing. SAG is the corresponding author for this study. All authors read and approved the final manuscript.

Competing interests

The authors declare that they have no competing interests.

Author details

[1]Department of Anesthesiology, Duke University, DUMC 3094, Durham, NC 27710, USA. [2]Department of Surgery, Duke University, Durham, USA.

References

Aarts M-A, Okrainec A, Glicksman A, Pearsall E, Charles Victor J, McLeod RS. Adoption of enhanced recovery after surgery (ERAS) strategies for colorectal surgery at academic teaching hospitals and impact on total length of hospital stay. Surg Endosc. 2012;26(2):442–50.

Adam MA, Lee LM, Kim J, Shenoi M, Mallipeddi M, Aziz H, et al. Alvimopan provides additional improvement in outcomes and cost savings in enhanced recovery colorectal surgery. Ann Surg. 2015 Oct 22; [Epub ahead of print]. Accessed on 16 Mar 2016. Available at: http://journals.lww.com/annalsofsurgery/Citation/2016/07000/Alvimopan_Provides_Additional_Improvement_in.23.aspx

Bakker N, Cakir H, Doodeman HJ, Houdijk APJ. Eight years of experience with enhanced recovery after surgery in patients with colon cancer: impact of measures to improve adherence. Surgery. 2015;157(6):1130–6.

Bellomo R, Ronco C, Kellum JA, Mehta RL, Palevsky P. Acute renal failure—definition, outcome measures, animal models, fluid therapy and information technology needs: the second international consensus conference of the Acute Dialysis Quality Initiative (ADQI) group. Crit Care. 2004;8(4):R204–12.

Brunkhorst FM, Engel C, Bloos F, Meier-Hellmann A, Ragaller M, Weiler N, Moerer O, Gruendling M, Oppert M, Grond S, et al. Intensive insulin therapy and pentastarch resuscitation in severe sepsis. NEJM. 2008;358:125–39.

Clemente A, Carli F. The physiological effects of thoracic epidural anesthesia and analgesia on the cardiovascular, respiratory and gastrointestinal systems. Minerva Anestesiol. 2008;74(10):549–63.

Dhruva Rao PK, Howells S, Haray PN. Does an enhanced recovery programme add value to laparoscopic colorectal resections? Int J Color Dis. 2015;30(11):1473–7.

ERAS Compliance Group. The impact of enhanced recovery protocol compliance on elective colorectal cancer resection: results from an international registry. Ann Surg. 2015;261(6):1153–9.

Fearon KCH, Ljungqvist O, Von Meyenfeldt M, Revhaug A, Dejong CHC, Lassen K, et al. Enhanced recovery after surgery: a consensus review of clinical care for patients undergoing colonic resection. Clin Nutr. 2005;24(3):466–77.

Gillissen F, Hoff C, Maessen JMC, Winkens B, Teeuwen JHFA, von Meyenfeldt MF, et al. Structured synchronous implementation of an enhanced recovery program in elective colonic surgery in 33 hospitals in the Netherlands. World J Surg. 2013;37(5):1082–93.

Gravante G, Elmussareh M. Enhanced recovery for colorectal surgery: practical hints, results and future challenges. World J Gastrointest Surg. 2012;4(8):190–8.

Greco M, Capretti G, Beretta L, Gemma M, Pecorelli N, Braga M. Enhanced recovery program in colorectal surgery: a meta-analysis of randomized controlled trials. World J Surg. 2014;38(6):1531–41.

Gupta R, Gan TJ. Peri-operative fluid management to enhance recovery. Anaesthesia. 2016;71(Suppl 1):40–5.

Gustafsson UO, Hausel J, Thorell A, Ljungqvist O, Soop M, Nygren J, et al. Adherence to the enhanced recovery after surgery protocol and outcomes after colorectal cancer surgery. Arch Surg. 2011;146(5):571–7.

Hübner M, Lovely JK, Huebner M, Slettedahl SW, Jacob AK, Larson DW. Intrathecal analgesia and restrictive perioperative fluid management within enhanced recovery pathway: hemodynamic implications. J Am Coll Surg. 2013;216(6):1124–34.

Huebner M, Hübner M, Cima RR, Larson DW. Timing of complications and length of stay after rectal cancer surgery. J Am Coll Surg. 2014;218(5):914–9.

Ihedioha U, Esmail F, Lloyd G, Miller A, Singh B, Chaudhri S. Enhanced recovery programmes in colorectal surgery are less enhanced later in the week: an observational study. JRSM Open. 2015;6(2):2054270414562983.

Lopes JA, Jorge S. The RIFLE and AKIN classifications for acute kidney injury: a critical and comprehensive review. Clin Kidney J. 2013;6(1):8–14.

Lv L, Shao Y, Zhou Y. The enhanced recovery after surgery (ERAS) pathway for patients undergoing colorectal surgery: an update of meta-analysis of randomized controlled trials. Int J Color Dis. 2012;27(12):1549–54.

Lyon A, Payne CJ, MacKay GJ. Enhanced recovery programme in colorectal surgery: does one size fit all? World J Gastroenterol. 2012;18(40):5661–3.

Marret E, Remy C, Bonnet F. Postoperative pain forum group. Meta-analysis of epidural analgesia versus parenteral opioid analgesia after colorectal surgery. Br J Surg. 2007;94(6):665–73.

Masoomi H, Carmichael JC, Dolich M, Mills S, Ketana N, Pigazzi A, Stamos MJ. Predictive factors of acute renal failure in colon and rectal surgery. Am Surg. 2012;78(10):1019–23.

Miller TE, Roche AM, Mythen M. Fluid management and goal-directed therapy as an adjunct to Enhanced Recovery After Surgery (ERAS). Can J Anaesth. 2015;62(2):158–68.

Miller TE, Thacker JK, White WD, Mantyh C, Migaly J, Jin J, et al. Reduced length of hospital stay in colorectal surgery after implementation of an enhanced recovery protocol. Anesth Analg. 2014;118(5):1052–61.

Rawlinson A, Kang P, Evans J, Khanna A. A systematic review of enhanced recovery protocols in colorectal surgery. Ann R Coll Surg Engl. 2011;93(8):583–8.

Ren L, Zhu D, Wei Y, Pan X, Liang L, Xu J, et al. Enhanced Recovery After Surgery (ERAS) program attenuates stress and accelerates recovery in patients after radical resection for colorectal cancer: a prospective randomized controlled trial. World J Surg. 2012;36(2):407–14.

Schortgen F, Lacherade JC, Bruneel F, Cattaneo I, Hemery F, Lemaire F, Brochard L. Effects of hydroxyethylstarch and gelatin on renal function in severe sepsis: a multicentre randomised study. Lancet. 2001;357:911–6.

Shida D, Tagawa K, Inada K, Nasu K, Seyama Y, Maeshiro T, et al. Enhanced recovery after surgery (ERAS) protocols for colorectal cancer in Japan. BMC Surg. 2015;15(1):1–6.

Spanjersberg WR, van Sambeeck JDP, Bremers A, Rosman C, van Laarhoven CJHM. Systematic review and meta-analysis for laparoscopic versus open colon surgery with or without an ERAS programme. Surg Endosc. 2015;29(12):3443–53.

Steinbrook RA. Epidural anesthesia and gastrointestinal motility. Anesth Analg. 1998;86(4):837–44.

Varadhan KK, Neal KR, Dejong CHC, Fearon KCH, Ljungqvist O, Lobo DN. The enhanced recovery after surgery (ERAS) pathway for patients undergoing major elective open colorectal surgery: a meta-analysis of randomized controlled trials. Clin Nutr. 2010;29(4):434–40.

Zhuang C-L, Ye X-Z, Zhang X-D, Chen B-C, Yu Z. Enhanced recovery after surgery programs versus traditional care for colorectal surgery. Dis Colon rectum. 2013;56(5):667–78.

10

Fluid resuscitation practices in cardiac surgery patients in the USA: a survey of health care providers

Solomon Aronson[1*], Paul Nisbet[2] and Martin Bunke[3]

Abstract

Background: Fluid resuscitation during cardiac surgery is common with significant variability in clinical practice. Our goal was to investigate current practice patterns of fluid volume expansion in patients undergoing cardiac surgeries in the USA.

Methods: We conducted a cross-sectional online survey of 124 cardiothoracic surgeons, cardiovascular anesthesiologists, and perfusionists. Survey questions were designed to assess clinical decision-making patterns of intravenous (IV) fluid utilization in cardiovascular surgery for five types of patients who need volume expansion: (1) patients undergoing cardiopulmonary bypass (CPB) without bleeding, (2) patients undergoing CPB with bleeding, (3) patients undergoing acute normovolemic hemodilution (ANH), (4) patients requiring extracorporeal membrane oxygenation (ECMO) or use of a ventricular assist device (VAD), and (5) patients undergoing either off-pump coronary artery bypass graft (OPCABG) surgery or transcatheter aortic valve replacement (TAVR). First-choice fluid used in fluid boluses for these five patient types was requested. Descriptive statistics were performed using Kruskal-Wallis test and follow-up tests, including *t* tests, to evaluate differences among respondent groups.

Results: The most commonly preferred indicators of volume status were blood pressure, urine output, cardiac output, central venous pressure, and heart rate. The first choice of fluid for patients needing volume expansion during CPB without bleeding was crystalloids, whereas 5% albumin was the most preferred first choice of fluid for bleeding patients. For volume expansion during ECMO or VAD, the respondents were equally likely to prefer 5% albumin or crystalloids as a first choice of IV fluid, with 5% albumin being the most frequently used adjunct fluid to crystalloids. Surgeons, as a group, more often chose starches as an adjunct fluid to crystalloids for patients needing volume expansion during CPB without bleeding. Surgeons were also more likely to use 25% albumin as an adjunct fluid than were anesthesiologists. While most perfusionists reported using crystalloids to prime the CPB circuit, one third preferred a mixture of 25% albumin and crystalloids. Less interstitial edema and more sustained volume expansion were considered the most important colloid traits in volume expansion.

Conclusions: Fluid utilization practice patterns in the USA varied depending on patient characteristics and clinical specialties of health care professionals.

Keywords: Fluid resuscitation, Colloids, Crystalloids, Albumin, Cardiovascular surgery, Intraoperative volume expansion, Cardiopulmonary bypass, Survey

* Correspondence: arons002@mc.duke.edu
[1]Department of Anesthesiology, Duke University, 201 Trent Drive, 101 Baker House, Durham, NC 27710, USA
Full list of author information is available at the end of the article

Background

Cardiac surgeries are commonly performed procedures that almost universally require fluid resuscitation during the intraoperative and perioperative period (Lange et al. 2011; Hirleman and Larson 2008; Verheij et al. 2006). The effects of fluid type, fluid amount, timing of fluid administration, and techniques for determining fluid responsiveness are actively debated topics (Lange et al. 2011; Cherpanath et al. 2014; van Haren and Zacharowski 2014). Specific disease and/or conditions of surgery involving cardiopulmonary bypass (CPB) and related patient pathophysiology have become increasingly recognized as key determinants for successful fluid resuscitation. For example, the balance between the hydrostatic pressure gradient which pushes water outward into the interstitial space and the colloid oncotic pressure (COP) which pulls water inward into the vessel (classic Starling's Principle believed to govern fluid movement across the capillary wall) does not fully apply to conditions involving systemic inflammation and vascular barrier damage (Aditianingsih and George 2014; Jacob and Chappell 2013). Moreover, the endothelial glycocalyx layer (EGL), which comprises membrane-bound glycoproteins and proteoglycans with side chains of heparan sulfate, chondroitin, and dermatan sulfate, is recognized as an important factor in vascular barrier function (Jacob and Chappell 2013; Weinbaum et al. 2007; Becker et al. 2010; Myburgh and Mythen 2013). Whereas large molecules (e.g., albumin in colloid solutions) are retained inside the vessel, generating COP in the intravascular compartment (Aditianingsih and George 2014; Jacob and Chappell 2013; Myburgh and Mythen 2013); small molecules (e.g., electrolytes in crystalloid solutions) can travel freely through the vessel wall and thus can draw water into the interstitial space. Cardiopulmonary bypass can produce changes in fluid physiology and fluid responsiveness in patients (Lange et al. 2011; Hirleman and Larson 2008; Verheij et al. 2006), characterized by increased interstitial fluid as a consequence of decreased COP, damaged EGL, and inflammatory changes (Lange et al. 2011; Hirleman and Larson 2008; Jacob and Chappell 2013; Hoeft et al. 1991; Ortega-Loubon et al. 2015). This shift of fluid from the intravascular space to the interstitial space, in addition to blood and fluid losses during the surgical procedure, can result in an intravascular hypovolemia that requires fluid resuscitation.

A survey of current fluid usage by health care professionals (HCPs) involved in cardiovascular surgeries in the USA was developed to (a) examine the use of different fluid types for resuscitation (i.e., crystalloids, plasma-derived colloid [albumin], synthetic colloids [hydroxyethyl starches, HES]) in patients undergoing cardiovascular surgery, (b) determine whether certain patient characteristics and/or practice settings influence the type of fluid utilized for resuscitation, (c) determine whether the fluid selected for resuscitation varies by clinical specialties of the treating HCPs, and (d) determine the fluids used to prime the CPB circuit in patients undergoing on-pump procedures.

Methods
Study design

This study was cross-sectional and collected survey data from 124 cardiothoracic surgeons, cardiovascular anesthesiologists, and perfusionists to investigate the patterns of fluid utilization in cardiovascular surgery. The online survey was conducted November 4 through 17, 2015, with an average survey completion time of 9 min. The 38-item self-administered questionnaire (Additional file 1) obtained information on fluids used for hemodynamic management in the operating room and in the first 24-h postoperative period, as well as on volume status indicators most often used to determine volume expansion needs. Survey participants were presented with five different hypothetical patient scenarios encountered frequently in cardiovascular surgery and asked to identify their first choice of fluid for volume expansion for each patient type from a list of colloid and crystalloid fluids. The five patient scenarios were:

(1) Volume expansion during CPB when not experiencing significant blood loss
(2) Volume expansion in the presence of blood loss during CPB when blood transfusion is not indicated (adequate hemoglobin [Hb])
(3) Volume maintenance during acute normovolemic hemodilution (ANH, autologous blood collection)
(4) Volume expansion while patients were supported with extracorporeal membrane oxygenation (ECMO) or a ventricular assist device (VAD)
(5) Intraoperative volume expansion for off-pump coronary artery bypass graft (OPCABG) surgery or transcatheter aortic valve replacement (TAVR)

The six types of fluids were crystalloids, 5% albumin, 25% albumin, first-generation HES or HES 450/600 (e.g., 6% HES 450/0.70 and 6% HES 600/0.75), third-generation HES or HES 130 (e.g., 6% HES 130/0.4), and blood-derived blood products other than albumin. The participants rated the frequency with which they used various fluid types for volume expansion using a 5-point scale (from 1 for "always" to 5 for "never"). Participants were also asked to indicate the bolus volumes (mL) of the crystalloids and of colloids that they typically use for volume expansion. Participants rated the importance of certain colloid characteristics (e.g., more sustained volume expansion, faster volume expansion) and non-oncotic properties of albumin (e.g., transport of metabolites, free radical scavenging) on the patient treatment decision-making process using a 5-point scale (from 1 for "not important" to 5 for "absolutely essential"). Four of the 38 questions addressed pump priming preferences for CPB circuits and were asked of perfusionists only.

Participants

A total of 124 participants were recruited from the e-Rewards Medical panel. e-Rewards Medical is a leading provider of market research services to the professional health care community. The panel consists of HCPs who have opted to become members of the panel and were paid for their time. Email invitations for participation in this study were sent from e-Rewards to the non-probability sample of its panelists, meaning this sample set was not a random selection of all physicians. Of note, the panelists remained anonymous to the investigators in this study. The email invitation provided a general description of the survey topic (i.e., "Fluid and Hemodynamic Management") and a link by which to access the online survey. Each invitation contained a unique identifier that prevented any one respondent from taking the survey more than once. To qualify for participation, respondents had to specialize in cardiac surgery, adult cardiovascular anesthesiology, or be a perfusionist; had been in practice for at least 2 years since residency or training in the USA but not in the states of Minnesota, Vermont, West Virginia, Massachusetts, nor the District of Columbia as these states prohibit or limit compensation to physicians; and had performed or were involved in at least four cardiac bypass surgeries per month. Anesthesiologists who specialized in pediatrics were excluded because fluid management for pediatrics is different than for adults due to vast differences in the pathophysiology of their circulatory system. To ensure a minimum number of completed surveys were received from each group, subquotas were set for each clinical specialty: 50 surgeons, 50 anesthesiologists, and 50 perfusionists.

This research project involved obtaining the opinions of physicians and perfusionists about their choices for the use of various fluids for volume expansion in five different hypothetical patient situations. No patient data were obtained, and no questions were asked of the participants that would help in identifying them. All participant data were de-identified. Hence, this study was exempt from requiring institutional review board approval under United States Code of Federal Regulations Title 45 Part 46.101(b)(2) by Copernicus Group Independent Review Board (CGIRB). The study did receive a formal Letter of Exemption from the CGIRB.

Statistical analyses

Most questions were based on 5-point scales and provided ordinal data which, by definition, are not normally distributed. As such, descriptive statistics were performed using a Kruskal-Wallis test to evaluate differences among the respondent groups on the ordinal measures. Follow-up tests were conducted to evaluate differences within and between patient scenarios. T tests were used to evaluate differences across ratio variables (i.e., bolus volume). Statistical significance was assessed at the alpha level of less than 0.05. Descriptive analyses were performed using SPSS (Version 23.0).

Results

Participant characteristics

Of the 124 HCPs who completed the survey, 52 (41.9%) were anesthesiologists, 47 (37.9%) were surgeons, and 25 (20.2%) were perfusionists (Table 1). The primary practice setting for most HCPs was a non-university hospital (73.4%) followed by university hospital (26.6%). The average number of bypass surgeries that the HCPs participated in per month was 28.6 for surgeons, 24.7 for anesthesiologists, and 21.4 for perfusionists.

Survey data

The five most commonly used indicators of volume status were blood pressure (77%), urine output (76%), cardiac output (74%), central venous pressure (73%), and heart rate (61%) (Fig. 1). Pulmonary capillary wedge pressure was used by 53% of HCPs as indicators of volume status, and transesophageal echocardiography was used by 52%. A statistically significant difference for volume indicator use was found between surgeons and anesthesiologists for transesophageal echocardiography (26 vs 79%, respectively, $P < .001$), pulse pressure variation (26 vs 56%, respectively, $P = .002$), and stroke volume variation (15 vs 44%, respectively, $P = .001$).

The first choice of intravenous (IV) fluid for a patient needing volume expansion during CPB when not experiencing significant blood loss (scenario 1) was crystalloids, followed by 5% albumin and 25% albumin, respectively (Fig. 2). In this patient scenario, crystalloids were used more frequently as the fluid of first choice by anesthesiologists (58%) compared to surgeons (38%, $P = 0.054$). Higher percentages of surgeons than anesthesiologists chose HES and blood-derived products other than albumin, while no perfusionists chose any of those fluid types. The most frequently used adjunct fluid to crystalloids was 5% albumin (Additional file 2: Figure S1).

For patients needing volume expansion in the presence of blood loss during CPB when blood transfusion is not indicated (adequate Hb, scenario 2), HCPs chose 5% albumin most frequently as the first choice of IV fluid

Table 1 Characteristics of survey respondents ($n = 124$)

	Anesthesiologists[A]	Surgeons[S]	Perfusionists[a]
	($n = 52$)	($n = 47$)	($n = 25$)
No. of cardiac bypass per month, mean (STD)	24.7 (21.1)	28.6 (20.2)	21.0 (13.5)
Median	17.5	25.0	20.0
(Range)	(4–100)	(8–100)	(7–60)
Primary practice setting			
Non-university hospital, %	78.8%	68.1%	72.0%
University hospital, %	21.2%	31.9%	28.0%
No. of beds in primary hospital, mean (STD)	476 (234.0)	486 (215.3)	513 (362.1)
Median	400	450	425
(Range)	(99–1500)	(150–1000)	(200–2000)
Years since residency/training, mean (STD)	14.3 (7.5)	20.6[A] (10.7)	22.1 (7.8)
Median	13.5	20.0	24.0
(Range)	(3–37)	(3–50)	(10–37)

Superscripts A and S denote differences between anesthesiologists and surgeons that are statistically significant at $P < .05$
[a]Statistical tests were not performed on data for perfusionists due to small sample size

(Fig. 3). Crystalloid was the second most frequently chosen fluid, followed by 25% albumin. Surgeons chose 25% albumin significantly more often than anesthesiologists (19 vs 2%, respectively, $P < .05$), while no HCP chose HES 130. When the first fluid choice was 5% albumin, the most frequently chosen adjunct fluid was crystalloids (Additional file 3: Figure S2).

Similar to scenario 1, the first choice of IV fluid for volume maintenance during ANH (scenario 3) was crystalloids, followed by 5% albumin and then 25% albumin (Fig. 4). Anesthesiologists chose crystalloids significantly more often than surgeons did (81 vs 36%, respectively, $P < .05$) for volume maintenance during ANH. Again, 5% albumin was the most frequently used adjunct fluid to crystalloids (Additional file 4: Figure S3).

For volume expansion, while patients were supported by ECMO or a VAD (scenario 4), HCPs preferred 5% albumin and crystalloids equally as the first choice of IV fluid (Fig. 5). While anesthesiologists seemed to prefer 5% albumin more often than surgeons (35 vs 17%, respectively, $P < .05$), more surgeons preferred 25% albumin than anesthesiologists (21 vs 4%, respectively, $P < .05$). Only surgeons utilized HES fluids for this scenario. When the first fluid choice was 5% albumin, crystalloid was the most frequently chosen adjunct fluid (Additional file 5: Figure S4A), and 5% albumin was the most frequently chosen adjunct fluid

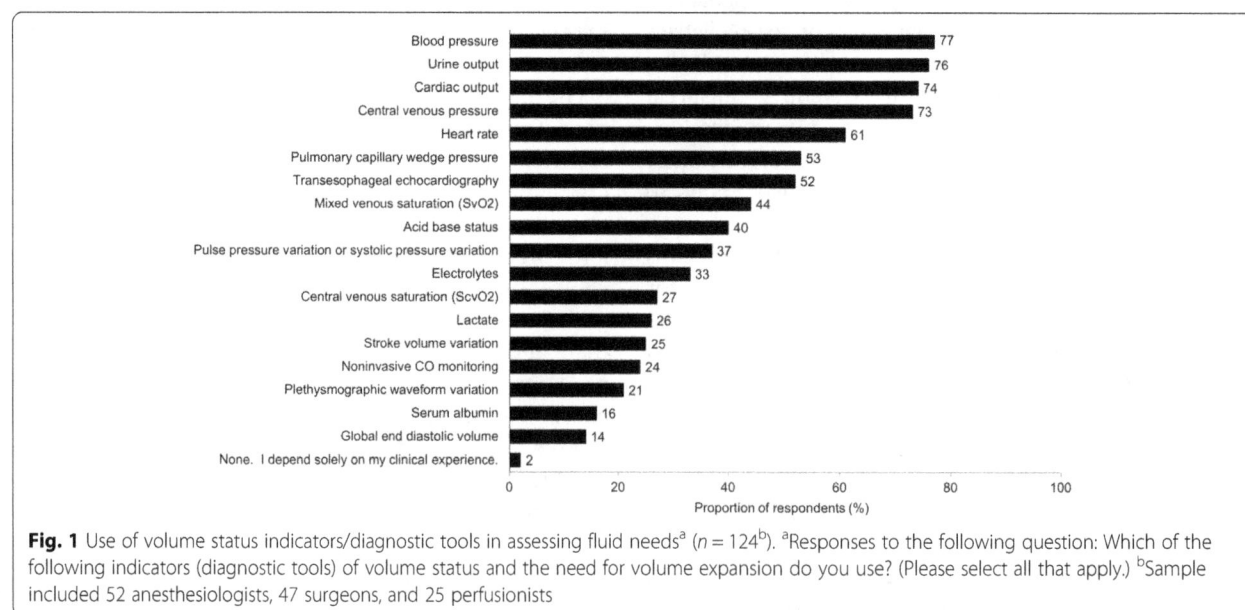

Fig. 1 Use of volume status indicators/diagnostic tools in assessing fluid needs[a] ($n = 124$[b]). [a]Responses to the following question: Which of the following indicators (diagnostic tools) of volume status and the need for volume expansion do you use? (Please select all that apply.) [b]Sample included 52 anesthesiologists, 47 surgeons, and 25 perfusionists

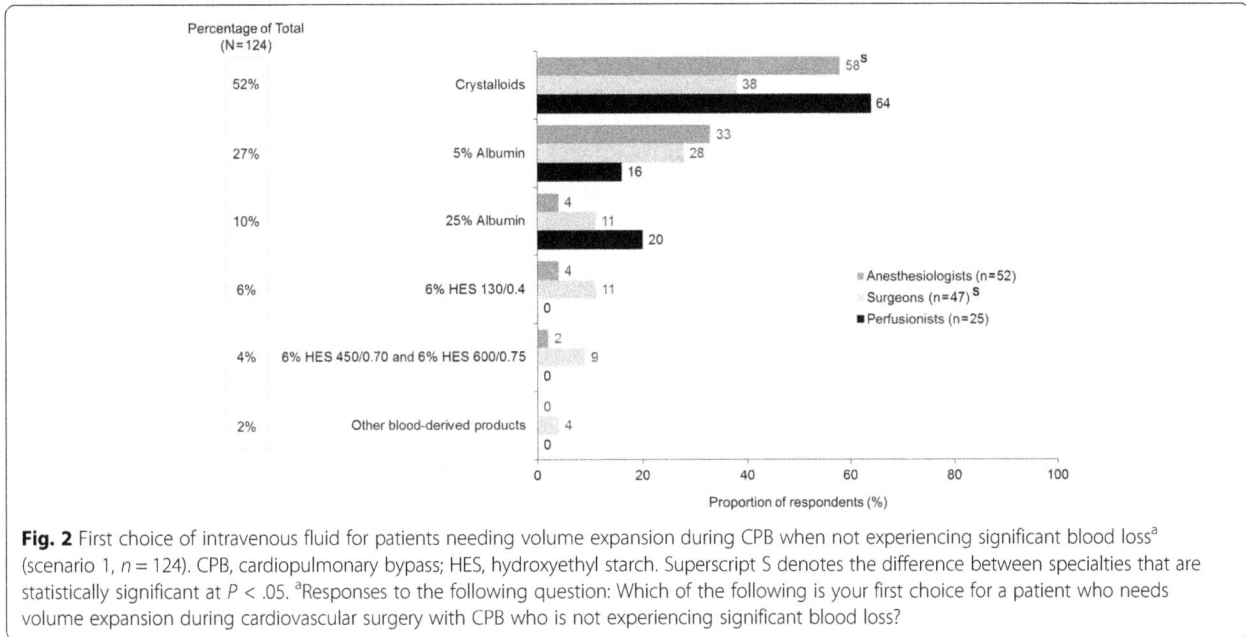

Fig. 2 First choice of intravenous fluid for patients needing volume expansion during CPB when not experiencing significant blood loss[a] (scenario 1, n = 124). CPB, cardiopulmonary bypass; HES, hydroxyethyl starch. Superscript S denotes the difference between specialties that are statistically significant at $P < .05$. [a]Responses to the following question: Which of the following is your first choice for a patient who needs volume expansion during cardiovascular surgery with CPB who is not experiencing significant blood loss?

when crystalloid was the first fluid choice (Additional file 5: Figure S4B). It is worth noting that 18% of the clinical practices in this survey did not utilize ECMO or VADs (Fig. 5).

As was seen in scenarios 1 and 3, a similar trend was observed for intraoperative volume expansion during OPCABG or TAVR (scenario 5). Crystalloid fluid was the most preferred first choice of IV fluid, followed by 5% albumin and then 25% albumin (Fig. 6), and 5% albumin was the adjunct fluid of choice when the first fluid choice was crystalloids (Additional file 6: Figure S5).

The most important colloid traits that influenced the decision to use colloids for volume expansion seemed to be "less interstitial edema" and "more sustained volume expansion" (Fig. 7). Most perfusionists (60%) preferred crystalloids as the priming solution for the CPB circuit, and approximately one third chose a mixture of 25% albumin and crystalloids (Fig. 8). One in five perfusionists have never used albumin to prime the CPB. The average volume of priming solution used by perfusionists was 1085 mL (median 1000 mL; range 500–2000 mL). In general, physicians reported the

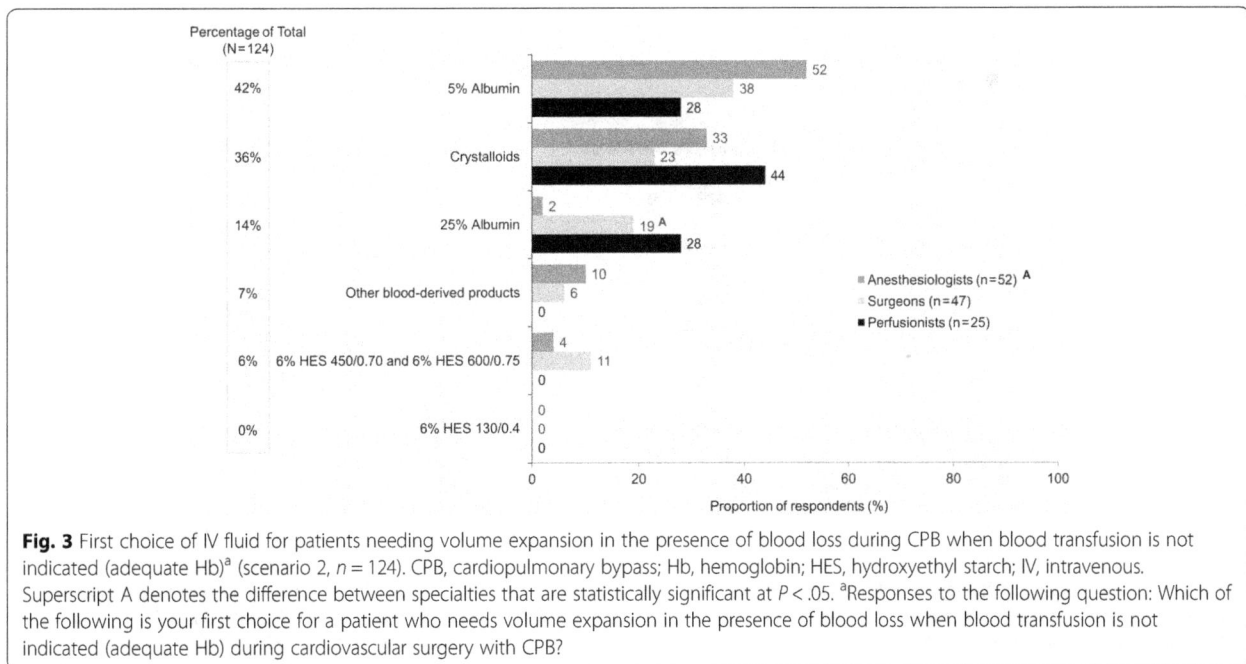

Fig. 3 First choice of IV fluid for patients needing volume expansion in the presence of blood loss during CPB when blood transfusion is not indicated (adequate Hb)[a] (scenario 2, n = 124). CPB, cardiopulmonary bypass; Hb, hemoglobin; HES, hydroxyethyl starch; IV, intravenous. Superscript A denotes the difference between specialties that are statistically significant at $P < .05$. [a]Responses to the following question: Which of the following is your first choice for a patient who needs volume expansion in the presence of blood loss when blood transfusion is not indicated (adequate Hb) during cardiovascular surgery with CPB?

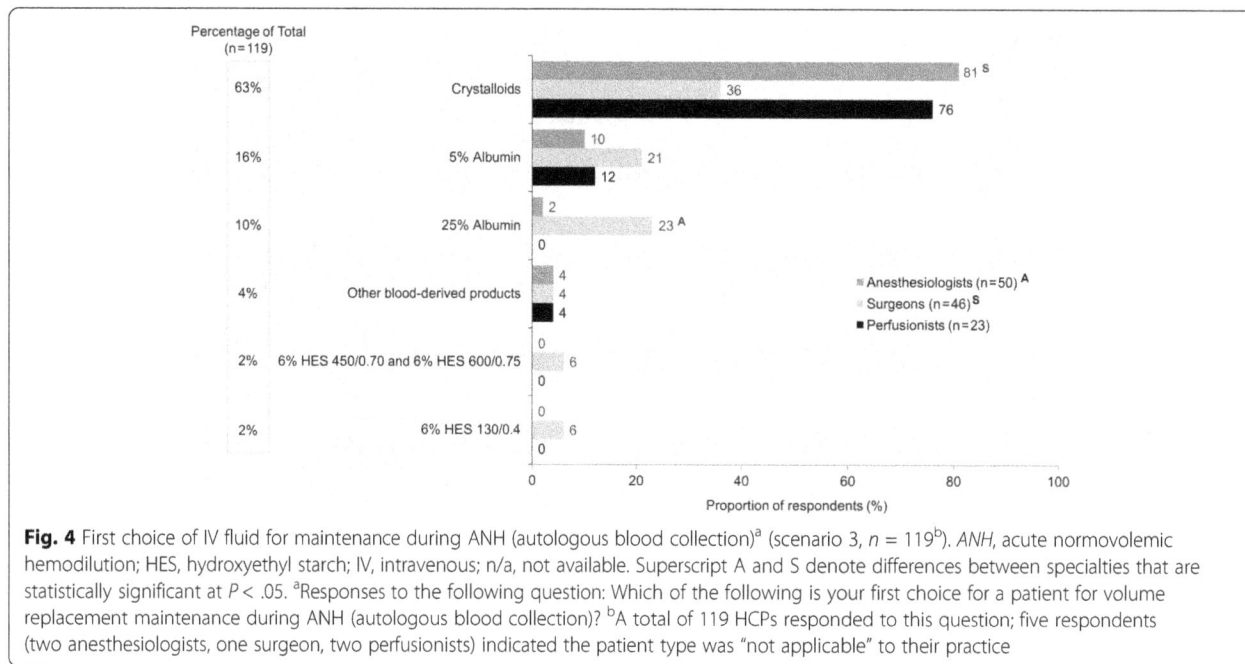

Fig. 4 First choice of IV fluid for maintenance during ANH (autologous blood collection)[a] (scenario 3, n = 119[b]). *ANH*, acute normovolemic hemodilution; *HES*, hydroxyethyl starch; *IV*, intravenous; *n/a*, not available. Superscript A and S denote differences between specialties that are statistically significant at *P* < .05. [a]Responses to the following question: Which of the following is your first choice for a patient for volume replacement maintenance during ANH (autologous blood collection)? [b]A total of 119 HCPs responded to this question; five respondents (two anesthesiologists, one surgeon, two perfusionists) indicated the patient type was "not applicable" to their practice

typical volume of colloid bolus as smaller (413–514 mL) than the volume of crystalloid bolus (620–670 mL). Physicians also reported having a higher level of influence (42–43%) on the decision to use albumin for volume expansion than perfusionists did (20%). The most common reasons given by physicians for not using 5% albumin were that it has a relatively higher cost relative to other fluids and that there is a lack of evidence for greater efficacy with albumin than with crystalloids. Perfusionists frequently mentioned that 5% albumin is often not available in their practices.

Discussion

This cross-sectional study provided insights on the patterns of fluid utilization in cardiovascular surgery from a survey of 52 cardiovascular anesthesiologists, 47 cardiothoracic surgeons, and 25 perfusionists in the USA. This survey examined the fluids chosen for volume resuscitation by these 124 HCPs to treat five different hypothetical patient scenarios. The 25 perfusionists were surveyed to determine the solutions that they utilized to prime the CPB circuit. There were remarkable variability in clinical practice and a lack of consensus

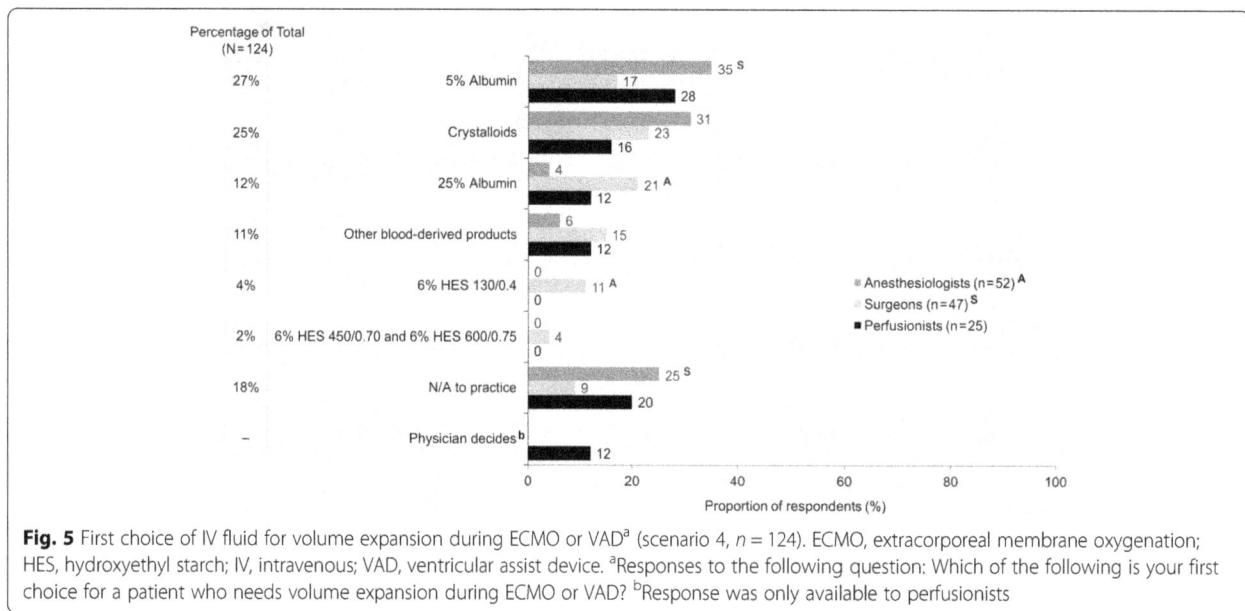

Fig. 5 First choice of IV fluid for volume expansion during ECMO or VAD[a] (scenario 4, n = 124). *ECMO*, extracorporeal membrane oxygenation; *HES*, hydroxyethyl starch; *IV*, intravenous; *VAD*, ventricular assist device. [a]Responses to the following question: Which of the following is your first choice for a patient who needs volume expansion during ECMO or VAD? [b]Response was only available to perfusionists

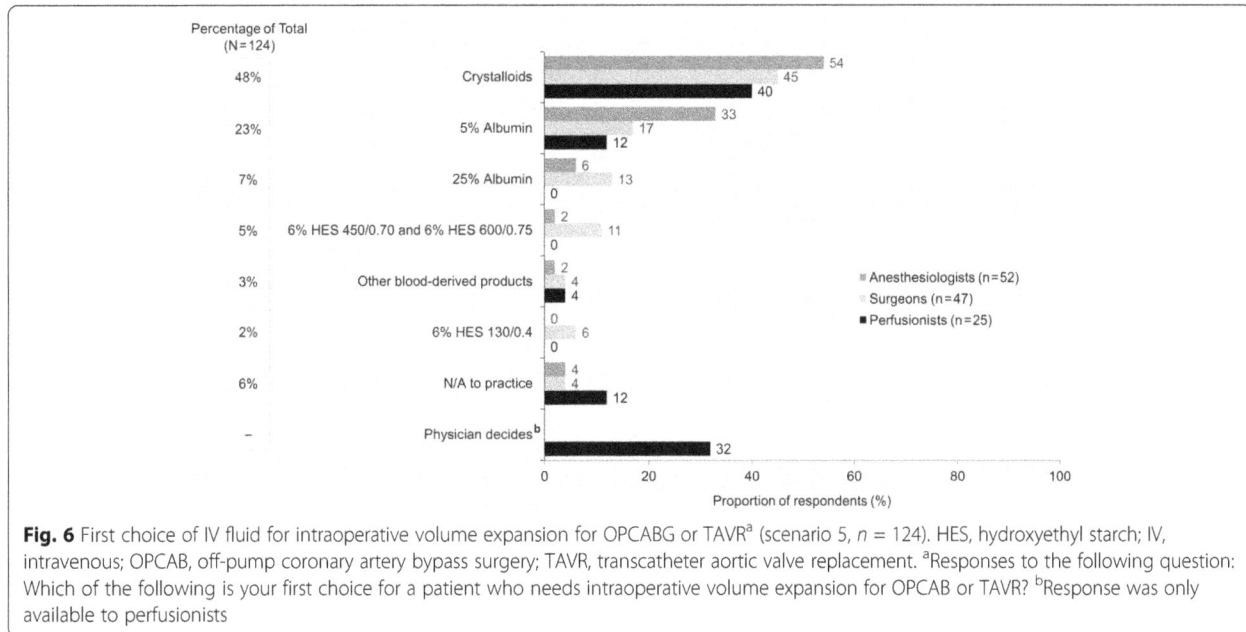

Fig. 6 First choice of IV fluid for intraoperative volume expansion for OPCABG or TAVR[a] (scenario 5, n = 124). HES, hydroxyethyl starch; IV, intravenous; OPCAB, off-pump coronary artery bypass surgery; TAVR, transcatheter aortic valve replacement. [a]Responses to the following question: Which of the following is your first choice for a patient who needs intraoperative volume expansion for OPCAB or TAVR? [b]Response was only available to perfusionists

about the use of various fluid types in cardiovascular surgery patients.

In this survey, the most commonly preferred indicators of volume status were blood pressure, urine output, cardiac output, central venous pressure, and heart rate. Anesthesiologists preferred transesophageal echocardiography, pulse pressure variation, and stroke volume variation as indicators of volume status significantly more frequently than surgeons. Different fluid types were chosen as the first choice of IV fluids depending on

the clinical context of the patients. For example, crystalloid fluid was the predominant first choice for patients needing volume expansion during CPB without bleeding (scenario 1), for fluid maintenance during ANH (scenario 3), and for intraoperative volume expansion during OPCABG or TAVR (scenario 5). On the other hand, 5% albumin was the primary fluid choice for patients needing volume expansion in the presence of blood loss during CPB not requiring transfusion (scenario 2) or during ECMO or VAD (scenario 4).

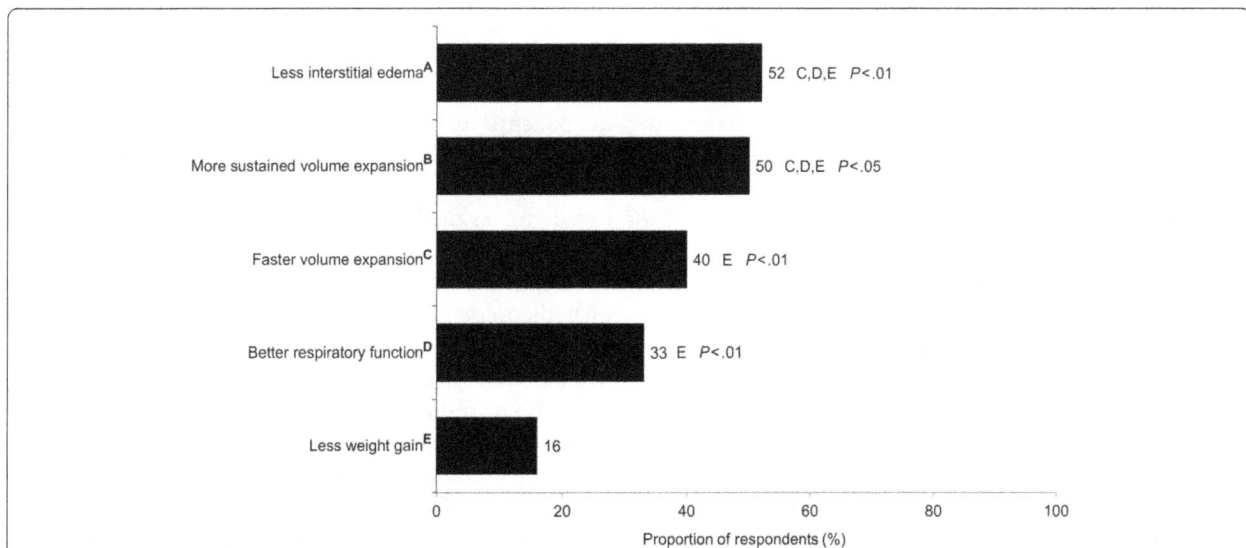

Fig. 7 Importance of colloid traits when colloids were used for volume expansion[a] (n = 124). Superscripts A–E on y-axis labels represent the respective trait for statistical comments. Letters following values represent the traits from which the trait's percentage differs significantly. [a]Responses to the following question: Using the scale below, please indicate how important each of the following is in terms of your reasons for using colloids for volume expansion (5-point scale: not important, somewhat important, important, very important, absolutely essential). Data presented in this graph are the proportions of respondents indicating colloid trait is "very important" or "absolutely essential" when used for volume expansion

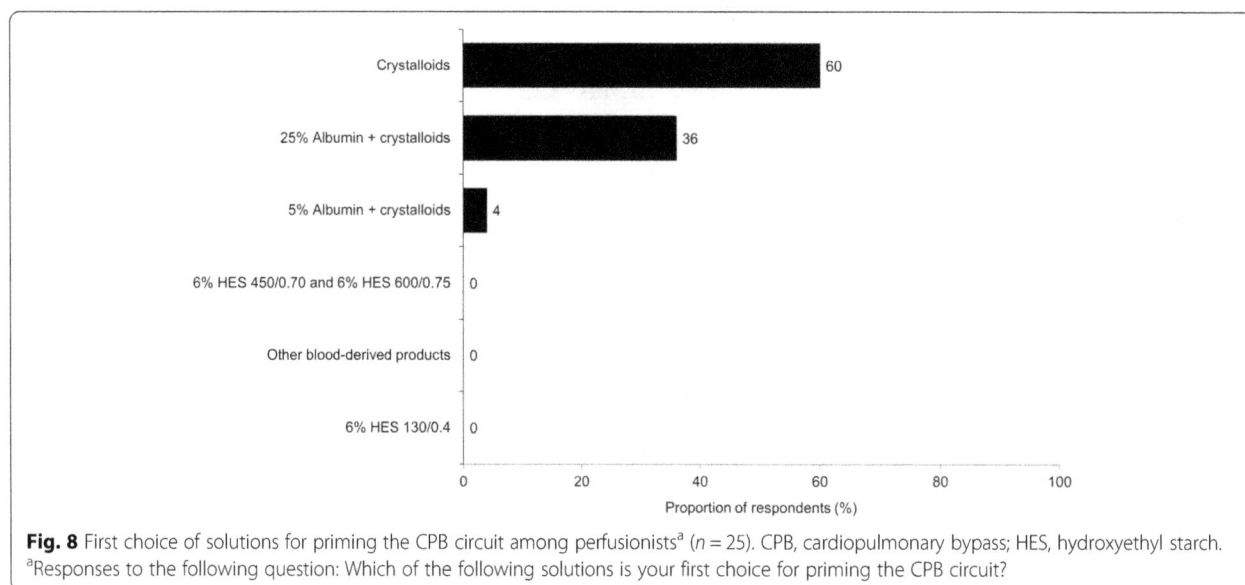

Fig. 8 First choice of solutions for priming the CPB circuit among perfusionists[a] (n = 25). CPB, cardiopulmonary bypass; HES, hydroxyethyl starch. [a]Responses to the following question: Which of the following solutions is your first choice for priming the CPB circuit?

When choosing colloids for volume expansion, HCPs felt that "less interstitial edema" and "more sustained volume expansion" were more important colloid traits than "faster volume expansion," "better respiratory function," and "less weight gain." "Other blood-derived products" were chosen infrequently (less than 10%) as the first choice for fluid resuscitation by both university- and non-university-affiliated physicians; the only situation in which it was chosen by more than 10% of the respondents was for patients on ECMO and VAD.

In addition, there were differences in practice patterns among the clinical specialties of the treating HCPs. Significantly larger numbers of surgeons, relative to anesthesiologists, preferred 25% albumin for patients who need volume expansion in the presence of blood loss (scenario 2), for fluid maintenance during ANH (scenario 3), and for volume expansion during EMCO or VAD (scenario 4). Sixty percent of the perfusionists in this study preferred to use only crystalloids for priming the CPB circuit, while the other 40% used a mixture of albumin and crystalloids. The data from this study demonstrate that volume repletion practices vary dramatically and clinical data do not allow for consensus recommendations. While there are no large, randomized trials available to inform HCPs of definitive protocols for optimal volume resuscitation during cardiovascular surgeries, it is well accepted that fluid overload increases the risk of major complications after CABG (Morin et al. 2011). Whereas several studies (Hoeft et al. 1991; Russell et al. 2004; Sade et al. 1985; Kuitunen et al. 2004) have suggested that the use of colloid fluids in the priming solution during CPB is beneficial for maintaining COP.

Additional data indicate that utilization of colloid fluid results in a larger intravascular volume expansion than an equal volume of crystalloid fluid (Verheij et al. 2006; Finfer et al. 2011; Jacob et al. 2012; Skhirtladze et al. 2014), and the role of the EGL may be important. Studies have suggested that the EGL becomes damaged in numerous systemic inflammatory states (i.e., ischemia-reperfusion injury (Rehm et al. 2007), trauma (Johansson et al. 2011), and sepsis (Steppan et al. 2011; Ait-Oufella et al. 2010)), which may lead to interstitial edema (Aditianingsih and George 2014; Myburgh and Mythen 2013). In such conditions, colloids may behave more like crystalloids when there is significant damage to the EGL, and several large studies (Finfer et al. 2011; Myburgh et al. 2012; Annane et al. 2013; Perner et al. 2012) have failed to show any benefit from colloids in this context. On the other hand, two randomized trials in patients undergoing cardiac surgery support the suggestion that smaller volumes of colloids (HES and albumin) are required for volume resuscitation when compared to crystalloid solutions (Verheij et al. 2006; Skhirtladze et al. 2014). In this context, it has been argued that the addition of colloids to crystalloid mixture may theoretically have benefits over crystalloids alone (Roger et al. 2014). In a retrospective, hospital-discharge database study of 19,578 cardiac surgery patients, albumin administration for volume expansion during CABG appeared to be associated with a 25% reduction in postoperative mortality, relative to other non-protein colloids (Sedrakyan et al. 2003). However, a recent retrospective study of one cardiac surgery program comparing outcomes from 9 months before vs 3 months after its protocol changed to restrict the use of albumin in patients who required more than 3-L crystalloids within the first 24 h, had an albumin concentration < 3.0 g/dL, or had volume overload, found that there was no difference in morbidity or mortality between the two groups (Rabin et al. 2017). Both of these studies have all the shortcomings of being retrospective. Of note, a recent single-center, double-blind, randomized, controlled trial of albumin administration for a serum albumin level of less than 4.0 g/dL prior to OPCABG revealed a significant decrease in stage 1 acute kidney injury in the albumin group (Lee et al. 2016).

A well-designed, prospective, randomized trial would be required to address the question of whether albumin has a benefit on patient outcomes in cardiac surgery.

While this survey cannot elucidate the reasons behind why clinicians preferred a particular fluid type over another, the respondents did refer to "a more sustained volume response" as one of the major reasons for choosing a colloid for volume expansion.

It is noteworthy that more surgeons than anesthesiologists in this survey preferred HES solutions for patients needing volume expansion during CPB without bleeding (scenario 1). HES should be given with caution or possibly avoided altogether due to warnings from the FDA (United States Food and Drug Administration 2013), European Medicines Agency (2013), and Surviving Sepsis Campaign (Dellinger et al. 2013). In a recently published survey of fluid management in cardiac surgery that was conducted in 18 European countries, it was noted that the use of HES products has decreased dramatically in the last several years (Protsyk et al. 2017). The most commonly used fluids for intraoperative and postoperative fluid management were crystalloids, and if colloids were used, the colloids were used in combination with crystalloids. The colloids that were used most frequently in this recent European survey were the gelatins, followed by HES and albumin. The warnings about the risks of HES use in critically ill patients issued by the FDA and EMA may have had an effect on the use of HES in the USA as well. In the present survey, which was performed about 2 years after the regulatory agency warnings, HES was chosen as the fluid of first choice by less than 10% of the respondents in most of the clinical scenarios. In agreement with the European survey, crystalloids were the most commonly chosen first fluid choice in three of the five clinical scenarios. However, in the USA, gelatins are not available and the only non-HES colloid that is easily available is albumin.

Limitations

A limitation of this study is that it describes current practices of fluid volume expansion in cardiovascular surgeries conducted only in the United States; these study results cannot be generalized to other countries in the rest of the world. We did not report on clinical outcomes, as this study is based on a survey of HCP preferences. We also recognize that the decision-making processes of HCPs are complex and may vary from the situations we put forth in

the survey. While our study design cannot provide details on the underlying reasons for treatment decisions, the results allow HCPs to compare their own practice patterns to those of their colleagues, which could be helpful given the lack of expert consensus on fluid resuscitation in patients undergoing cardiovascular surgeries. The results in this survey also provide basic background information for the design of future trials that address complicated issues, such as fluid volume expansion strategies in the hypothetical scenarios we described.

Conclusions

This study examined current practice patterns of fluid volume expansion in patients undergoing cardiac surgeries in the USA and found that fluid utilization varied depending on patient characteristics and clinical specialties of HCPs. Crystalloid fluid was most commonly chosen as the first-choice fluid for volume expansion. The most frequently used adjunct fluid to crystalloids was 5% albumin, which was also the most frequent first choice of IV fluid for patients needing volume expansion in the presence of blood loss during CPB when blood transfusion is not indicated (adequate Hb). In addition, perfusionists predominately preferred crystalloids to prime the CPB circuit; one third of the perfusionists preferred 25% albumin mixed with crystalloids for priming.

Additional files

Additional file 1: Albumin Surgical Utilization Survey. (DOCX 415 kb)

Additional file 2: Figure S1. Frequency of adjunct fluid use for patients needing volume expansion during CPB when not experiencing significant blood loss when the first choice is crystalloids[a] (scenario 1, $n = 64$). CPB, cardiopulmonary bypass; HES, hydroxyethyl starch. [a]Responses to the following question: How often do you use each of the following as an adjunct to your first choice in a patient not experiencing significant blood loss when volume expansion is indicated during cardiovascular surgery with CPB? (JPEG 168 kb)

Additional file 3: Figure S2. Frequency of adjunct fluid use for patients needing volume expansion in the presence of blood loss during CPB when blood transfusion is not indicated (scenario 2) **a** when first fluid choice is 5% albumin[a] ($n = 52$) and **b** when first fluid choice is crystalloids[b] ($n = 39$). CPB cardiopulmonary bypass; Hb, hemoglobin; HES, hydroxyethyl starch. [a]Responses to the following question: How often do you use each of the following as an adjunct to your first choice in a patient not experiencing significant blood loss when volume expansion is indicated during cardiovascular surgery with CPB? [b]Responses to the following question: How often do you use each of the following as an adjunct to your first choice in a patient for volume expansion in the presence of blood loss when blood transfusion is not indicated (adequate Hb) during cardiovascular surgery with CPB? (ZIP 186 kb)

Additional file 4: Figure S3. Frequency of adjunct fluid use for patients needing volume maintenance during acute normovolemic hemodilution when first fluid choice is crystalloids[a] (scenario 3, $n = 78$). HES, hydroxyethyl starch. [a]Responses to the following question: How often do you use the following as an adjunct to your first choice for a patient for volume maintenance during acute normovolemic hemodilution (autologous blood collection)? (JPEG 167 kb)

Additional file 5: Figure S4. Frequency of adjunct fluid use for expansion during ECMO or VAD (scenario 4) **a** when first fluid choice is albumin 5%[a]

($n = 33^b$) and **b** when first fluid choice is crystalloids[a] ($n = 31^b$). ECMO, extracorporeal membrane oxygenation; HES, hydroxyethyl starch; VAD, ventricular assist device. [a]Responses to the following question: How often do you use the following as an adjunct to your first choice for a patient who needs volume expansion during ECMO or VAD? [b]No statistical tests were performed due to small sample size. (ZIP 169 kb)

Additional file 6: Figure S5. Frequency of adjunct fluid use for intraoperative volume expansion for OPCABG or TAVR when first fluid choice is crystalloids[a] (scenario 5, $n = 59$). HES, hydroxyethyl starch; OPCAB, off-pump coronary artery bypass surgery; TAVR, transcatheter aortic valve replacement. [a]Responses to the following question: How often do you use the following as an adjunct to your first choice for a patient who needs intraoperative volume expansion for OPCAB or TAVR? (JPEG 167 kb)

Abbreviations

ANH: Acute normovolemic hemodilution; CABG: Coronary artery bypass graft surgery; COP: Colloid oncotic pressure; CPB: Cardiopulmonary bypass; ECMO: Extracorporeal membrane oxygenation; Hb: Hemoglobin; HCP: Health care professional; HES: Hydroxyethyl starches; ICU: Intensive care unit; IV: Intravenous; OPCABG: Off-pump coronary artery bypass graft surgery; TAVR: Transcatheter aortic valve replacement; VAD: Ventricular assist device

Acknowledgements

The authors wish to thank Tam Nguyen-Cao, PhD of Grifols for providing medical writing assistance under the direction of the authors and Kenichi Tanaka, MD of the University of Maryland School of Medicine for his assistance in the creation of the online questionnaire.

Funding

This study was funded by Grifols (Research Triangle Park, NC, USA), a manufacturer of albumin.

Authors' contributions

SA designed the study and generated the questionnaire. MB edited the questionnaire and provided a critical review of the manuscript. PN refined the questionnaire along with SA and KT and performed all data analyses. All authors reviewed the manuscript thoroughly and approved the final draft.

Competing interests

SA has received an honorarium as a medical advisor from Grifols. MB is an employee of Grifols, a manufacturer of albumin. PN has no competing interests relevant to this manuscript.

Author details

[1]Department of Anesthesiology, Duke University, 201 Trent Drive, 101 Baker House, Durham, NC 27710, USA. [2]One Research, LLC, 1150 Hungryneck Blvd. Suite C-303, Mt. Pleasant, SC 29464, USA. [3]Department of Medical Affairs, Grifols, 79 T.W. Alexander Drive, 4101 Research Commons, Research Triangle Park, Raleigh, NC 27709, USA.

References

Aditianingsih D, George YW. Guiding principles of fluid and volume therapy. Best Pract Res Clin Anaesthesiol. 2014;28(3):249–60.

Ait-Oufella H, Maury E, Lehoux S, Guidet B, Offenstadt G. The endothelium: physiological functions and role in microcirculatory failure during severe sepsis. Intensive Care Med. 2010;36(8):1286–98.

Annane D, Siami S, Jaber S, Martin C, Elatrous S, Declere AD, et al. Effects of fluid resuscitation with colloids vs crystalloids on mortality in critically ill patients presenting with hypovolemic shock: the CRISTAL randomized trial. JAMA. 2013;310(17):1809–17.

Becker BF, Chappell D, Jacob M. Endothelial glycocalyx and coronary vascular permeability: the fringe benefit. Basic Res Cardiol. 2010;105(6):687–701.

Cherpanath TG, Aarts LP, Groeneveld JA, Geerts BF. Defining fluid responsiveness: a guide to patient-tailored volume titration. J Cardiothorac Vasc Anesth. 2014;28(3):745–54.

Dellinger RP, Levy MM, Rhodes A, Annane D, Gerlach H, Opal SM, et al. Surviving Sepsis Campaign: international guidelines for management of severe sepsis and septic shock, 2012. Intensive Care Med. 2013;39(2):165–228.

European Medicines Agency. Hydroxyethyl-starch solutions (HES) no longer to be used in patients with sepsis or burn injuries or in critically ill patients. 2013. http://www.ema.europa.eu/docs/en_GB/document_library/Referrals_document/Solutions_for_infusion_containing_hydroxyethyl_starch/European_Commission_final_decision/WC500162361.pdf. Accessed 30 Jun 2016.

Finfer S, McEvoy S, Bellomo R, McArthur C, Myburgh J, Norton R. Impact of albumin compared to saline on organ function and mortality of patients with severe sepsis. Intensive Care Med. 2011;37(1):86–96.

Hirleman E, Larson DF. Cardiopulmonary bypass and edema: physiology and pathophysiology. Perfusion. 2008;23(6):311–22.

Hoeft A, Korb H, Mehlhorn U, Stephan H, Sonntag H. Priming of cardiopulmonary bypass with human albumin or Ringer lactate: effect on colloid osmotic pressure and extravascular lung water. Br J Anaesth. 1991;66(1):73–80.

Jacob M, Chappell D. Reappraising Starling: the physiology of the microcirculation. Curr Opin Crit Care. 2013;19(4):282–9.

Jacob M, Chappell D, Hofmann-Kiefer K, Helfen T, Schuelke A, Jacob B, et al. The intravascular volume effect of Ringer's lactate is below 20%: a prospective study in humans. Crit Care. 2012;16(3):R86.

Johansson PI, Stensballe J, Rasmussen LS, Ostrowski SR. A high admission syndecan-1 level, a marker of endothelial glycocalyx degradation, is associated with inflammation, protein C depletion, fibrinolysis, and increased mortality in trauma patients. Ann Surg. 2011;254(2):194–200.

Kuitunen AH, Hynynen MJ, Vahtera E, Salmenpera MT. Hydroxyethyl starch as a priming solution for cardiopulmonary bypass impairs hemostasis after cardiac surgery. Anesth Analg. 2004;98(2):291–7.

Lange M, Ertmer C, Van Aken H, Westphal M. Intravascular volume therapy with colloids in cardiac surgery. J Cardiothorac Vasc Anesth. 2011;25(5):847–55.

Lee EH, Kim WJ, Kim JY, Chin JH, Choi DK, Sim JY, et al. Effect of exogenous albumin on the incidence of postoperative acute kidney injury in patients undergoing off-pump coronary artery bypass surgery with a preoperative albumin level of less than 4.0 g/dl. Anesthesiology. 2016;124(5):1001–11.

Morin J-F, Mistry B, Langlois Y, Ma F, Chamoun P, Holcroft C. Fluid overload after coronary artery bypass grafting surgery increases the incidence of post-operative complications. World Journal of Cardiovascular Surgery. 2011;01(02):18–23.

Myburgh JA, Finfer S, Bellomo R, Billot L, Cass A, Gattas D, et al. Hydroxyethyl starch or saline for fluid resuscitation in intensive care. N Engl J Med. 2012;367(20):1901–11.

Myburgh JA, Mythen MG. Resuscitation fluids. N Engl J Med. 2013;369(13):1243–51.

Ortega-Loubon C, Hinojal YC, Carreras EF, Nunez GL, Pelaez PP, Saez MB, et al. Extracorporeal circulation in cardiac surgery inflammatory response, controversies and future directions. Intl Arch Med. 2015;8(19):1–13.

Perner A, Haase N, Guttormsen AB, Tenhunen J, Klemenzson G, Aneman A, et al. Hydroxyethyl starch 130/0.42 versus Ringer's acetate in severe sepsis. N Engl J Med. 2012;367(2):124–34.

Protsyk V, Rasmussen BS, Guarracino F, Erb J, Turton E, Ender J. Fluid management in cardiac surgery: results of a survey in European Cardiac Anesthesia Departments. J Cardiothorac Vasc Anesth. 2017 Apr 13; https://doi.org/10.1053/j.jvca.2017.04.017. [Epub ahead of print]

Rabin J, Meyenburg T, Lowery AV, Rouse M, Gammie JS, Herr D. Restricted albumin utilization is safe and cost effective in a cardiac surgery intensive care unit. Ann Thorac Surg. 2017;104(1):42–48.

Rehm M, Bruegger D, Christ F, Conzen P, Thiel M, Jacob M, et al. Shedding of the endothelial glycocalyx in patients undergoing major vascular surgery with global and regional ischemia. Circulation. 2007;116(17):1896–906.

Roger C, Muller L, Deras P, Louart G, Nouvellon E, Molinari N, et al. Does the type of fluid affect rapidity of shock reversal in an anaesthetized-piglet model of near-fatal controlled haemorrhage? A randomized study. Br J Anaesth. 2014;112(6):1015–23.

Russell JA, Navickis RJ, Wilkes MM. Albumin versus crystalloid for pump priming in cardiac surgery: meta-analysis of controlled trials. J Cardiothorac Vasc Anesth. 2004;18(4):429–37.

Sade RM, Stroud MR, Crawford FA Jr, Kratz JM, Dearing JP, Bartles DM. A prospective randomized study of hydroxyethyl starch, albumin, and lactated Ringer's solution as priming fluid for cardiopulmonary bypass. J Thorac Cardiovasc Surg. 1985;89(5):713–22.

Sedrakyan A, Gondek K, Paltiel D, Elefteriades JA. Volume expansion with albumin decreases mortality after coronary artery bypass graft surgery. Chest. 2003; 123(6):1853–7.

Skhirtladze K, Base EM, Lassnigg A, Kaider A, Linke S, Dworschak M, et al. Comparison of the effects of albumin 5%, hydroxyethyl starch 130/0.4 6%, and Ringer's lactate on blood loss and coagulation after cardiac surgery. Br J Anaesth. 2014;112(2):255–64.

Steppan J, Hofer S, Funke B, Brenner T, Henrich M, Martin E, et al. Sepsis and major abdominal surgery lead to flaking of the endothelial glycocalix. J Surg Res. 2011;165(1):136–41.

United States Food and Drug Administration. FDA Safety Communication: Boxed Warning on increased mortality and severe renal injury, and additional warning on risk of bleeding, for use of hydroxyethyl starch solutions in some settings 2013. http://www.fda.gov/biologicsbloodvaccines/safetyavailability/ucm358271.htm. Accessed 9 Jun 2016.

van Haren F, Zacharowski K. What's new in volume therapy in the intensive care unit? Best Pract Res Clin Anaesthesiol. 2014;28(3):275–83.

Verheij J, van Lingen A, Beishuizen A, Christiaans HM, de Jong JR, Girbes AR, et al. Cardiac response is greater for colloid than saline fluid loading after cardiac or vascular surgery. Intensive Care Med. 2006;32(7):1030–8.

Weinbaum S, Tarbell JM, Damiano ER. The structure and function of the endothelial glycocalyx layer. Annu Rev Biomed Eng. 2007;9:121–67.

11

Impact of ASA score misclassification on NSQIP predicted mortality

Alex Helkin[†], Sumeet V. Jain[*†], Angelika Gruessner, Maureen Fleming, Leslie Kohman, Michael Costanza and Robert N. Cooney

Abstract

Background: The ASA physical classification score has a major impact on the observed/expected (O/E) mortality ratio in the NSQIP General Vascular Mortality Model. The difference in predicted mortality is greatest between ASAs 3 and 4. We hypothesized under-classified ASA scores significantly affect the O/E mortality.

Methods: We conducted a retrospective review of NSQIP essential surgery cases from January 2014 to December 2014 ($n = 1264$) with mortality sub-analysis ($n = 33$) at our institution. We recorded transfer and emergency status and independently calculated the ASA score for mortalities using published definitions. A random sample of 50 survivors and 10 emergency survivors were reviewed and ASA recalculated. We performed statistical modeling to simulate the effects of ASA misclassifications. Statistical analysis was performed using JMP 10 and SAS 9.4.

Results: ASA was under-classified in 18.2% of mortalities, most commonly ASAs 3 and 4. Sixteen percent of ASA 3 survivors were misclassified, including 60% in the emergency subgroup ($p < 0.05$ vs. elective cases). Patients transferred from other institutions were more likely to be emergency cases than non-transferred patients (43.5 vs. 7.84%, $p < 0.05$). Transferred patients had a higher proportion of ASAs 3–5 vs. ASAs 1–2 compared with non-transfers (84.38 vs. 49.76%, $p < 0.05$) Simulation data showed ASA misclassification underestimated predicted mortality by 2.5 deaths on average.

Conclusion: ASA misclassification significantly impacts O/E mortality. With accurate ASA classification, observed mortality would not have exceeded expected mortality in our institution. Education regarding the impact of ASA scoring is critical to ensure accurate O/E mortality data at hospitals using NSQIP to assess surgical quality.

Keywords: ASA, NSQIP, Predicted mortality

Background

A current focus of health care systems is to improve the cost and quality of patient care. The American College of Surgeons National Surgical Quality Improvement Program (NSQIP®) is commonly used to collect and report data on institution-specific, risk-adjusted surgical outcomes. A systematic sampling approach is used to determine which surgical cases are selected for abstraction (Shiloach et al. 2010) based on the hospital's specific program: Essentials, Procedure-Targeted, Small & Rural, or Pediatric. Participating institutions are provided with quarterly reports on risk-adjusted complication rates for a variety of postoperative occurrences including surgical site infections, renal failure, thromboembolic complications, cardiac events, readmission, and observed to expected (O/E) mortality. Institutional performance for specific complications are compared with other hospitals and assigned a decile rank. The ranking is reported as "Needs Improvement," "As Expected," or "Exemplary," when compared with expected complication rates using standardized models, such as the NSQIP General Vascular Mortality Model (GVMM) for O/E mortality. Institutions can then use the NSQIP's institution-specific benchmarking data to focus their quality improvement initiatives. NSQIP participation is effective in helping

* Correspondence: jainsu@upstate.edu
This manuscript has been accepted for poster presentation at the 2016 ACS NSQIP Annual Conference in San Diego, CA.
[†]Equal contributors
Department of Surgery, SUNY Upstate Medical University, 750 East Adams Street, Syracuse, NY 13206, USA

institutions identify potential problems in surgical care (Steinberg et al. 2008; Fink et al. 2002); however, in most instances, additional analyses by the participating hospitals are required to develop a better understanding of how best to prevent or decrease complications.(Schilling et al. 2008).

In 2014, our institution received a NSQIP report indicating a higher than expected observed-to-expected 30-day mortality rate and was subsequently assigned a "Needs Improvement" status. We routinely review all major surgical complications and mortalities through our surgical Morbidity and Mortality conference and were surprised to learn we ranked in the lowest decile for this category. Focusing on mortality, we first reviewed the surgical literature to aid in identifying factors that might impact predicted mortality (Fink et al. 2002) and then did chart reviews of all surgical mortalities in 2014. We initially abstracted data to get a better understanding of patient-specific risk factors and process-of-care variables that might affect mortality including transfer status, need for emergency surgery, use and timing of "do not resuscitate" (DNR) status, "procedure risk" (low, medium, or high), NSQIP and University Hospital Consortium predicted mortality, and finally the American Society of Anesthesia (ASA) physical status classification system.

Based on our initial review, we turned our focus to the ASA score (Table 1) (Durham et al. 2006) as a potential contributor to our higher than expected O/E mortality rate. The ASA score is assigned by the anesthesia team and provides a baseline metric for the fitness of a patient prior to undergoing surgery. The ASA score is an important predictor of mortality in surgical patients (Davenport et al. 2006; Davenport et al. 2005) and has been specifically validated for use in the NSQIP GVMM. The NSQIP rules for data entry require the SCR to use the ASA score recorded by the anesthesia team but allow the SCR to add the suffix E in cases where the surgical team documents the emergent nature of the surgical procedure, if not already documented in the "anesthesia assigned" ASA score. During our chart review of the 2014 mortalities, we identified several misclassified ASA scores, which greatly altered predicted mortality according to the NSQIP online preoperative risk calculator. Based on this finding, we hypothesized misclassified ASA scores falsely decreased the expected mortality and contributed to the increased 2014 NSQIP O/E mortality at our institution.

Methods

The study was approved by our institutional review board for exemption from review because it used retrospective, de-identified data. At our institution, 1264 general and vascular surgical cases were reported to NSQIP in 2014, which included 33 mortalities. The medical records of these 33 patients were reviewed by two surgery residents (AH and SJ) independently, who did not participate in any of the cases. ASA score was independently calculated by each reviewer and then discussed together to reach consensus based on published guidelines on the ASA website (asahq.org). In addition to ASA score, the following data were abstracted: transfer from another institution, the need for emergency surgery, DNR status and timing relative to death, and procedure risk. To determine factors significantly affecting

Table 1 American Society of Anesthesiologists physical classification system (Durham et al. 2006)

ASA physical status classification	Definition	Examples, including, but not limited to
ASA I	A normal healthy patient	Healthy, non-smoking, no or minimal alcohol use
ASA II	A patient with mild systemic disease	Mild diseases only without substantive functional limitations. Examples include (but not limited to) current smoker, social alcohol drinker, pregnancy, obesity (30 < BMI < 40), well-controlled DM/HTN, and mild lung disease
ASA III	A patient with severe systemic disease	Substantive functional limitations: one or more moderate to severe diseases. Examples include (but not limited to) poorly controlled DM or HTN, COPD, morbid obesity (BMI ≥ 40), active hepatitis, alcohol dependence or abuse, implanted pacemaker, moderate reduction of ejection fraction, ESRD undergoing regularly scheduled dialysis, premature infant PCA < 60 weeks, and history (> 3 months) of MI, CVA, TIA, or CAD/stents
ASA IV	A patient with severe systemic disease that is a constant threat to life	Examples include (but not limited to) recent (< 3 months) MI, CVA, TIA, or CAD/stents, ongoing cardiac ischemia or severe valve dysfunction, severe reduction of ejection fraction, sepsis, DIC, and ARD or ESRD not undergoing regularly scheduled dialysis
ASA V	A moribund patient who is not expected to survive without the operation	Examples include (but not limited to) ruptured abdominal/thoracic aneurysm, massive trauma, intracranial bleeding with mass effect, and ischemic bowel in the face of significant cardiac pathology or multiple organ/system dysfunction
ASA VI	A declared brain-dead patient whose organs are being removed for donor purposes	

predicted mortality, all patient factors that are part of the NSQIP online calculator were reviewed including procedure, age, gender, functional status, emergency status, wound class, steroid use, ascites present within 30 days of surgery, systemic sepsis present within 30 days of surgery, diabetes, hypertension, previous cardiac events, congestive heart failure, dyspnea on presentation, tobacco use, history of COPD, dialysis, acute renal failure, ventilator dependence, disseminated cancer, body mass index, and reclassification of the ASA score using the American Society of Anesthesiologists published guidelines (Table 1) (Durham et al. 2006). This analysis determined ASA was the major factor in NSQIP modeling, and discrepancies in classification lead to substantially different outcomes, specifically changes from ASA 3 to ASA 4. Changes from ASA 2 to ASA 3 or ASA 4 to ASA 5 did not impact mortality predictions as expected.

To understand the impact of ASA misclassification, we needed to develop a global estimate of ASA misclassification incidence for the entire NSQIP population, not just the mortalities. As the differential impact between ASAs 2 and 3, and between 4 and 5, was negligible compared to that between ASAs 3 and 4, our study focused on ASA 3 cases only. To objectively estimate the incidence of misclassified ASA 3 patients, a random sample of 50 patients was selected from the 2014 elective NSQIP surgical cases with charted ASA 3 classifications. Additionally, 10 patients of the total 74 emergency cases who were initially charted ASA 3 were randomly selected. These samples were used to estimate the frequency of ASA 3 over- and under-classification. Patient selection was performed by random number generating software (SAS 9.4, Cary, NC).

After correcting the misclassified ASA scores of the random samples, SAS 9.4 was used to simulate the number of expected deaths using the odds ratios for mortality in the published 2014 GVMM and adjusted for the new rates of each ASA class. Both over- and under-classifications were included in the model. The simulation was run 1000 times. As the entered data represented the probabilities of a particular outcome, each run of the simulation generates a number of predicted deaths.

Statistical analyses were performed using JMP 10 and SAS 9.4 (Cary, NC). Contingency analysis using the chi-square test was performed for categorical variables.

Results

The patient characteristics of our study populations (all cases and mortalities) are shown in Table 2. Patients who died were older and more likely to be outside transfers and emergencies ($p < 0.05$). In addition, certain surgical populations, namely, breast and endocrine surgery patients, had no observed mortality. Characteristics such as gender, race, and Hispanic ethnicity were not different

Table 2 Patient Characteristics of the Study Population

Demographics		All cases % (no.)	Mortalities % (no.)	p value
Age		56.5 ± 0.47	71 ± 3	< 0.001
Gender	Male	45.3% (573)	57.6% (19)	0.215
	Female	54.7% (691)	42.4% (14)	
Race	White	82.2% (1039)	84.8% (28)	0.896
	Black	10.4% (132)	12.1% (4)	
	American Indian	1.1% (14)	0.0% (0)	
	Asian	1.1% (14)	0.0% (0)	
	Unknown	5.1% (65)	3.0% (1)	
Hispanic ethnicity		3.4% (43)	0.0% (0)	0.624
Emergency		12.1% (153)	70.0% (23)	< 0.001
Transfer		12.1% (153)	60.6% (20)	< 0.001
Surgery type	General surgery	41.0% (518)	51.5% (17)	0.046
	Breast/endocrine	21.5% (272)	0.0% (0)	
	Vascular	18.4% (233)	27.3% (9)	
	Colorectal	10.1% (128)	15.2% (5)	
	Hepatobiliary	5.8% (73)	6.1% (2)	
	Bariatric	3.2% (40)	0.0% (0)	

between groups. When evaluating NSQIP variables, the mortality group also had a greater incidence of partially dependent functional status, disseminated cancer, diabetes, hypertension, tobacco use, chronic obstructive pulmonary disease, acute renal failure, dirty wounds, ascites, and ventilator use at the time of surgery (Table 3, $p < 0.05$). A total of 1264 NSQIP essential cases were performed during 2014. Patients transferred from other institutions were more likely to be emergency cases compared with patients who were not transfers (43.5 vs. 7.84%, $p < 0.05$), and transferred patients had a higher proportion of ASAs 3–5 vs. ASAs 1–2 compared with non-transfers (84.38 vs. 49.76%, $p < 0.05$). When comparing our study population to the NSQIP reported total population ($n = 768,612$), our study population had a higher proportion of transferred patients for mortalities (57.6 vs. 29.9%, $p < 0.05$) and survivors (11 vs. 3.9%, $p < 0.05$). Additionally, our study population had a higher number of patients with 3+ risk factors in both mortalities (87.9 vs. 60.1%, $p < 0.05$) and survivors (23 vs. 11.6%, $p < 0.05$) than the NSQIP comparison population.

Our initial medical record review of 33 mortalities showed 18.2% of ASA scores were misclassified, mostly in patients originally scored ASA 3 or ASA 4. 12.1% were under-classified (initially received a lower ASA), and 6.1% were over-classified. Discrepancies between recorded and reclassified ASA scores appeared to be the greatest contributor to the NSQIP predicted mortality

Table 3 NSQIP risk factors in the study population

NSQIP variables		All cases % (no.)	Mortalities % (no.)	p value
Functional status	Independent	96.2% (1216)	87.9% (29)	0.013
	Partially dependent	3.2% (40)	12.1% (4)	
	Totally dependent	0.6% (8)	0.0% (0)	
Wound class	Clean	55.0% (695)	33.3% (11)	0.003
	Clean/ contaminated	27.3% (345)	27.3% (9)	
	Contaminated	7.9% (100)	12.1% (4)	
	Dirty	9.8% (124)	27.3% (9)	
Steroid		4.1% (52)	12.1% (4)	0.050
Ascites		0.5% (6)	9.1% (3)	0.001
Sepsis	SIRS	6.6% (84)	21.2% (7)	< 0.001
	Sepsis	4.7% (59)	18.2% (6)	
	Septic shock	1.0% (13)	24.2% (8)	
Ventilator		1.3% (16)	27.3% (9)	< 0.001
Disseminated cancer		4.2% (53)	24.2% (8)	< 0.001
Diabetes		20.1% (254)	39.4% (13)	0.014
Hypertension		48.7% (616)	75.8% (25)	0.002
CHF		0.6% (8)	3.0% (1)	0.208
Dyspnea	At rest	0.6% (7)	3.0% (1)	0.069
	Moderate exertion	8.4% (106)	15.2% (5)	
	None	91.1% (1151)	81.8% (27)	
Smoker		31.3% (396)	39.4% (13)	0.039
COPD		7.5% (95)	27.3% (9)	< 0.001
Dialysis		2.4% (30)	6.1% (2)	0.194
ARF		0.6% (8)	6.1% (2)	0.025
BMI		30.4 ± 0.24	27.5 ± 1.54	0.054

Table 4 Reasons for ASA misclassification in the study population

2014 mortalities

Patient	Charted ASA	Recalculated ASA	Reason for change
1	4	5	Ruptured abdominal aortic aneurysm with intraoperative cardiac arrest
2	3E	5E	Superior mesenteric artery occlusion with bowel ischemia
3	Not recorded	5	Perforated colon with sepsis. Moribund
4	4	3	Reviewer used subsequent cases after complications instead of index case
5	4	3	Several severe systemic comorbidities (poorly controlled diabetes, chronic obstructive pulmonary disease, asthma), but none were a constant threat to life
6	3	4	Active congestive heart failure

2014 all cases sample

Patient	Charted ASA	Recalculated ASA	Reason for change
1	3	2	Controlled hypertension and asthma, otherwise healthy. Localized Hurthle cell cancer
2	3	4	Stroke within 3 months
3	3	4	Myocardial infarction within 3 months with 14% left ventricular ejection fraction on echocardiogram
4	3E	4E	Perforated small bowel with sepsis
5	3E	2E	Infected thigh hematoma, but not septic. Remote history of supraventricular tachycardia, but otherwise healthy and not on medications
6	3E	4E	Perforated viscus with sepsis
7	3E	4E	Bowel necrosis present on colonoscopy prior to operation

2014 emergency cases sample

Patient	Charted ASA	Recalculated ASA	Reason for change
1	3E	4E	Perforated viscus
2	3E	5E	Ruptured abdominal aortic aneurysm
3	3E	4E	Perforated diverticulitis
4	3E	4E	Perforated small bowel with sepsis
5	3E	4E	Ongoing crescendo transient ischemic attacks
6	3E	2E	Appendicitis, not septic and no major medical problems

(compared to all other factors on the online NSQIP model) particularly when ASA 4 and 5 cases were under-classified as ASA 3. Emergency cases were more likely to have a higher ASA score ($p < 0.05$) and were more likely to be misclassified ($p < 0.05$). Table 4 lists the reclassified ASA scores and the medical rationale for reclassifying the ASA score.

To determine if ASA scores were also systematically misclassified in the all cases population, we reviewed medical records of 50 randomly chosen survivors initially assigned an ASA score of 3. In this random sample, the ASA was misclassified in 16% of patients with five under-classified and two over-classified. A random sample of 10 patients who underwent emergency surgery was also analyzed. Six of these patients had ASA scores that were misclassified ($p < 0.05$) including one over-classification. Table 4 summarizes the factors that led to ASA reclassification.

Predicted mortality simulations were then performed using the misclassification rates discovered above. Figure 1 shows the distribution of the results of the simulation model for the ASA 3 misclassifications.

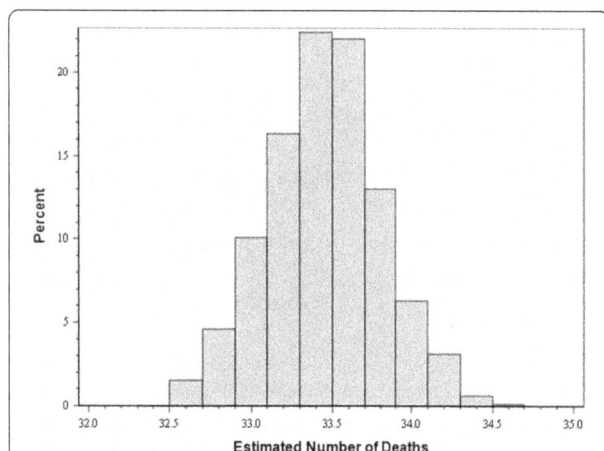

Fig. 1 Simulated predicted death adjusting for ASA misclassification. When adjusting for re-classified ASA scores in the sample populations, simulations using the odds ratio of mortality based on the GVMM reports predicted increased mortality matching our institutions observed mortality. Histogram bars depict the percentage of simulations that resulted in the mortality rates shown on the x-axis. The number of deaths with the greatest likelihood based on the simulation model was 33.5. The simulation was run 1000 times. Both over-classification and under-classification rates were included in the model

Ultimately, the simulation shows the number of predicted deaths was 33.46 (95% CI 33.44–33.48), determined by the median of the curve generated by the histogram. Based upon the simulated estimated deaths, our O/E mortality rate would be 0.9864 (95% CI 0.9858–0.9871), essentially identical to the number of observed deaths in 2014 (33 deaths), whereas the NSQIP report only predicted 30.6 deaths (O/E mortality 1.0784).

Discussion

Quality improvement initiatives such as the NSQIP and the University Hospital Consortium (UHC) databases are important benchmarking resources, which allow participating hospital systems to assess the quality of care provided at their institutions (Fink et al. 2002). However, when specific quality scoring systems are used to evaluate patient care, it is assumed that the data used to assess patient acuity and outcomes are accurate. The UHC quality benchmarking process utilizes administrative data to "risk-stratify" patient outcomes. Administrative databases require accurate documentation of patient's medical diagnoses in the medical record to accurately "risk-stratify" patient outcomes. Abstracted databases like NSQIP are assumed to be more accurate in patient risk factor stratification (Steinberg et al. 2008). However, as with any "scoring system," the users must understand the strengths and weakness of the system to use it properly. NSQIP is designed to predict the risk of complications and mortality based on information about the

patients and their medical conditions that is available prior to performing surgery. Consequently, misrepresentation of these variables, such as failure to recognize sepsis or misclassifying the ASA, can significantly underestimate predicted mortality and thereby inaccurately categorize hospitals as being poor performers.

We discovered that at our institution, an academic medical center with many trainees, ASA misclassifications were relatively common (16%), especially in emergencies (60%). Under-classification of ASA scores 4 and 5 as ASA 3 was unexpected. The statistical model we created suggests that with proper ASA classification, our institution's predicted mortality would have matched our observed mortality. In addition, emergency surgical procedures were most commonly misclassified and transferred patients were most often emergency cases. Thus, the predicted mortality of institutions with a high volume of transferred emergency surgical cases, such as ours, may be artificially reduced from underestimated ASA classifications. This is consistent with data suggesting that emergency cases are prone to high O/E ratios and risk under-classification in general (Hyder et al. 2015).

The reasons why so many ASA scores were misclassified are unclear. As a teaching hospital, it is tempting to assume that junior anesthesia trainees were not as familiar with the ASA score calculation as they should be, or that emergency cases performed on nights and weekends were prone to "erroneous ASA classification" (Gawande et al. 2003). However, Tables 3 and 4 offer some additional insights. First, many patients who were misclassified as ASA 3, when they should have been ASA 4, presented with sepsis or perforated viscus. In reviewing their charts, some of these patients appeared quite well on initial examination; however, their vital signs, laboratory values, and imaging met the Systemic Inflammatory Response Syndrome criteria for sepsis. In addition, all of the ASA 5 patients misclassified as ASA 3 presented with ruptured abdominal aortic aneurysm. On presentation and initial exam, because they were "contained ruptures," these patients also appeared quite well with minimal abnormalities in their vitals or laboratory values. However, while these patients were clinically well appearing, ruptured aortic aneurysms are by definition granted an ASA 5 on the ASA guidelines, as the natural history for these cases is quick propagation to overt rupture and death. A few under-classified patients had medical histories consistent with ASA 4 as well, such as myocardial infarction within 3 months or ongoing transient ischemic attacks prior to surgery. As such, there appeared to be an over reliance on the subjective physical appearance of the patient at the time of examination, as opposed to factors such as the natural history of their disease process and previous medical history.

The ASA score is a subjective measure of baseline patient illness; however, it is critical that all providers who assign ASAs are doing so in a consistent manner. Our study provides evidence ASA misclassification can significantly impact predicted mortality and supports continued education regarding the potential impact of ASA scoring on O/E mortality in surgical patients. To address this concern, we communicated our findings on ASA misclassification to both the surgery and anesthesia departments and provided education regarding the ASA score and its importance in calculating predicted mortality. We also modified our institutional procedure verification and time out policy by incorporating the ASA score into the surgical time out. Our revised policy requires the attending anesthesiologist to communicate the ASA score to the surgical team as part of the time out. The attending surgeon is required to acknowledge the assigned ASA score prior to starting the operation and initiate a discussion about it if there are concerns about the assigned score. In addition, surgical residents are required to use the online NSQIP calculator for all cases presented in the weekly morbidity and mortality conference. A future study will reevaluate the incidence of misclassified ASAs after such education has been instituted.

There are several limitations to this study. First, it is a single-center retrospective review of NSQIP mortalities in a large academic medical center. Consequently, the results may not apply to participating NSQIP institutions of varying size and type. Future studies being considered include expansion of the current study to multiple institutions, as well as revisiting our ASA misclassification rate after education. Second, the actual model used to calculate NSQIP predicted mortality is proprietary, so we are unable to report exact statistical change in predicted mortality. In the future, NSQIP plans to be increasingly robust. For example, NSQIP models will improve with specific variables collected for complex hepatobiliary cases.

Conclusion

ASA misclassification significantly impacts observed/expected mortality ratio, and thus, how a particular institution's safety is viewed. In our review, misclassification, particularly in emergency cases, underestimated the number of predicted deaths by up to 9%. With accurate ASA classification, observed mortality would not have exceeded expected mortality in our institution. Continued education regarding the impact of ASA scoring is essential to ensure accurate O/E mortality data is being used to assess surgical quality at participating NSQIP institutions. Our institution has since instituted a policy that the ASA must be announced during the pre-procedure time out and agreed upon or discussed prior to incision.

Abbreviations

ASA: American Society of Anesthesia; DNR: Do not resuscitate; GVMM: General Vascular Mortality Model; NSQIP: National Surgical Quality Improvement Project; O/E: Observed to expected; UHC: University Hospital Consortium

Funding

This research was not funded by any funding body. The design, data collection, analysis, and interpretation were all done by the authors alone.

Authors' contributions

AH, SVJ, and RNC were responsible for the study conception and design. AH, SVJ, and MF were responsible for the data acquisition. All authors contributed to the analysis and interpretation of the data. The manuscript was drafted by AH, SVJ, AG, LK, MC, and RNC. Critical revision was performed by all authors. All authors read and approved the final manuscript.

Competing interests

SVJ has been invited to speak by Draeger Medical at conferences without expenses paid. LK has received travel expenses for consultations with Carefusion and the American Cancer Society. She also has received a grant for an after-market analysis of a tunneled pleural catheter. RNC has received less than $5000 for expert testimony provided for a malpractice case, as well as a stipend from the NIH for review panel service. All other others have no competing interests to disclose.

References

Davenport DL, Bowe EA, Henderson WG, Khuri SF, Mentzer RM Jr. National Surgical Quality Improvement Program (NSQIP) risk factors can be used to validate American Society of Anesthesiologists Physical Status Classification (ASA PS) levels. Ann Surg. 2006;243(5):636–41. discussion 641-634

Davenport DL, Henderson WG, Khuri SF, Mentzer RM Jr. Preoperative risk factors and surgical complexity are more predictive of costs than postoperative complications: a case study using the National Surgical Quality Improvement Program (NSQIP) database. Ann Surg. 2005;242(4):463–8. discussion 468-471

Durham R, Pracht E, Orban B, Lottenburg L, Tepas J, Flint L. Evaluation of a mature trauma system. Ann Surg. 2006;243(6):775–83. discussion 783-775

Fink AS, Campbell DA Jr, Mentzer RM Jr, et al. The National Surgical Quality Improvement Program in non-veterans administration hospitals: initial demonstration of feasibility. Ann Surg. 2002;236(3):344–53. discussion 353-344

Gawande AA, Zinner MJ, Studdert DM, Brennan TA. Analysis of errors reported by surgeons at three teaching hospitals. Surgery. 2003;133(6):614–21.

Hyder JA, Reznor G, Wakeam E, Nguyen LL, Lipsitz SR, Havens JM. Risk prediction accuracy differs for emergency versus elective cases in the ACS-NSQIP. Ann Surg. 2015;264(6):959-65.

Schilling PL, Dimick JB, Birkmeyer JD. Prioritizing quality improvement in general surgery. J Am Coll Surg. 2008;207(5):698–704.

Shiloach M, Frencher SK Jr, Steeger JE, et al. Toward robust information: data quality and inter-rater reliability in the American College of Surgeons National Surgical Quality Improvement Program. J Am Coll Surg. 2010;210(1):6–16.

Steinberg SM, Popa MR, Michalek JA, Bethel MJ, Ellison EC. Comparison of risk adjustment methodologies in surgical quality improvement. Surgery. 2008; 144(4):662–7. discussion 662-667

12

Rationale for and approach to preoperative opioid weaning: a preoperative optimization protocol

Heath McAnally[1,2] (iD)

Abstract: The practice of chronic opioid prescription for chronic non-cancer pain has come under considerable scrutiny within the past several years as mounting evidence reveals a generally unfavorable risk to benefit ratio and the nation reels from the grim mortality statistics associated with the opioid epidemic. Patients struggling with chronic pain tend to use opioids and also seek out operative intervention for their complaints, which combination may be leading to increased postoperative "acute-on-chronic" pain and fueling worsened chronic pain and opioid dependence.

Besides worsened postoperative pain, a growing body of literature, reviewed herein, indicates that preoperative opioid use is associated with significantly worsened surgical outcomes, and severely increased financial drain on an already severely overburdened healthcare budget. Conversely, there is evidence that preoperative opioid reduction may result in substantial improvements in outcome. In the era of accountable care, efforts such as the Enhanced Recovery After Surgery (ERAS) protocol have been introduced in an attempt to standardize and facilitate evidence-based perioperative interventions to optimize surgical outcomes. We propose that addressing preoperative opioid reduction as part of a targeted optimization approach for chronic pain patients seeking surgery is not only logical but mandatory given the stakes involved. Simple opioid reduction/abstinence however is not likely to occur in the absence of provision of viable and palatable alternatives to managing pain, which will require a strong focus upon reducing pain catastrophization and bolstering self-efficacy and resilience.

In response to a call from our surgical community toward that end, we have developed a simple and easy-to-implement outpatient preoperative optimization program focusing on gentle opioid weaning/elimination as well as a few other high-yield areas of intervention, requiring a minimum of resources.

Keywords: Preoperative, Chronic pain, Opioid, Weaning, Optimization, Outcomes, Length of stay, Prehabilitation, Opioid-induced hyperalgesia, Biopsychosocial

Background

America's opioid problem remains unrelenting, insidious, and without a clear solution in sight. One particular arena where aggressive intervention may have significant impact is the perioperative period. Within the surgical population, a large proportion of patients (as many as 33–70% (Tye et al. 2017)) seeking elective operations are already using chronic prescription opioids. These patients have been shown to demand greater doses and duration of opioid therapy postoperatively (VanDenKerkhof et al. 2012;

Correspondence: hmcan@uw.edu
[1]Northern Anesthesia & Pain Medicine, LLC, 10928 Eagle River Rd #240, Eagle River, AK 99577, USA
[2]Department of Anesthesiology and Pain Medicine, University of Washington, Box 356540, Seattle, WA 98195-6540, USA

Carroll et al. 2012; Hah et al. 2015; Rozet et al. 2014; Lawrence et al. 2008b; Armaghani et al. 2014). This may simply represent the presence of more serious "pain generators" leading to greater opioid consumption both pre- and postoperatively, or may represent a more complex scenario with compromised resilience and self-efficacy, increased underlying emotional and psychological distress, and frank opioid dependence driving the process. Chronic opioid use also reliably confers tolerance to the agent's analgesic properties (Collett 1998; Adriaensen et al. 2003; Chang et al. 2007; Williams et al. 2013) leading to less effective perioperative pain management and often disproportionate pain. Furthermore, there is growing evidence that chronic opioid use increases pain sensitivity—currently labeled opioid-induced hyperalgesia (OIH)—thus leading to a pernicious cycle of increased demand for mu-receptor agonism/narcotization which in turn increases pain which increases demand (Angst and Clark 2006; Lee et al. 2011).

Seasoned surgeons of all disciplines have learned that the risk to benefit ratio of surgery may lie toward the harmful for elective procedures in patients who are morbidly obese, nutritionally deficient, deconditioned/"sarcopenic", tobacco users, etc. A growing body of evidence (reviewed below) indicates that even after adjusting for many of these obvious confounders, chronic opioid use also predisposes to poor surgical outcomes including immediate postoperative complications such as infection and other physiologic perturbation (e.g., ileus and respiratory suppression with atelectasis and pneumonia) but also long-term issues such as compromised wound healing and reduced arthroplasty or intervertebral fusion success.

We propose that bringing opioid-dependent patients to the operating room for elective surgery carries an unacceptably high risk of conferring "acute-on-chronic pain" much like unaddressed hypovolemia in the chronic renal-insufficient patient invites acute-on-chronic renal failure. We also propose that among numerous high-yield targets for optimizing surgical outcome (e.g., tobacco cessation and nutritional prehabilitation), opioid reduction or elimination deserves particular consideration in the context of the growing public health problem of misuse, abuse, and dependence. Finally, we propose that deferring elective surgery until adequate preoperative optimization (i.e., reduction or elimination if possible) of opioid use, just like delaying for body mass index (BMI) improvements or tobacco cessation, comprises wise stewardship of private and public monies funding healthcare.

Survey

We surveyed 62 local surgeons (with 48 respondents) from the disciplines of general surgery, gynecology, neurosurgery, ophthalmology, orthopedics, otolaryngology, plastic surgery, and urology to see how long they would be willing to defer elective operations in unprepared patients, and also what the top three to five issues (modifiable risk factors) were they would like to see optimized prior to elective surgery. The results are shown in Figs. 1 and 2. The range of perceived acceptable preoperative delay for non-urgent problems ranged from 4 weeks to indefinite, with the majority of surgeons favoring waiting longer than 2–3 months if necessary to optimize their patients. Among the common modifiable risk factors that our surgeons prioritized for preoperative optimization, the most frequently identified issues were tobacco use, opioid use, obesity, unrealistic expectations and other psychological factors, deconditioning, and diabetes or other systemic diseases.

A weighted value ("optimization importance factor") was created for each variable reported by our surgeon population by multiplying the number of surgeons reporting it by

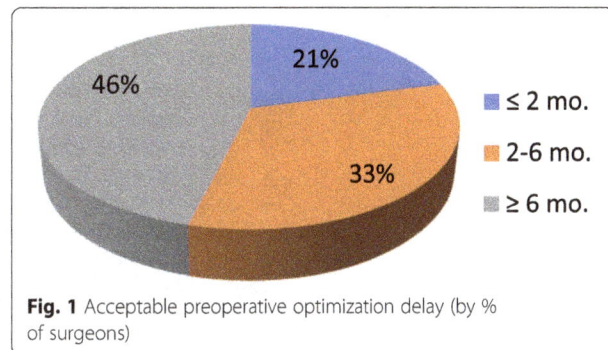

Fig. 1 Acceptable preoperative optimization delay (by % of surgeons)

a numeric scale ranking (in descending order from 5 to 1) of prioritization.

Literature review

Over the past 10 years, multiple reports (Armaghani et al. 2014; Lawrence et al. 2008a; Anderson et al. 2009; Roullet et al. 2009; Zywiel et al. 2011; Raebel et al. 2013; Pivec et al. 2014; Menendez et al. 2015; Morris et al. 2015; Hina et al. 2015; Aasvang et al. 2016; Morris et al. 2016; Sing et al. 2016; Zarling et al. 2016; Nguyen et al. 2016; Faour et al. 2017; Ben-Ari et al. 2017; Villavicencio et al. 2017; Waljee et al. 2017; Smith et al. 2017; Rozell et al. 2017; Chan et al. 2017; Cheah et al. 2017) have noted a generally consistent association between preoperative chronic opioid use and worsened postoperative outcomes. These studies are summarized in Table 1, and individual studies of interest are briefly presented below. A negative study is discussed first, however, along with criticism.

Kelly et al.'s (2015) retrospective cohort study indicated no evident difference in pain or disability 2 years out from cervical disc replacement or interbody fusion patients stratified into those using "weak" (n = 762) vs. "strong" (n = 226) opioids. A third control arm comprised only 16 individuals who were opioid-naïve going into surgery. The opioid categorization however was arbitrary and did not accurately reflect potency (e.g., meperidine which is considerably less potent than hydromorphone was placed in the "strong opioid" group whereas hydrocodone, essentially equipotent to morphine, was placed in the "weak opioid" group). Furthermore, there was undoubtedly considerable overlap between the two groups in terms of actual equivalent opioid dosage. This study must then be interpreted with considerable skepticism.

Menendez et al. (2015) performed a tremendously powered retrospective analysis of 15,901 opioid-dependent individuals undergoing various arthroplasties or spinal fusion operations, compared to over 9 million controls. After adjusting for demographic, comorbidity, hospital, and operative variables, they noted that opioid dependence was statistically significantly associated with increased morbidity and mortality. Increased hospital length of stay (LOS) and

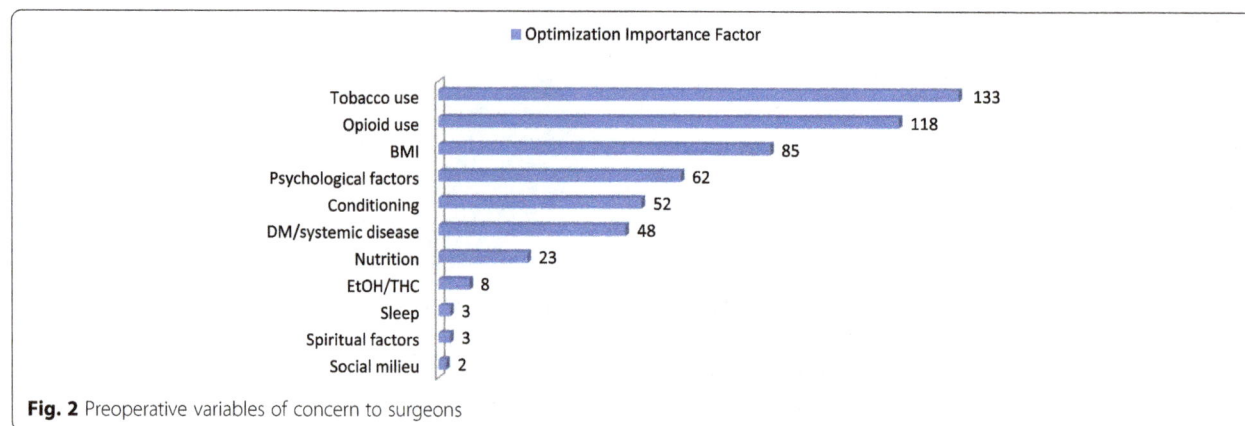

Fig. 2 Preoperative variables of concern to surgeons

discharge to rehabilitation facilities also correlated with opioid dependence.

A small but interesting study by Hina et al. (2015) adds to the literature on opioid-induced hyperalgesia and demonstrated that preoperative opioid use is associated with demonstrable OIH prior to operation, and despite a more aggressive intraoperative anesthetic approach (e.g., inclusion of ketamine into the anesthetic), patients using chronic preoperative opioids displayed greater postoperative pain and increased opioid demand, consistent with the experience of most clinicians and the literature.

Sing et al. (2016) in a subgroup analysis examined the negative consequences of preoperative extended-release/long-term opioid use in relation to postoperative outcomes. They reported that of 116 total knee and hip arthroplasty patients using preoperative opioids, there was a trend noted for more severe outcomes (increased postoperative pain and opioid consumption, increased hospital LOS, increased admission to rehabilitation facilities, worsened surgical outcomes including arthrofibrosis and periprosthetic fractures) in the extended-release/long-acting opioid-using subgroup compared to the immediate-release opioid-using group.

Ben-Ari et al. (2017) in another highly powered study demonstrated that 12,772 patients undergoing total knee arthroplasty who had been using chronic preoperative opioids were significantly more likely to undergo revision arthroplasty compared to 19,864 controls, results echoed by other studies as listed in Table 1.

A few studies have examined the associated between preoperative opioid use and economic outcomes. Waljee et al. (2017) performed a retrospective analysis of nearly 200,000 patients undergoing various general surgical operations and hysterectomies. The patients using chronic preoperative opioids (n = 17,577) had significantly longer hospital LOS, increased incidence of discharge to rehabilitation facilities and hospital readmission, and generated greater than double the financial costs than 182,428 controls, after adjusting for numerous psychosocial variables. Faour et al.

(2017) and Tye et al. (2017) have demonstrated that cervical and lumbar spine surgical patients, respectively, who used chronic preoperative opioids had significantly lower incidence of return to work than matched cohorts who did not use chronic preoperative opioids.

Finally, a very interesting study by Nguyen et al. (2016) suggests that preoperative opioid reduction may prove protective against these negative outcomes. Forty-one patients who successfully weaned their opioid burden prior to surgery by at least 50% were compared to 41 opioid-dependent patients who did not, and 41 opioid-naïve controls. The intervention group had outcomes comparable to the opioid-naïve group, with both of those two groups demonstrating significantly improved pain and functional outcomes compared to the patient group that did not reduce their opioid use preoperatively. This is the first study to demonstrate efficacy of preoperative opioid reduction.

Discussion

The International Association for the Study of Pain has labeled 2017 the Global Year Against Pain After Surgery (International Association for the Study of Pain 2017). This laudable, ambitious approach highlights well-accepted and traditional objectives such as aggressive perioperative multimodal analgesia, and its goals are echoed in the philosophy of constructs such as Toronto's Transitional Pain Service and the American Society of Anesthesiologists' Perioperative Surgical Home (Katz et al. 2015; Desebbe et al. 2016). As important as such diversification of response is, it still comprises response and is thus at least theoretically inferior to an approach of proactive "pain prehabilitation," certainly within the chronic pain patient population.

The biologic complexity of chronic pain, and opioid-induced hyperalgesia

Pain is a complex and subjective experience now well-known to occur outside of the context of nociception, and with considerable potential for both amplification and suppression from the central nervous system (Latremoliere

Table 1 Studies reporting outcomes following preoperative opioid use

Authors	Year	Discipline	Findings
Lawrence et al.	2008	Spine	47 chronic opioid-using patients experienced significantly worsened outcomes of pain and disability postoperatively compared to 44 non-opioid-using patients
Anderson et al.	2009	Spine	Logistical regression model of 488 ACDF patients revealed "weak" preoperative opioid use as an independently significant negative predictive variable for postoperative neck disability
Roullet et al.	2009	Orthopedics	12 chronic preoperative opioid-using patients had greater postoperative opioid consumption and phantom limb pain than 10 non-opioid-using controls
Zywiel et al.	2011	Orthopedics	45 TKA patients using opioids preoperatively had significantly greater postoperative dysfunction and complications including need for revision compared to non-opioid-using controls
Raebel et al.	2013	Bariatric surgery	77% of 933 chronic opioid-using bariatric surgery patients continued to use opioids at 12-month postoperative follow-up and generally at higher doses
Pivec et al.	2014	Orthopedics	54 THA patients using opioids preoperatively had significantly greater postoperative pain and opioid consumption, increased hospital LOS, worsened postoperative function and increased arthroplasty failure compared to non-opioid-using controls
Armaghani et al.	2014	Spine	Logistic regression model of 583 patients demonstrated that of 321 patients using chronic preoperative opioids, "increasing preoperative use" correlated with ongoing opioid dependence 12 months postoperatively
Kelly et al.	2015		762 "weak opioid" (codeine, propoxyphene, hydrocodone), 226 "strong opioid" (meperidine, morphine, oxycodone) and 16 non-opioid-using patients showed no significant differences in pain and disability at 2-year follow-up
Menendez et al.	2015	Orthopedics	15,901 THA, TKA, TSA, and spine fusion patients with a diagnosis of opioid dependence or abuse had statistically significantly worsened morbidity and mortality outcomes than over 9 million controls
Hina et al.	2015	Orthopedics	28 opioid-using orthopedic patients displayed significantly greater hyperalgesia preoperatively, reported greater pain and consumed significantly more opioids postoperatively than 40 non-opioid-using controls
Morris et al.	2015	Orthopedics	32 Reverse TSA patients using chronic preoperative opioids had significantly worse outcomes of postoperative shoulder function including ROM compared to 36 controls
Morris et al.	2016	Orthopedics	60 TSA patients using chronic preoperative opioids had significantly worse outcomes of postoperative shoulder function including ROM and decreased satisfaction compared to 164 controls
Sing et al.	2016	Orthopedics	116 TKA and THA patients using preoperative opioids had significantly worse postoperative pain and increased opioid consumption, increased hospital LOS, admission to rehabilitation facilities, worsened surgical outcomes (including arthrofibrosis and periprosthetic fractures) compared to 58 non-opioid-using controls
Aasvang et al.	2016	Orthopedics	58 TKA patients using chronic preoperative opioids had significantly increased pain and opioid requirements within the first week of surgery compared to 57 non-opioid-using controls
Zarling et al.	2016	Orthopedics	106 TKA and THA using chronic preoperative opioids had greater likelihood of postoperative rehabilitation facility admission and significantly increased continued use of opioids 12 months postoperatively than 209 non-opioid-using controls
Nguyen et al.	2016	Orthopedics	
Faour et al.	2017	Spine	77 ACDF patients using chronic preoperative opioids had significantly lower incidence of return to work than 204 non-opioid-using controls
Tye et al.	2017	Spine	80 lumbar decompression patients from the worker's compensation population using chronic preoperative opioids greater than 3 months were significantly less likely to return to work than those ($n = 60$) using opioids less than 3 months preoperatively
Ben-Ari et al.	2017	Orthopedics	12,772 TKA patients using chronic preoperative opioids had significantly higher incidence of revision than 19,864 non-opioid-using controls

Table 1 Studies reporting outcomes following preoperative opioid use *(Continued)*

Authors	Year	Discipline	Findings
Smith et al.	2017	Orthopedics	36 TKA patients using chronic preoperative opioids had significantly worse pain 6 months postoperatively compared to 120 non-opioid-using controls
Waljee et al.	2017	General surgery	17,577 patients using chronic preoperative opioids had significantly longer hospital LOS, increased incidence of discharge to rehabilitation facilities and hospital readmission, and generated significantly higher financial expenditures than 182,428 controls
Villavicencio et al.	2017	Spine	60 TLIF patients using chronic preoperative opioids had significantly greater 12-month postoperative pain and disability compared to 33 non-opioid-using controls
Rozell et al.	2017	Orthopedics	275 TKA and THA patients using chronic preoperative opioids (compared to 527 controls) were shown in a regression model to be more likely to require increase perioperative opioids and increased hospital LOS as well as suffer higher incidence of complications
Chan et al.	2017	Orthopedics	36 TKA patients maintained on methadone preoperatively required greater postoperative opioids and inpatient pain management consultation, and had increased hospital LOS compared to 36 matched controls
Cheah et al.	2017	Orthopedics	138 TSA patients using chronic preoperative opioids had significantly greater postoperative pain and opioid use compared to 124 non-opioid-using controls

and Woolf 2009; Tracey and Mantyh 2007; Heinricher et al. 2009). While acute/nociceptive pain comprises a warning system alerting the organism to adopt avoidant behavior, it is now widely accepted (and supported by functional imaging evidence) that chronic pain for the most part represents maladaptive neuroplastic changes at the dorsal horn, and multiple higher (brain) centers including amygdala, hippocampus, insula, cingulate, and other parietal cortex areas and the prefrontal cortex (Flor et al. 1997; Tinazzi et al. 1998; Apkarian et al. 2004; Apkarian et al. 2005; Schmidt-Wilcke 2008; Rodriguez-Raecke et al. 2009; Baliki et al. 2010; Malinen et al. 2010; Apkarian et al. 2011; Farmer et al. 2012; Baliki et al. 2012).

Chronic opioid use is believed to reinforce this pathology, and again, functional neuroimaging studies seem to support shared neuroanatomic pathways and perturbances (Wanigasekera et al. 2011; Younger et al. 2011).

Chronic opioid use has also been shown to increase pain sensitivity via a process known as opioid-induced hyperalgesia (OIH). Distinct from tolerance, which represents an increasing threshold for analgesic responsiveness, OIH represents a reduced threshold for pain perception. Teleologically, the prolonged and imbalanced exogenous suppression of pain impulses to the brain should result in a reactionary increase in sensitivity to maintain homeostasis of this most critical protective sense. OIH is likely multifactorial with a host of postulated mechanisms including structural and functional alterations in opioid receptors, long-term potentiation at the dorsal horn, glial-mediated neuroinflammation, enhanced descending pain facilitation, and epigenetic factors (Lee et al. 2011; Roeckel et al. 2016; Weber et al. 2017). Once thought to require months of exposure to opioids, it is now recognized from animal and human investigations that OIH may occur with exposure as brief as days (Angst and Clark 2006; Compton et al. 2003;

Cooper et al. 2012) and the recent widespread use of intraoperative remifentanil infusions has demonstrated that exposure on the order of hours is sufficient (Guignard et al. 2000; Angst et al. 2003). There may be a dose-response effect (Salengros et al. 2010; Fechner et al. 2013; Fletcher and Martinez 2014; Mauermann et al. 2016).

A specific association between chronic preoperative opioid use and postoperative hyperalgesia has been demonstrated recently (Hina et al. 2015; Chapman et al. 2011). This may result from preoperative OIH persisting into the postoperative period or may be mediated more acutely by requisite increased intra- and postoperative opioid doses. The association may also be confounded in the perioperative setting by inadequate analgesia resulting from tolerance; increased immediate postoperative pain intensity has been shown to correlate with increased incidence of persistent postoperative hyperalgesia (Malik et al. 2017; Weinbroum 2017).

Regardless of the mechanisms involved, the study by Nguyen et al. (2016) showing improved pain and functional outcomes after even a 50% reduction in preoperative opioid burden argues convincingly in the context of the other literature reviewed herein for a concerted effort toward preoperative opioid reduction if not elimination. Additional supporting evidence for this tactic comes from the recent demonstration that downtitration of remifentanil infusion rates is associated with a lower incidence of OIH (Comelon et al. 2016).

The psychosocial complexity of chronic pain and opioid misuse

Chronic pain is also associated with psychological distress such as anxiety, post-traumatic stress disorder, borderline personality disorders, and to a lesser degree depression (Fishbain et al. 1998; Von Korff et al. 2005;

Gureje et al. 2008; Bushnell et al. 2013; Simons et al. 2014). The reported severity of such chronic pain has been shown to correlate much more closely with these psychosocial variables than with somatic contributors including injury severity, which has in fact been shown in several studies to be non-predictive (Harris et al. 2007; Jenewein et al. 2009; Trevino et al. 2013). These psychological/behavioral comorbidities have also been shown to predict chronic postoperative pain specifically (Kleiman et al. 2011; Theunissen et al. 2012; Attal et al. 2014; Hoofwijk et al. 2015).

The distinct construct of pain catastrophizing has received significant attention recently in the arenas of pain management and perioperative medicine. Pain catastrophizing is defined as persistent negative cognitive and affective responses to actual or anticipated pain (Quartana et al. 2009) and incorporates various degrees of magnification, rumination, and perception of helplessness (Sullivan et al. 1995). Pain catastrophizing and learned helplessness correlate with many of the underlying psychiatric comorbidities mentioned above and also independently confer worsened postoperative pain (Theunissen et al. 2012; Ip et al. 2009; Khan et al. 2011; Vissers et al. 2012; Denison et al. 2004) and surgical outcomes (Abbot et al. 2011, Coronado et al. 2015, Teunis et al. 2015)

All of these behavioral comorbidities are strongly associated with chronic opioid use, misuse, and dependence (Turk et al. 2008; Becker et al. 2008; Goldner et al. 2014; Gross et al. 2016; Arteta et al. 2016; McAnally 2017) and in fact have been shown repeatedly to be the most robust predictors (Martins et al. 2012; Katz et al. 2013; Blanco et al. 2013).

A final consideration related to the complex association of psychopathology, chronic pain, opioid use, and the perioperative arena is that patients suffering with chronic pain are more likely to seek not only opioid prescriptions, but also operative intervention. Among those patients struggling with chronic pain is a disproportionate number of individuals plagued with catastrophic thinking regarding pain, as well as poor self-efficacy. To quote Beth Darnall, a leading contemporary researcher in the field, "pain catastrophizing may speed the path to surgery while simultaneously undermining surgical response" (Darnall 2016). In other words, the path to the operating room may be disproportionately self-selected by the very people who are least likely to benefit from it, or who are the least prepared at any rate.

Over-eager desire for surgical intervention and persistent seeking of opioid prescriptions are both more likely to be associated with an external locus of control. While impossible to measure objectively, this lack of self-efficacy may in fact be the most important independent variable.

The rationale for preoperative opioid cessation and an effective biopsychosocial substitute

An increasing number of publications as well as our local survey of surgeons indicate the importance of preoperative opioid reduction. The survey results may be biased somewhat in terms of the importance associated to preoperative opioid reduction or elimination given our reputation and that of our preoperative optimization program within the community. Nonetheless, the literature does support both plausibility and rationality of this objective, and at an anecdotal level, anyone involved in perioperative care for more than a handful of years has learned the challenges involved in rendering opioid-tolerant patients comfortable in the post-anesthesia care unit and the ward, and surgeons and pain physicians are well aware of the difficulties they face afterward. As discussed above, there is growing recognition also that chronic preoperative opioid use confers postoperative problems beyond simple analgesic compromise. However, answering the question at hand, whether preoperative opioid reduction/elimination is beneficial in terms of outcome may be more difficult than appears on the surface. First of all, randomization is almost certainly not going to occur—patients either are or are not willing to reduce or eliminate their opioids preoperatively. Second, blinding would be nearly impossible in that the high probability of withdrawal symptoms would likely unmask treatment arms. Whether or not preoperative opioid reduction is beneficial must then most likely be judged from non-randomized prospective or retrospective studies, the plausibility of compelling "reverse" evidence such as the studies discussed herein, and common sense given the known associations between chronic opioid use and its harms.

Beyond mere opioid reduction/cessation, in view of the complex risk factors for chronic pain discussed briefly above, it stands to reason (and has been advocated by numerous experts, consensus groups, and clinical practice guidelines) (Veterans Health Administration and Department of Defense 2002; Chou et al. 2007; Federation of State Medical Boards 2013; United States Department of Health and Human Services 2016; Manchikanti et al. 2017) that a biopsychosocial-spiritual paradigm with particular focus upon enhancing resilience and diversify coping skills is required. Simply removing opioids without providing effective substitute coping mechanisms will invariably lead to non-compliance and dropout. A systematic, rigorous (e.g., weekly visit) program of opioid reduction/withdrawal palliation needs to be coupled with basic preoperative counseling addressing the replacement of multifactorial "wellness-killers" (e.g., poor self-valuation and esteem, unaddressed psychopathology, poor sleep, poor nutrition, sedentary lifestyle, tobacco use) with proactive steps supporting personal responsibility for health and wellness.

Growing recognition of the disproportionate impact of chronic pain syndromes upon operative outcomes in Canada has led to the establishment of what appears to be a promising, comprehensive approach to perioperative pain management for chronic pain patients with the Toronto General Transitional Pain Service (TPS) (Katz et al. 2015). The current iteration of the TPS involves five anesthesiology-based pain physicians, a palliative care specialist/family physician, two clinical psychologists and trainees, three acute pain nurse practitioners, two physical therapists with expertise in acupuncture, an exercise physiologist, and administrative staff (Katz et al. 2015).

The American Society of Anesthesiologists, among other organizations, has championed the concept of a Perioperative Surgical Home (PSH) (Desebbe et al. 2016) which is intended to address multiple perioperative health deficits at an institutional level. One of the theoretical functions of a PSH would be to address perioperative chronic pain management optimization including opioid reduction (Vetter and Kain 2017). A significant practical barrier however in the USA (with payer source fragmentation and limitations of reimbursement allocation) is actually coming up with the resources for such an effort. As noted by Vetter and Kain,

> How will an organization finance these additional resources necessary for a Transitional Pain Service? … A small community hospital may be hard-pressed to mobilize the comprehensive services and personnel required to successfully implement a full-scale perioperative Transitional Pain Service.

We propose that moving such perioperative chronic pain optimization functions outside of the institution to a smaller, leaner paradigm shaped by market pressures including outcomes-driven referral patterns will result in more efficient use of resources and improved care. Toward that end, we have created and begun implementation of a multidisciplinary preoperative optimization program for chronic pain patients focusing on a few high-yield areas of intervention, with opioid reduction and pain catastrophizing as two of the top priorities (as well as tobacco cessation and diet and activity improvements). The current iteration of the program comprises a 10–12-week course and incorporates traditional preoperative assessment and consultation issues (e.g., cardiac clearance and endocrinologic optimization) into a basic "wellness program" with simple, graded, measurable objectives including gentle opioid weaning along the lines of the fairly standard 10% per week paradigm (Manchikanti et al. 2017). Evidence from the behavioral world indicates that it takes at least 12 weeks to change habits (Lally et al. 2010);

moving such "pain prehabilitation" into the outpatient realm and allowing for adequate optimization time beforehand allows for such and furthermore overcomes the institutional-level problem of lack of resources by placing this critical component of healthcare into the hands of invested providers. While the cost of a dozen or so outpatient follow-up visits may seem formidable up front, it is exceeded by the cost of a single extra day in the hospital and pales in comparison to a canceled operation, or worst of all an adverse outcome.

Conclusions

The literature increasingly supports an association between preoperative opioid use and worsened postoperative pain, surgical outcomes, length of stay, and financial costs. Conversely, there is evidence that preoperative opioid reduction may result in substantial improvements in outcomes. In order to optimize chronic pain patients seeking surgery, we propose that addressing preoperative opioid reduction (among a handful of high-yield risk factors) is not only logical but also imperative. Simple opioid reduction/abstinence however is not likely to occur in the absence of provision of viable and palatable alternatives to managing pain, which will require a strong focus upon reducing pain catastrophization and bolstering self-efficacy and resilience, and nurturing a commitment to overall biopsychosocial-spiritual health. We have developed a simple and easy-to-implement outpatient preoperative optimization program focusing on gentle opioid weaning/elimination along with tobacco cessation, "de-catastrophization" and expectation management, and nutritional, sleep, and conditioning "prehabilitation." This 3-month program requires a minimum of resources and promises a good return on investment for chronic pain patients willing to exert a nominal degree of effort toward improving their surgical experience and outcome.

Abbreviations
BMI: Body mass index; ERAS: Enhanced Recovery After Surgery; LOS: Length of stay; OIH: Opioid-induced hyperalgesia; PSH: Perioperative Surgical Home; TPS: Transitional Pain Service

Acknowledgements
Jeanne Chapman, RN assisted in gathering of local surgeon data.

Funding
Not applicable.

Authors' contributions
The entire article was conceived and written by Dr. McAnally along with gathering of local surgeon data.

Competing interests

Dr. McAnally is the Medical Director of Northern Anesthesia & Pain Medicine, LLC, which is one of the two organizations that have created, copyrighted, and implemented the Valeras© Preoperative Optimization Program described herein.

References

Aasvang EK, Lunn TH, Hansen TB, Kristensen PW, Solgaard S, Kehlet H. Chronic pre-operative opioid use and acute pain after fast-track total knee arthroplasty. Acta Anaesthesiol Scand. 2016;60:529–36.

Abbott AD, Tyni-Lenne R, Hedlund R. Leg pain and psychological variables predict outcome 2–3 years after lumbar fusion surgery. Eur Spine J. 2011;20:1626–34.

Adriaensen H, Vissers K, Noorduin H, Meert T. Opioid tolerance and dependence: an inevitable consequence of chronic treatment? Acta Anaesthesiol Belg. 2003;54:37–47.

Anderson PA, Subach BR, Riew KD. Predictors of outcome after anterior cervical discectomy and fusion: a multivariate analysis. Spine (Phila Pa 1976). 2009;34:161–6.

Angst MS, Clark JD. Opioid-induced hyperalgesia: a qualitative systematic review. Anesthesiology. 2006;104:570–87.

Angst MS, Koppert W, Pahl I, Clark DJ, Schmelz M. Short-term infusion of the mu-opioid agonist remifentanil in humans causes hyperalgesia during withdrawal. Pain. 2003;106:49–57.

Apkarian AV, Bushnell MC, Treede RD, Zubieta JK. Human brain mechanisms of pain perception and regulation in health and disease. Eur J Pain. 2005;9:463–84.

Apkarian AV, Hashmi JA, Baliki MN. Pain and the brain: specificity and plasticity of the brain in clinical chronic pain. Pain. 2011;152(3 Suppl):S49–64.

Apkarian AV, Sosa Y, Sonty S, Levy RE, Harden RN, Parrish TB, et al. Chronic back pain is associated with decreased prefrontal and thalamic gray matter density. J Neurosci. 2004;24:10410–5.

Armaghani SJ, Lee DS, Bible JE, Archer KR, Shau DN, Kay H, et al. Preoperative opioid use and its association with perioperative opioid demand and postoperative opioid independence in patients undergoing spine surgery. Spine (Phila Pa 1976). 2014;39(25):E1524–30. https://doi.org/10.1097/BRS.0000000000000622.

Arteta J, Cobos B, Hu Y, Jordan K, Howard K. Evaluation of how depression and anxiety mediate the relationship between pain catastrophizing and prescription opioid misuse in a chronic pain population. Pain Med. 2016;17:295–303.

Attal N, Masselin-Dubois A, Martinez V, Jayr C, Albi A, Fermanian J, et al. Does cognitive functioning predict chronic pain? Results from a prospective surgical cohort. Brain. 2014;137:904–17.

Baliki MN, Geha PY, Fields HL, Apkarian AV. Predicting value of pain and analgesia: nucleus accumbens response to noxious stimuli changes in the presence of chronic pain. Neuron. 2010;66(1):149–60. https://doi.org/10.1016/j.neuron.2010.03.002.

Baliki MN, Petre B, Torbey S, Herrmann KM, Huang L, Schnitzer TJ, et al. Corticostriatal functional connectivity predicts transition to chronic back pain. Nat Neurosci. 2012;15:1117–9.

Becker WC, Sullivan LE, Tetrault JM, Desai RA, Fiellin DA. Non-medical use, abuse and dependence on prescription opioids among U.S. adults: psychiatric, medical and substance use correlates. Drug Alcohol Depend. 2008;94:38–47.

Ben-Ari A, Chansky H, Rozet I. Preoperative opioid use is associated with early revision after total knee arthroplasty: a study of male patients treated in the veterans affairs system. J Bone Joint Surg Am. 2017;99:1–9.

Blanco C, Rafful C, Wall MM, Jin CJ, Kerridge B, Schwartz RP. The latent structure and predictors of non-medical prescription drug use and prescription drug use disorders: a national study. Drug Alcohol Depend. 2013;133:473–9.

Bushnell MC, Ceko M, Low LA. Cognitive and emotional control of pain and its disruption in chronic pain. Nat Rev Neurosci. 2013;14:502–11.

Carroll I, Barelka P, Wang CK, Wang BM, Gillespie MJ, McCue R. A pilot cohort study of the determinants of longitudinal opioid use after surgery. Anesth Analg. 2012;115:694–702.

Chan FJ, Schwartz AM, Wong J, Chen C, Tiwari B, Kim SJ. Use of chronic methadone before total knee arthroplasty. J Arthroplast. 2017;32:2105–7.

Chang G, Chen L, Mao J. Opioid tolerance and hyperalgesia. Med Clin North Am. 2007;91:199–211.

Chapman CR, Davis J, Donaldson GW, Naylor J, Winchester D. Postoperative pain trajectories in chronic pain patients undergoing surgery: the effects of chronic opioid pharmacotherapy on acute pain. J Pain. 2011;12:1240–6.

Cheah JW, Sing DC, McLaughlin D, Feeley BT, Ma CB, Zhang AL. The perioperative effects of chronic preoperative opioid use on shoulder arthroplasty outcomes. J Shoulder Elb Surg. 2017; https://doi.org/10.1016/j.jse.2017.05.016.

Chou R, Qaseem A, Snow V, Casey D, Cross JT Jr, Shekelle P, et al. Diagnosis and treatment of low back pain: a joint clinical practice guideline from the American College of Physicians and the American Pain Society. Ann Intern Med. 2007;147:478–91. Erratum in: Ann Intern Med. 2008;148:247-8

Collett BJ. Opioid tolerance: the clinical perspective. Br J Anaesth. 1998;81:58–68.

Comelon M, Raeder J, Stubhaug A, Nielsen CS, Draegni T, Lenz H, Colvin L. Gradual withdrawal of remifentanil infusion may prevent opioid-induced hyperalgesia. Br J Anaesth. 2016;116:524–30.

Compton P, Athanasos P, Elashoff D. Withdrawal hyperalgesia after acute opioid physical dependence in nonaddicted humans: a preliminary study. J Pain. 2003; 4:511–9.

Cooper ZD, Sullivan MA, Vosburg SK, Manubay JM, Haney M, Foltin RW, et al. Effects of repeated oxycodone administration on its analgesic and subjective effects in normal, healthy volunteers. Behav Pharmacol. 2012;23:271–9.

Coronado RA, George SZ, Devin CJ, et al. Pain sensitivity and pain catastrophizing are associated with persistent pain and disability after lumbar spine surgery. Arch Phys Med Rehabil. 2015;96:1763–70.

Darnall BD. Pain psychology and pain catastrophizing in the perioperative setting: a review of impacts, interventions and unmet needs. Hand Clin. 2016;32:33–9.

Denison E, Åsenlöf P, Lindberg P. Self-efficacy, fear avoidance, and pain intensity as predictors of disability in subacute and chronic musculoskeletal pain patients in primary health care. Pain. 2004;111:245–52.

Desebbe O, Lanz T, Kain Z, Cannesson M. The perioperative surgical home: an innovative, patient-centred and cost-effective perioperative care model. Anaesth Crit Care Pain Med. 2016;35:59–66.

Faour M, Anderson JT, Haas AR, Percy R, Woods ST, Ahn UM, Ahn NU. Neck pain, preoperative opioids, and functionality after cervical fusion. Orthopedics. 2017;40:25–32.

Farmer MA, Baliki MN, Apkarian AV. A dynamic network perspective of chronic pain. Neurosci Lett. 2012;520:197–203.

Fechner J, Ihmsen H, Schuttler J, Jeleazcov C. The impact of intraoperative sufentanil dosing on postoperative pain, hyperalgesia and morphine consumption after cardiac surgery. Eur J Pain. 2013;17:562–70.

Federation of State Medical Boards. Model policy on the use of opioid analgesics in the treatment of chronic pain. 2013 Downloaded from http://www.fsmb.org/Media/Default/PDF/FSMB/Advocacy/pain_policy_july2013.pdf. Accessed 6 Aug 2017

Fishbain DA, Cutler BR, Rosomoff HL, Rosomoff RS. Comorbidity between psychiatric disorders and chronic pain. Curr Rev Pain. 1998;2:1–10.

Fletcher D, Martinez V. Opioid-induced hyperalgesia in patients after surgery: a systematic review and a meta-analysis. Br J Anaesth. 2014;112:991–1004.

Flor H, Braun C, Elbert T, Birbaumer N. Extensive reorganization of primary somatosensory cortex in chronic back pain patients. Neurosci Lett. 1997;224:5–8.

Goldner EM, Lusted A, Roerecke M, Rehm J, Fischer B. Prevalence of Axis-1 psychiatric (with focus on depression and anxiety) disorder and symptomatology among non-medical prescription opioid users in substance use treatment: systematic review and meta-analyses. Addict Behav. 2014;39:520–31.

Gross R, Long D, Cox S. (197) Predicting opioid misuse with a brief screener of catastrophizing. J Pain. 2016;17(4S):S25.

Guignard B, Bossard AE, Coste C, Sessler DI, Lebrault C, Alfonsi P, et al. Acute opioid tolerance: intraoperative remifentanil increases postoperative pain and morphine requirement. Anesthesiology. 2000;93:409–17.

Gureje O, Von Korff M, Kola L, Demyttenaere K, He Y, Posada-Villa J, et al. The relation between multiple pains and mental disorders: results from the world mental health surveys. Pain. 2008;135:82–91.

Hah JM, Sharifzadeh Y, Wang BM, Gillespie MJ, Goodman SB, Mackey SC, et al. Factors associated with opioid use in a cohort of patients presenting for surgery. Pain Res Treat. 2015;2015:829696. https://doi.org/10.1155/2015/829696.

Harris IA, Young JM, Rae H, Jalaludin BB, Solomon MJ. Factors associated with back pain after physical injury: a survey of consecutive major trauma patients. Spine (Phila Pa 1976). 2007;32:1561–5.

Heinricher MM, Tavares I, Leith JL, Lumb BM. Descending control of nociception: specificity, recruitment and plasticity. Brain Res Rev. 2009;60:214–25.

Hina N, Fletcher D, Poindessous-Jazat F, Martinez V. Hyperalgesia induced by low-dose opioid treatment before orthopaedic surgery: an observational case-control study. Eur J Anaesthesiol. 2015;32:255–61.

Hoofwijk DM, Fiddelers AA, Peters ML, Stessel B, Kessels AG, Joosten EA, et al. Prevalence and predictive factors of chronic postsurgical pain and poor global recovery one year after outpatient surgery. Clin J Pain. 2015; Epub

International Association for the Study of Pain. IASP sponsors global year against pain after surgery. 2017. Available at: https://www.iasp-pain.org/files/2017GlobalYear/News%20Release%20for%202017%20Global%20Year.pdf. Accessed 4 Aug 2017.

Ip HY, Abrishami A, Peng PW, et al. Predictors of postoperative pain and analgesic consumption: a qualitative systematic review. Anesthesiology. 2009;111:657–77.

Jenewein J, Moergeli H, Wittmann L, Büchi S, Kraemer B, Schnyder U. Development of chronic pain following severe accidental injury. Results of a 3-year follow-up study. J Psychosom Res. 2009;66:119–26.

Katz C, El-Gabalawy R, Keyes KM, Martins SS, Sareen J. Risk factors for incident nonmedical prescription opioid use and abuse and dependence: results from a longitudinal nationally representative sample. Drug Alcohol Depend. 2013; 132:107–13.

Katz J, Weinrib A, Fashler SR, Katznelson R, Shah BR, Ladak SS, et al. The Toronto General Hospital Transitional Pain Service: development and implementation of a multidisciplinary program to prevent chronic postsurgical pain. J Pain Res. 2015;8:695–702.

Kelly MP, Anderson PA, Sasso RC, Riew KD. Preoperative opioid strength may not affect outcomes of anterior cervical procedures: a post hoc analysis of 2 prospective, randomized trials. J Neurosurg Spine. 2015;23:484–9.

Khan RS, Ahmed K, Blakeway E, et al. Catastrophizing: a predictive factor for postoperative pain. Am J Surg. 2011;201:122–31.

Kleiman V, Clarke H, Katz J. Sensitivity to pain traumatization: a higher-order factor underlying pain-related anxiety, pain catastrophizing and anxiety sensitivity among patients scheduled for major surgery. Pain Res Manag. 2011;16:169–77.

Lally P, van CHM J, HWW P, Wardle J. How are habits formed: modelling habit formation in the real world. Eur J Soc Psychol. 2010;40:998–1009.

Latremoliere A, Woolf CJ. Central sensitization: a generator of pain hypersensitivity by central neural plasticity. J Pain. 2009;10:895–926.

Lawrence JT, London N, Bohlman HH, Chin KR. Preoperative narcotic use as a predictor of clinical outcome: results following anterior cervical arthrodesis. Spine (Phila Pa 1976). 2008a;(33):2074–8.

Lawrence JTR, London N, Bohlman HH, Chin KR. Preoperative narcotic use as a predictor of clinical outcome: results following anterior cervical arthrodesis. Spine. 2008b;33:2074–8.

Lee M, Silverman SM, Hansen H, Patel VB, Manchikanti L. A comprehensive review of opioid-induced hyperalgesia. Pain Physician. 2011;14:145–61.

Malik OS, Kaye AD, Urman RD. Perioperative hyperalgesia and associated clinical factors. Curr Pain Headache Rep. 2017;21:4.

Malinen S, Vartiainen N, Hlushchuk Y, Koskinen M, Ramkumar P, Forss N, et al. Aberrant temporal and spatial brain activity during rest in patients with chronic pain. Proc Natl Acad Sci U S A. 2010;107:6493–7.

Manchikanti L, Kaye AM, Knezevic NN, McAnally H, Slavin K, Trescot AM, et al. Responsible, safe, and effective prescription of opioids for chronic non-cancer pain: American Society of Interventional Pain Physicians (ASIPP) guidelines. Pain Physician. 2017;20(2S):S3–S92.

Martins SS, Fenton MC, Keyes KM, Blanco C, Zhu H, Storr CL. Mood/anxiety disorders and their association with non-medical prescription opioid use and prescription opioid use disorder: longitudinal evidence from the National Epidemiologic Study on alcohol and related conditions. Psychol Med. 2012;42:1261–72.

Mauermann E, Filitz J, Dolder P, Rentsch KM, Bandschapp O, Ruppen W. Does Fentanyl lead to opioid-induced hyperalgesia in healthy volunteers?: a double-blind, randomized. Crossover Trial Anesthesiology. 2016;124:453–63.

McAnally HB. Opioid dependence risk factors and risk assessment. In: McAnally HB, opioid dependence: a clinical and epidemiologic approach. New York: Springer. p. 2017.

Menendez ME, Ring D, Bateman BT. Preoperative opioid misuse is associated with increased morbidity and mortality after elective orthopaedic surgery. Clin Orthop Relat Res. 2015;473:2402–12.

Morris BJ, Laughlin MS, Elkousy HA, Gartsman GM, Edwards TB. Preoperative opioid use and outcomes after reverse shoulder arthroplasty. J Shoulder Elb Surg. 2015;24:11–6.

Morris BJ, Sciascia AD, Jacobs CA, Edwards TB. Preoperative opioid use associated with worse outcomes after anatomic shoulder arthroplasty. J Shoulder Elb Surg. 2016;25:619–23.

Nguyen LC, Sing DC, Bozic KJ. Preoperative reduction of opioid use before total joint arthroplasty. J Arthroplast. 2016;31(9 Suppl):282–7.

Pivec R, Issa K, Naziri Q, Kapadia BH, Bonutti PM, Mont MA. Opioid use prior to total hip arthroplasty leads to worse clinical outcomes. Int Orthop. 2014;38: 1159–65.

Quartana PJ, Campbell CM, Edwards RR. Pain catastrophizing: a critical review. Expert Rev Neurother. 2009;9:745–58.

Raebel MA, Newcomer SR, Reifler LM, Boudreau D, Elliott TE, DeBar L, et al. Chronic use of opioid medications before and after bariatric surgery. JAMA. 2013;310:1369–76.

Rodriguez-Raecke R, Niemeier A, Ihle K, Ruether W, May A. Brain gray matter decrease in chronic pain is the consequence and not the cause of pain. J Neurosci. 2009;29:13746–50.

Roeckel LA, Le Coz GM, Gavériaux-Ruff C, Simonin F. Opioid-induced hyperalgesia: cellular and molecular mechanisms. Neuroscience. 2016;338: 160–82.

Roullet S, Nouette-Gaulain K, Biais M, Bernard N, Bénard A, Revel P, et al. Preoperative opioid consumption increases morphine requirement after leg amputation. Can J Anaesth. 2009;56:908–13.

Rozell JC, Courtney PM, Dattilo JR, Wu CH, Lee GC. Preoperative opiate use independently predicts narcotic consumption and complications after total joint arthroplasty. J Arthroplast. 2017; https://doi.org/10.1016/j.arth.2017.04.002.

Rozet I, Nishio I, Robbertze R, Rotter D, Chansky H, Hernandez AV. Prolonged opioid use after knee arthroscopy in military veterans. Anesth Analg. 2014; 119:454–9.

Salengros J-C, Huybrechts I, Ducart A, Faraoni D, Marsala C, Barvais L, et al. Different anesthetic techniques associated with different incidences of chronic post-thoracotomy pain: low dose remifentanil plus pre-surgical epidural analgesia is preferable to high dose remifentanil with postsurgical epidural analgesia. J Cardiothorac Vasc Anesth. 2010;24:608–16.

Schmidt-Wilcke T. Variations in brain volume and regional morphology associated with chronic pain. Curr Rheumatol Rep. 2008;10:467–74.

Simons LE, Elman I, Borsook D. Psychological processing in chronic pain: a neural systems approach. Neurosci Biobehav Rev. 2014;39:61–78.

Sing DC, Barry JJ, Cheah JW, Vail TP, Hansen EN. Long-acting opioid use independently predicts perioperative complication in total joint arthroplasty. J Arthroplast. 2016;31(9 Suppl):170–4.

Smith SR, Bido J, Collins JE, Yang H, Katz JN, Losina E. Impact of preoperative opioid use on total knee arthroplasty outcomes. J Bone Joint Surg Am. 2017; 99:803–8.

Sullivan MJL, Bishop SR, Pivik J. The pain catastrophizing scale: development and validation. Psychol Assess. 1995;7:524–32.

Teunis T, Bot AG, Thornton ER, Ring D. Catastrophic thinking is associated with finger stiffness after distal radius fracture surgery. J Orthop Trauma. 2015 Oct; 29(10):e414–20.

Theunissen M, Peters ML, Bruce J, Gramke HF, Marcus MA. Preoperative anxiety and catastrophizing: a systematic review and meta-analysis of the association with chronic postsurgical pain. Clin J Pain. 2012;28:819–41.

Tinazzi M, Zanette G, Volpato D, Testoni R, Bonato C, Manganotti P, Miniuissi C, Fiachi A. Neurophysiological evidence of neuroplasticity at multiple levels of the somatosensory system in patients with carpal tunnel syndrome. Brain. 1998;121:1785–94.

Tracey I, Mantyh PW. The cerebral signature for pain perception and its modulation. Neuron. 2007;2:377–91.

Trevino CM, deRoon-Cassini T, Brasel K. Does opiate use in traumatically injured individuals worsen pain and psychological outcomes? J Pain. 2013;14:424–30.

Turk DC, Swanson KS, Gatchel RJ. Predicting opioid misuse by chronic pain patients: a systematic review and literature synthesis. Clin J Pain. 2008;24:497–508.

Tye EY, Anderson J, Faour M, Haas A, Percy R, Woods ST, Ahn UM, Ahn N. Prolonged preoperative opioid therapy in patients with degenerative lumbar stenosis in a workers' compensation setting. Spine (Phila Pa 1976). 2017; https://doi.org/10.1097/BRS.0000000000002112.

United States Department of Health and Human Services. National Pain Strategy: a comprehensive population health-level strategy for pain. 2016 Downloaded from https://iprcc.nih.gov/sites/default/files/HHSNational_Pain_Strategy_508C.pdf. Accessed 6 Aug 2017.

VanDenKerkhof EG, Hopman WM, Goldstein DH, Wilson RA, Towheed TE, Lam M, et al. Impact of perioperative pain intensity, pain qualities, and opioid use on chronic pain after surgery: a prospective cohort study. Reg Anesth Pain Med. 2012;37:19–27.

Veterans Health Administration and Department of Defense. VHA/DoD clinical practice guideline for the management of postoperative pain. 2002. Downloaded from https://www.healthquality.va.gov/guidelines/Pain/pop/pop_fulltext.pdf. Accessed 4 Aug 2017.

Vetter TR, Kain ZV. Role of the perioperative surgical home in optimizing the perioperative use of opioids. Anesth Analg. 2017; https://doi.org/10.1213/ANE.0000000000002280. [Epub ahead of print]

Villavicencio AT, Nelson EL, Kantha V, Burneikiene S. Prediction based on preoperative opioid use of clinical outcomes after transforaminal lumbar interbody fusions. J Neurosurg Spine. 2017;26:144–9.

Vissers MM, Bussmann JB, Verhaar JA, Busschbach JJ, Bierma-Zeinstra SM, Reijman M. Psychological factors affecting the outcome of total hip and knee arthroplasty: a systematic review. Semin Arthritis Rheum. 2012;41:576–88.

Von Korff N, Crane P, Lane M, Miglioretti DL, Simon G, Saunders K, et al. Chronic spinal pain and physical–mental comorbidity in the United States: results from the national comorbidity survey replication. Pain. 2005;113:331–9.

Waljee JF, Cron DC, Steiger RM, Zhong L, Englesbe MJ, Brummett CM. Effect of preoperative opioid exposure on healthcare utilization and expenditures following elective abdominal surgery. Ann Surg. 2017;265:715–21.

Wanigasekera V, Lee MC, Rogers R, Hu P, Tracey I. Neural correlates of an injury-free model of central sensitization induced by opioid withdrawal in humans. J Neurosci. 2011;31:2835–42.

Weber L, Yeomans DC, Tzabazis A. Opioid-induced hyperalgesia in clinical anesthesia practice: what has remained from theoretical concepts and experimental studies? Curr Opin Anaesthesiol. 2017;30:458–65.

Weinbroum AA. Postoperative hyperalgesia—a clinically applicable narrative review. Pharmacol Res. 2017;120:188–205.

Williams JT, Ingram SL, Henderson G, Chavkin C, von Zastrow M, Schulz S, et al. Regulation of μ-opioid receptors: desensitization, phosphorylation, internalization, and tolerance. Pharmacol Rev. 2013;65:223–54.

Younger JW, Chu LF, D'Arcy NT, Trott KE, Jastrzab LE, Mackey SC. Prescription opioid analgesics rapidly change the human brain. Pain. 2011;152:1803–10.

Zarling BJ, Yokhana SS, Herzog DT, Markel DC. Preoperative and postoperative opiate use by the arthroplasty patient. J Arthroplast. 2016;31:2081–4.

Zywiel MG, Stroh DA, Lee SY, Bonutti PM, Mont MA. Chronic opioid use prior to total knee arthroplasty. J Bone Joint Surg Am. 2011;93:1988–93.

13

The evaluation of risk prediction models in predicting outcomes after bariatric surgery

David Andrew Gilhooly[1,2,3*], Michelle Cole[3] and Suneetha Ramani Moonesinghe[1,4]

Abstract

Background: As the prevalence of obesity is increasing, the number of patients requiring surgical intervention for obesity-related illness is also rising. The aim of this pilot study was to explore predictors of short-term morbidity and longer-term poor weight loss after bariatric surgery.

Methods: This was a single-centre prospective observational cohort pilot study in patients undergoing bariatric surgery. We assessed the accuracy (discrimination and calibration) of two previously validated risk prediction models (the Physiological and Operative Severity Score for the enumeration of Morbidity and Mortality, POSSUM score, and the Obesity Surgical Mortality Risk Score, OS-MS) for postoperative outcome (postoperative morbidity defined using the Post Operative Morbidity Survey). We then tested the relationship between postoperative morbidity and longer-term weight loss outcome adjusting for known patient risk factors.

Results: Complete data were collected on 197 patients who underwent surgery for obesity or obesity-related illnesses between March 2010 and September 2013. Results showed POSSUM and OS-MRS were less accurate at predicting Post Operative Morbidity Survey (POMS)-defined morbidity on day 3 than defining prolonged length of stay due to poor mobility and/or POMS-defined morbidity. Having fewer than 28 days alive and out of hospital within 30 days of surgery was predictive of poor weight loss at 1 year, independent of POSSUM-defined risk (odds ratio 2.6; 95% confidence interval 1.28–5.24).

Conclusions: POSSUM may be used to predict patients who will have prolonged postoperative LOS after bariatric surgery due to morbidity or poor mobility. However, independent of POSSUM score, having less than 28 days alive and out of hospital predicted poor weight loss outcome at 1 year. This adds to the literature that postoperative complications are independently associated with poor longer-term surgical outcomes.

Keywords: Morbid obesity, Postoperative complications, Bariatric surgery, Risk assessment

Background

Obesity is one of the twenty-first century's pre-eminent public health problems. The World Health Organization (WHO) estimates that there are 2.3 billion overweight people globally, of which 700 million are obese (W.H.O

2018). A report by the UN Food and Agriculture Organization in 2013 showed that 24.9% of people in the United Kingdom (UK) were considered obese and that the UK was at the top of Europe's obesity league table (The State of Food and Agriculture 2013). In the United States of America (USA), the prevalence is even higher with data showing that more than one in three adults are considered obese (Flegal et al. 2012).

High levels of obesity put significant burden on health services as a result of associated comorbidities. It has been estimated that the direct cost to the NHS of

* Correspondence: davidg115@hotmail.com
[1]UCLH NIHR Surgical Outcomes Research Centre, Department of Anaesthesia and Perioperative Medicine, University College Hospital, London NW1 2BU, UK
[2]Department of Applied Health and Research, 1-19 Torrington Place, London WE1C 7HB, UK
Full list of author information is available at the end of the article

treating overweight and obese people was £4.2 billion in 2007 (Butland et al. 2007). The UK's National Bariatric Register shows that 53.9% of men and 41.4% of women had four or more obesity-related diseases at the time of primary surgery (Welbourn et al. 2014). However, significant improvement, if not resolution, of comorbidities can occur within 2 years of bariatric surgery (Welbourn et al. 2014; Arterburn and Courcoulas 2014; Colquitt et al. 2014) with long-term cost savings due to treatment of not just obesity, but obesity-related illnesses ((UK) NCGC 2014).

The UK second National Bariatric Register report has shown that 16,956 primary bariatric surgical procedures were performed between 2001 and 2013, 95% of which were performed laparoscopically. In this cohort, surgical complication rates were 2.9% and observed in-hospital mortality 0.07% (Welbourn et al. 2014). With such low mortality rates, monitoring morbidity or complications may provide clinicians and patients with more useful information on quality and variation in standards of care and provide a greater opportunity for performance improvement.

Although weight loss is not considered to be the most important outcome of bariatric surgery (rather, the aim is to support resolution of obesity-related illnesses), it is nevertheless an important proxy of surgical effectiveness (Welbourn et al. 2014). Factors that have been found to influence various outcomes include higher body mass index (BMI), age, increase in number of comorbidities and American Society of Anesthesiologists'-Physical Status (ASA-PS) (Colquitt et al. 2014; Abraham et al. 2015). Of note, postoperative complications can vary in incidence depending on the definition of complication being used.

Finding an accurate risk stratification tool is important so that patients at higher risk of postoperative morbidity can be identified and their perioperative pathway optimised to drive better surgical outcomes. Studies have previously looked at the OS-MRS as a tool for prediction of perioperative outcome with variable results (Coblijn et al. 2016; Lorente et al. 2014), but this scoring system was designed and validated as a predictor of mortality and not morbidity (DeMaria et al. 2007). The Physiology and Operative Severity Score for the enUmeration of Morbidity and Mortality has been previously suggested as the most well-validated risk stratification model for predicting morbidity in heterogeneous patient populations (Moonesinghe et al. 2013), but previous research in bariatric surgery found it overestimated postoperative morbidity (Charalampakis et al. 2014).

The aim of this study was to evaluate two previously developed and validated scores, the POSSUM and OS-MRS scores, for the prediction of postoperative morbidity and longer-term weight loss at 1 year. In addition, we also evaluated independent predictors for poor weight loss using multivariable analysis.

Methods

This single-centre observational cohort pilot study was approved by the University College London Hospitals NHS Foundation Trust's (UCLH) Research and Development office as a service evaluation. Between 01 March 2010 and 30 September 2013, data were collected prospectively on consecutive adult (> 18 years) patients undergoing bariatric surgery which included sleeve gastrectomy and laparoscopic Roux-en-Y gastric by-pass (RYGB) procedures at University College Hospital, a London teaching hospital.

Patient pathway

Patients initially attended a combined bariatric outpatient clinic where they were seen by the dietician, bariatric nurse specialist, bariatric surgeon and endocrinologist. Initial weights of patients were documented. Cases were then reviewed at a multidisciplinary meeting, and suitable cases were listed for surgery. After discharge from hospital, patients were followed up by the surgical bariatric team for outcomes and complications (Grocott et al. 2007) at regular intervals of 6 weeks and 3, 6, 12 and 18 to 24 months. Outpatient clinic weight measurements were routinely taken during follow-up appointments, and incidence of all complications were determined by case note review.

Predictor variables

Data were collected by a trained research team working within the UCLH NIHR Surgical Outcomes Research Centre (SOuRCe). Demographics collected on all patients included age, weight, BMI, ethnicity, gender, attendance to pre-assessment, comorbidities, American Society of Anesthesiologists' Physical Status, grade of attending surgeon and anaesthetist, operation performed, postoperative care ward and necessary investigations to calculate POSSUM and OS-MRS scores. The POSSUM score is calculated using a combination of 12 physiological and 6 operative data variables for each patient to calculate percentage risk. Originally developed in 1991 by Copeland et al. (Copeland et al. 1991), it has been evaluated widely, including in orthopaedic, vascular, head and neck and colorectal surgeries (Mohamed et al. 2002; Prytherch et al. 2001; Myers 1993; Griffiths et al. 2002; Tekkis et al. 2000). The OS-MRS uses a binary point scoring system based on five variables to stratify patients into three main groups (DeMaria et al. 2007). It is currently the most commonly used risk stratification tool for bariatric surgery (Daniel Guerron and Portenier 2016) and has been shown to be a useful tool for morbidity prediction as well (Lorente et al. 2014; Pinho et al. 2015).

Outcome measures

The primary outcome was poor weight loss, defined as < 50% percentage of excess body weight loss (EBWL) at 1 year postoperatively. Secondary outcomes included in-patient postsurgical morbidity, measured using the Post Operative Morbidity Survey (POMS) on day 3 after surgery (Grocott et al. 2007), and length of hospital stay. The POMS has been previously validated as a measure of morbidity which necessitates hospital admission (Grocott et al. 2007; Davies et al. 2013; Goodman et al. 2015). Day 3 POMS-defined morbidity was selected as the primary outcome measure as the national UK average postoperative stay has been reported as 2.7 days (Welbourn et al. 2014), and therefore, we hypothesised that day 3 morbidity would represent a departure from the usual postoperative pathway. If a patient was already discharged from hospital by day 3, the patient was recorded as being morbidity free, as previously described (Grocott et al. 2007). In order to capture the impact of serious adverse events occurring after the initial discharge from hospital, such as short-term mortality and hospital readmissions, we also report the composite endpoint of days alive and hospital free at 30 days postsurgery—this has been colloquially termed 'happy days' (Moonesinghe et al. 2017).

Statistical analysis

Continuous variables are presented as mean (SD) when normally distributed and median (range) when not (normality was assessed using the Stata 'sktest' for skewness and kurtosis in large sample sizes). Categorical variables are presented as n (%). Both POMS-defined morbidity according to the originally defined 9 physiological domains and prolonged length of stay due to failure to return to preoperative level of mobility were recorded and analysed separately. We tested the predictive accuracy (discrimination and calibration) of the ASA-PS score, (Saklad 1941) OS-MRS and POSSUM morbidity equation for predicting prolonged length of stay with morbidity defined using the POMS. Discrimination was assessed by analysing the area under the receiver-operator-characteristic curve (AUROC) and calibration measured, using the Hosmer-Lemeshow (HL) chi-squared statistic. A priori, we determined that AUROC > 0.9 would indicate good discrimination, 0.6–0.9 would indicate moderate and < 0.6 would indicate poor performance (Swets 1988). Calibration gives an estimation of how good the model is at predicting the probability of the event occurring across the full range of outcomes in that population. We assessed the calibration of the

POSSUM score, using the Hosmer-Lemeshow chi-squared statistic, with significance set at $p > 0.05$.

The morbidity prediction model with the highest discrimination was then used to adjust for patient risk factors in an analysis, which tested the independent relationship between postoperative morbidity and poor longer-term outcome (defined by EBWL less than 50% at 1 year follow-up).

Results (Fig. 1)

Baseline patient characteristics

Two hundred and thirty-one patients underwent bariatric surgery during the study period and had demographics collected by the SOuRCe team. This was then collated with the surgical postoperative database. One hundred and ninety-seven patients were included in the analyses. Demographics are shown in Table 1. All 197 patients had their weight recorded at 1 year.

POSSUM scores were calculated for all patients and divided into physiological, operative and total POSSUM scores. The median POSSUM physiology score was 14 (IQR 13–15), the median POSSUM operative score was 9 (IQR 9–9) and total POSSUM median score was 22 (IQR 22–24).

The most common procedure was a laparoscopic sleeve gastrectomy, (59.9%), followed by laparoscopic Roux-en-Y gastric by-pass procedures (38%). Of the remaining procedures, one was converted from a sleeve

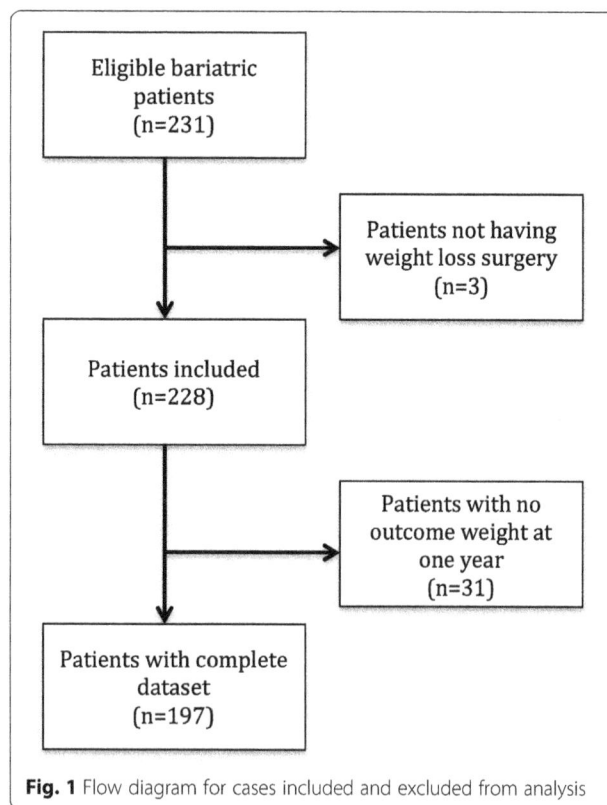

Fig. 1 Flow diagram for cases included and excluded from analysis

Table 1 Characteristics of patients with complete data collected

Characteristics	Complete data n = 197	No outcome weight n = 34	p
Mean age (SD)	45 years (12.8)	44.34 (11.6)	p = 0.63
Sex			
Male	21.3%	22.9%	p = 1.0
Female	79.7%	77.1%	
Ethnicity			
White British	68.5%	68.6%	p = 1.0
Other	31.5%	31.4%	
Attended pre-assessment	96.5%	91.4%	p = 0.072
Smoker			p = 0.199
Current	12.7%	11.4%	
Ex-smoker	25.4%	40%	
Non-smoker	61.9%	48.6%	
Alcohol			p = 0.251
Current drinker	52.2%	50%	
Non-drinker	47.8%	50%	
ASA-PS			p = 0.892
ASA 1	13.7%	8.5%	
ASA 2	67%	68.6%	
ASA 3	19.3%	20.0%	
ASA 4	0%	2.8%	
Diabetic			p = 0.73
Insulin controlled	3.6%	5.7%	
Tablet controlled	24.9%	17.1%	
Diet controlled	2%	2.9%	
Non-diabetic	69.5%	74.3%	
Other comorbidities			p < 0.001
Ischaemic heart disease	3%	0%	
Liver disease	1.5%	0%	
OS-MRS mean (SD)	1.09 (0.77)	1.17 (0.98)	p = 0.564
POSSUM physiology mean (SD)	14.48 (2.63)	15.6 (2.24)	p = 0.013
POSSUM operative mean (SD)	9.11 (0.64)	8.34 (0.94)	p < 0.001 95% CI (0.52–1.02)
Postoperative destination			p = 0.42
Intensive care	0.5%	0%	
Post anaesthetic care unit (PACU)	36.6%	45.7%	
Ward	62.9%	54.3%	

gastrectomy to a RYGB, one had a cholecystectomy with the procedure, one had a hiatus hernia repair and one was converted to an open procedure.

Postoperative outcomes

Postoperatively, 124 patients were admitted to the general ward (62.9%); 72 were admitted to post anaesthetic care unit (PACU) (36.5%), a high dependency unit designated for post surgical patients; and one was admitted to ICU. The median length of stay (LOS) was 2 days postoperatively (IQR range 2–3 days).

There were two inpatient hospital deaths (mortality = 0.85%); all patients who were discharged went home to their usual residence. Seventeen patients (8.6%) were readmitted within 30 days of hospital discharge, of whom seven had a readmission stay longer than 3 days. The date of readmission varied between 1 and 30 days post-discharge (median 4, IQR 2–19.5). The most common reason for re-admission was abdominal pain (8 patients—47% of readmissions or 4% of the total cohort), and 3 patients (17.6% of readmissions, 1.5% of the total cohort) had an anastomotic leak.

The mean %EBWL at 12 months was 56.86%, (SD 19.9%). Seventy-nine patients (40.1%) had an EBWL less than 50% at 1-year follow-up.

One hundred thirty-eight patients were discharged by day 3; thus, 59 patients (30%) remained in hospital and had day 3 POMS data collected. Table 2 shows the POMS-defined morbidity on days 3, 5, 7, 14 and 21.

Risk prediction according to POSSUM and OS-MRS
Both POSSUM and OS-MRS were less accurate in predicting POMS-defined morbidity on day 3 than predicting the composite of prolonged length of stay due to poor mobility and/or POMS-defined morbidity. Neither of these tools reached moderate predictive accuracy for predicting POMS-defined morbidity on day 3, but both were moderately accurate for predicting inpatient stay ≥ 3 days due to morbidity or poor mobility. In order to be able to evaluate the predictive accuracy of 'happy days' for poor weight loss at 1 year, we converted this into a binary variable for the purpose of estimating AUROC by assigning a poor outcome to patients who had less than 28 days alive and out of hospital (as the median length of stay of the primary admission was 2 days). In multivariable analysis, considering POSSUM-defined risk, age, and whether or not the patient had < 28 days alive and out of hospital by 30 days post-discharge, the only independent predictor of a poor EBWL outcome at 1 year

was having less than 28 days alive and out of hospital (odds ratio (OR) 2.6; 95% confidence interval (95% CI 1.28–5.24)) followed by age (OR 1.03; 95% CI 1.00–1.06) (Table 3).

Discussion
In this study, we report the accuracy of POSSUM and OS-MRS in predicting postoperative morbidity in patients undergoing bariatric surgery. Both were shown to be poor predictors of POMS-defined morbidity on day 3 but showed moderate accuracy at predicting inpatient LOS ≥ 3 days due to morbidity or poor mobility. The average LOS of bariatric patients postoperatively has been reported nationally as 2.7 days (Welbourn et al. 2014), so these tools may be useful in predicting patients who are at risk of increased resource utilization. In this analysis, the strongest independent predictor of poor weight loss at 1 year (< 50% EBLW) was the failure to have > 28 days alive and out of hospital within the first 30 days of surgery—a composite endpoint of death, length of hospital stay and readmission to hospital.

It is important to risk stratify patients for bariatric surgery in order to facilitate optimal allocation of resources. There is no previously validated risk tool for sleeve gastrectomies and RYGB procedures, which comprise the majority of bariatric procedures. Three US studies have evaluated morbidity risk prediction models for bariatric surgery, all of which used the American College of Surgeons National Surgical Quality Improvement Program (ACS-NSQIP) as their source of data. Turner et al. reviewed data from 2005 to 2008 and derived a normogram based on four factors (age, BMI, albumin and functional status); the C-statistic (which is equal to the

Table 2 Number (and percentage) of patients with POMS-defined morbidity for each collection day and the total inpatient number on that day (denominator 197 patients)

	POD 3 (%)	POD 5 (%)	POD 7 (%)	POD 14 (%)	POD 21 (%)
Number of patients in hospital	59 (30.0)	9 (4.6)	5 (2.5)	2 (1.0)	1 (0.5)
Number of patients POMS + (excluding mobility)	51 (25.9)	7 (3.5)	5 (2.5)	2 (1.0)	1 (0.5)
Respiratory	7 (3.5)	5 (2.5)	2 (1.0)	0	0
Infection	5 (2.5)	4 (2.0)	4 (2.0)	0	0
Renal	7 (3.5)	3 (1.5)	2 (1.0)	0	0
Gastrointestinal	48 (24.4)	3 (1.5)	3 (1.5)	1 (0.5)	0
Cardiovascular	3 (1.5)	0	0	0	1 (0.5)
Wound	3 (1.5)	3 (1.5)	1 (0.5)	0	0
Haematological	4 (2.0)	0	0	0	0
Neurological	0	0	0	0	0
Pain	9 (4.6)	2 (1.0)	1 (0.5)	1 (0.5)	0
Mobility	59 (29.9)	3 (1.5)	0	0	0

Note that mobility is not part of the original POMS domains but is widely used to help define reasons for continued hospital stay other than morbidity
POD postoperative day

Table 3 Discrimination and calibration of risk prediction tools for morbidity outcomes

	AUROC POMS-defined morbidity on D3: AUROC (95% CI; standard error)	HL statistic (p value)	AUROC POMS-defined morbidity or failure to return to preoperative mobility on D3	HL statistic (p value)	EBWL < 50% at 1 year	HL statistic (p value)	AUROC: < 28 days alive and out of hospital	HL statistic (p value)
POSSUM	0.60 (0.50–0.69; 0.04)	1.85 (0.87)	0.63 (0.55–0.72)	1.36 (0.93)	0.60 (0.52–0.69; 0.04)	11.64 (0.04)	0.66 (0.58–0.74; 0.04)	19.74 (0.47)
OS-MRS	0.62 (0.53–0.70; 0.05)	NA	0.63 (0.55–0.71)	NA	0.59 (0.50–0.67; 0.04)	NA	0.62 (0.55 0.70; 0.04)	NA

Note: No HL statistics calculated for the OS-MRS as this is an ordinal scale rather than providing a percentage prediction of the outcome
POSSUM Physiology and Operative Severity Score for the enUmeration of Morbidity and Mortality, OS-MRS Obesity Surgery Mortality risk Score, AUROC area under the receiver-operator-characteristic curve, HL statistic Hosmer-Lemeshow chi-squared statistic, POMS Post Operative Morbidity Survey, EBWL excess body weight loss

AUROC) in the validation cohort was 0.629 (Turner et al. 2011). Although this study analysed over 32,000 bariatric procedures, these did not include sleeve gastrectomies (Gupta et al. 2011). Gupta et al. derived a risk prediction model based on six factors using the 2007 ACS-NSQIP dataset: the variables included recent myocardial infarction/angina, functional status, stroke, bleeding disorder, hypertension, BMI and type of bariatric surgery. The C-statistic for this model was 0.66 (Gupta et al. 2011) with almost a third of the cases were gastric band procedures, which are less commonly performed now. More recently, Aminian et al. used the 2012 ACS-NSQIP dataset to develop a model for laparoscopic sleeve resections comprising seven variables (congestive heart failure, chronic steroid use, male sex, diabetes, preoperative serum bilirubin, BMI and preoperative haematocrit). This model appeared to be the most promising, with a C-statistic of 0.682 (Aminian et al. 2015).

Our analyses found that POSSUM and OS-MRS were moderately accurate for predicting stay ≥ 3 days due to morbidity and poor mobility, with AUROC 0.63 for both. They were less accurate in predicting POMS-defined morbidity on day 3. Although they have not been shown to be a significant predictor of EBWL at 1 year, they do predict increased length of stay in hospital. Using one of these systems in the preoperative assessment clinic may support clinicians in identifying patients who may benefit from admission to the PACU (Daniel Guerron and Portenier 2016) or more intensive after-care pathways, including physiotherapy and occupational therapy. Preoperative optimization of these patients, or pre-habilitation, may be also of benefit to this demographic as it can improve physical fitness, which can help to improve outcomes (West et al. 2015; Bond et al. 2015).

Independent of the patient's preoperative health status, a complicated postoperative course predicted poor weight loss at 1 year. This observation adds to the body of evidence that postoperative morbidity may have lasting impact on patient outcomes, which outlast the resolution of the overt complication, and which makes the prevention of postoperative morbidity an important goal of quality improvement (Moonesinghe et al. 2014; Khuri et al. 2005). Weight loss after bariatric surgery is not a certainty and requires the patient to be supported by a multidisciplinary team to achieve this. Patients require regular follow-up in the first 2 years post-surgery to ensure lifestyle changes occur, continued nutritional support and identify any maladaptive eating disorders (Metcalf et al. 2005). Postoperative surgical complications and prolonged recovery also have been shown to have an adverse effect on patient psychology (Pinto et al. 2016). Together, these factors may contribute to a poor outcome through lack of engagement and inability to access the necessary postoperative support as a result of their morbidity. In a patient population already at risk of depression (Carey et al. 2014), the added stress of complications may compound this risk and added to probable immobility as a result of postoperative complications, may result in a more sedentary lifestyle.

We also found an association between age and EBWL at 1 year, with a 3% increase in the risk of not achieving target weight loss, per year of advancing age. Previous analyses from large US cohorts have found conflicting evidence on this. A prospective observational study of 4776 patients evaluating 30-day outcomes (Flum et al. 2009) found no association between age and morbidity or mortality. A subsequent retrospective cohort analysis of 48,378 patients who underwent bariatric surgery in the 2005–2009 American College of Surgeons National Surgical Quality Improvement program (ACS-NSQIP) (Dorman et al. 2012) found older age was associated with prolonged LOS but not major adverse events. However, two more recent publications from the ACS-NSQIP of 44,408 (Khan et al. 2013) and 20,308 (Sanni et al. 2014) patients respectively showed an association between increasing age and morbidity and mortality. The latter study found that the odds of postoperative complications increased by 2% with each additional year of age. An analysis of 8945 patients from the Bariatric Outcome Longitudinal Database found that women and younger patients had significantly more weight loss (Van De Laar 2014).

Finally, comparing the POSSUM and OS-MRS, both show similar low accuracy in predicting postoperative morbidity at day 3 and moderate accuracy for predicting prolonged LOS due to morbidity or poor mobility, or 'happy days'. As there is no tool for prediction of morbidity related to current bariatric surgery practices, either of these could act as a tool. This paper also highlights the need for a larger study to define a risk prediction tool for morbidity in bariatric surgery.

Clinical implications

From this study, we can hypothesise that patients with a higher POSSUM score and older patients may benefit from more intensive perioperative care. Candidate interventions might include those which have been found to be associated with improved outcomes in other settings, such as goal-directed therapy, (Grocott et al. 2013; Hamilton et al. 2011), enhanced recovery (Grocott et al. 2012; Barreca et al. 2015) or admitting these patients to a critical care setting after surgery (Alfa Wali et al. 2014). However, randomised trials of these interventions in bariatric surgical patients are required to answer these questions.

Limitations

This study was undertaken at a single centre, and this may affect the generalizability of our findings. The psychological status of the patient plays an important role in the final surgical outcome after bariatric surgery; in our analyses, this factor was not taken into account for two reasons: not all patients had a psychological assessment prior to surgery and results of such an assessment can be difficult to describe quantitatively.

In our study, the postoperative morbidity rates appear much higher than those quoted from our national register (33 vs 2.9%). It has been shown that morbidity can vary widely between different studies, depending, at least in part, on how you classify complications (Colquitt et al. 2014). The comparatively high morbidity rate in our study is likely to be because the POMS include relatively minor morbidities; an alternative definition might be to describe this as 'absence of full recovery'. The most common type of morbidity on D3 was gastrointestinal, and in most cases, this was due to nausea, vomiting or abdominal distension—which would not commonly appear as a 'complication' in other classification systems.

Conclusion

As the demand for surgery to treat the obesity epidemic increases, it will become increasingly important to risk stratify patients in order to effectively plan perioperative care. The mortality associated with surgery is very low but there is a need to reduce postoperative morbidity, which can have an effect on hospital resource utilization and is associated with reduced postoperative weight loss. Although the POSSUM and OS-MRS scores have been shown in this study only to be moderately effective at predicting outcome for both sleeve gastrectomies and RYGB procedures, they are equivalent to previously published analyses of other models in large US cohorts (Turner et al. 2011; Gupta et al. 2011; Aminian et al. 2015). Further, none of these US models have been validated on populations of patients undergoing the two most common bariatric procedures undertaken currently. Validation of our findings in multi-centre cohorts would be of value.

Abbreviations

ACS-NSQIP: American College of Surgeons National Surgical Quality Improvement Program; ASA-PS: American Society of Anesthesiologists'-Physical Status; AUROC: Area under the receiver-operator-characteristic curve; BMI: Body mass index; CI: Confidence interval; EBWL: Excess body weight loss; HL: Hosmer-Lemeshow; IQR: Inter quartile range; LOS: Length of stay; NA: Not applicable; NHS: National Health Service; NIHR: National Institute for Health Research; OR: Odds ratio; OS-MRS: Obesity Surgical Mortality Risk Score; POMS: Post Operative Morbidity Survey; POSSUM: Physiology and Operative Severity Score for the enUmeration of Morbidity and Mortality; RYGB: Roux-en-Y gastric by-pass; SD: Standard deviation; SOuRCe: Surgical Outcomes Research Centre; UCLH: University College London Hospitals; UN: United Nations; WHO: World Health Organization

Acknowledgements

The authors acknowledged the University College London Hospital Surgical Outcomes Research Centre research staff, Ernesto Bettini and Denise Wyndham, and the surgical and anaesthesia staff involved in the care of these patients, Andrew Jenkinson, Majid Hashemi, Marco Adamo, James Holding, Viki Mitchell and Maan Hasan.

Funding

The UCLH Surgical Outcomes Research Centre is funded through Research Capability Funding from the UCLH NIHR Biomedical Research Centre (BRC); SRM also receives RCF funding from the UCLH NIHR BRC.

Authors' contributions

SRM conceived the study; DG, MC and SRM analysed the data; DG wrote the initial draft of the manuscript, and SRM revised the manuscript. All authors approved the final version.

Competing interests

The authors declare that they have no competing interests.

Author details

UCLH NIHR Surgical Outcomes Research Centre, Department of Anaesthesia and Perioperative Medicine, University College Hospital, London NW1 2BU, UK. [2]Department of Applied Health and Research, 1-19 Torrington Place, London WE1C 7HB, UK. [3]Bariatric Fellow, UCL Centre for Anaesthesia, University College London Hospital, London NW1 2BU, UK. [4]NIAA Health Services Research Centre, Churchill House, 35 Red Lion Square, London WC1R 4SG, UK.

References

(UK) NCGC. (2014). Obesity. http://www.ncbi.nlm.nih.gov/pubmed/25535639.

Abraham CR, Werter CR, Ata A, Hazimeh YM, Shah US, Bhakta A, et al. Predictors of hospital readmission after bariatric surgery. J Am Coll Surg. 2015;221: 220–7. https://doi.org/10.1016/j.jamcollsurg.2015.02.018.

Alfa Wali M, Ashrafian H, Schofield KL, Harling L, Alkandari A, Darzi A, et al. Is social deprivation associated with weight loss outcomes following bariatric surgery? A 10-year single institutional experience. Obes Surg. 2014;24:2126–32.

Aminian A, Brethauer SA, Sharafkhah M, Schauer PR. Development of a sleeve gastrectomy risk calculator. Surg Obes Relat Dis. 2015;11:758–64.

Arterburn DE, Courcoulas AP. Bariatric surgery for obesity and metabolic conditions in adults. BMJ. 2014;349:g3961.

Barreca M, Renzi C, Tankel J, Shalhoub J, Sengupta N. Is there a role for enhanced recovery after laparoscopic bariatric surgery? Preliminary results from a specialist obesity treatment center. Surg Obes Relat Dis. 2015; https://doi.org/10.1016/j.soard.2015.03.008.

Bond DS, Thomas JG, King WC, Vithiananthan S, Trautvetter J, Unick JL, et al. Exercise improves quality of life in bariatric surgery candidates: results from the Bari-Active trial. Obesity (Silver Spring). 2015;23:536–42. https://doi.org/10.1002/oby.20988.

Butland B, Jebb S, Kopelman P, McPherson K, Thomas S, Mardell J, et al. Foresight tackling obesities: future choices—project report, 2nd Edition p. 40. Gov Off Sci. 2007:1–161.

Carey M, Small H, Yoong SL, Boyes A, Bisquera A, Sanson-Fisher R. Prevalence of comorbid depression and obesity in general practice: a cross-sectional survey. Br J Gen Pract. 2014;64:e122–7.

Charalampakis V, Wiglesworth A, Formela L, Senapati S, Akhtar K, Ammori B. POSSUM and p-POSSUM overestimate morbidity and mortality in laparoscopic bariatric surgery. Surg Obes Relat Dis. 2014;10:1147–53.

Coblijn UK, Lagarde SM, de Raaff CAL, de Castro SMM, van Tets WF, Bonjer HJ, et al. Evaluation of the Obesity Surgery Mortality Risk Score (OS-MRS) for the prediction of postoperative complications after primary and revisional laparoscopic Roux-en-Y gastric bypass. Surg Obes Relat Dis. 2016; https://doi.org/10.1016/j.soard.2016.04.003.

Colquitt JL, Pickett K, Loveman E, Frampton GK. Surgery for weight loss in adults. Cochrane Database Syst Rev. 2014;8:CD003641. https://doi.org/10.1002/14651858.CD003641.pub4.

Copeland GP, Jones D, Walters M. POSSUM: a scoring system for surgical audit. Br J Surg. 1991;78:355–60. https://doi.org/10.1002/bjs.1800780327.

Daniel Guerron A, Portenier DD. Patient selection and surgical management of high-risk patients with morbid obesity. Surg Clin North Am. 2016;96:743–62. https://doi.org/10.1016/j.suc.2016.03.009.

Davies SJ, Francis J, Dilley J, Wilson RJT, Howell SJ, Allgar V. Measuring outcomes after major abdominal surgery during hospitalization: reliability and validity of the Postoperative Morbidity Survey. Perioper Med (London, England). 2013;2:1. https://doi.org/10.1186/2047-0525-2-1.

DeMaria EJ, Murr M, Byrne TK, Blackstone R, Grant JP, Budak A, et al. Validation of the obesity surgery mortality risk score in a multicenter study proves it stratifies mortality risk in patients undergoing gastric bypass for morbid obesity. Ann Surg. 2007;246:578–82. 584

Dorman RB, Abraham AA, Al-Refaie WB, Parsons HM, Ikramuddin S, Habermann EB. Bariatric surgery outcomes in the elderly: an ACS NSQIP study. J Gastrointest Surg. 2012;16:35–44.

Flegal KM, Carroll MD, Kit BK, Ogden CL. Prevalence of obesity and trends in the distribution of body mass index among US adults, 1999-2010. JAMA. 2012;307:491–7. https://doi.org/10.1001/jama.2012.39.

Flum DR, Belle SH, King WC, Wahed AS, Berk P, Chapman W, et al. Perioperative safety in the longitudinal assessment of bariatric surgery. N Engl J Med. 2009;361:445–54. https://doi.org/10.1056/NEJMoa0901836.

Goodman BA, Batterham AM, Kothmann E, Cawthorn L, Yates D, Melsom H, et al. Validity of the Postoperative Morbidity Survey after abdominal aortic aneurysm repair-a prospective observational study. Perioper Med. 2015;4:10. https://doi.org/10.1186/s13741-015-0020-1.

Griffiths H, Cuddihy P, Davis S, Parikh S, Tomkinson A. Risk-adjusted comparative audit. Is Possum applicable to head and neck surgery? Clin Otolaryngol Allied Sci. 2002;27:517–20.

Grocott MPW, Browne JP, Van der Meulen J, Matejowsky C, Mutch M, Hamilton MA, et al. The Postoperative Morbidity Survey was validated and used to describe morbidity after major surgery. J Clin Epidemiol. 2007;60:919–28.

Grocott MPW, Dushianthan A, Hamilton MA, Mythen MG, Harrison D, Rowan K. Perioperative increase in global blood flow to explicit defined goals and outcomes after surgery: a Cochrane Systematic Review. Br J Anaesth. 2013;111:535–48.

Grocott MPW, Martin DS, Mythen MG. Enhanced recovery pathways as a way to reduce surgical morbidity. Curr Opin Crit Care. 2012;18:385–92. https://doi.org/10.1097/MCC.0b013e3283558968.

Gupta PK, Franck C, Miller WJ, Gupta H, Forse RA. Development and validation of a bariatric surgery morbidity risk calculator using the prospective, multicenter NSQIP dataset. J Am Coll Surg. 2011;212:301–9.

Hamilton MA, Cecconi M, Rhodes A. A systematic review and meta-analysis on the use of preemptive hemodynamic intervention to improve postoperative outcomes in moderate and high-risk surgical patients. Anesth Analg. 2011;112:1392–402.

Khan MA, Grinberg R, Johnson S, Afthinos JN, Gibbs KE. Perioperative risk factors for 30-day mortality after bariatric surgery: is functional status important? Surg Endosc. 2013;27:1772–7. https://doi.org/10.1007/s00464-012-2678-5.

Khuri SF, Henderson WG, DePalma RG, Mosca C, Healey NA, Kumbhani DJ, et al. Determinants of long-term survival after major surgery and the adverse effect of postoperative complications. Ann Surg. 2005;242:326–43. https://doi.org/10.1097/01.sla.0000179621.33268.83.

Lorente L, Ramón JM, Vidal P, Goday A, Parri A, Lanzarini E, et al. Obesity surgery mortality risk score for the prediction of complications after laparoscopic bariatric surgery. Cir Esp. 2014;92:316–23. https://doi.org/10.1016/j.ciresp.2013.09.014.

Metcalf B, Rabkin RA, Rabkin JM, Metcalf LJ, Lehman-Becker LB. Weight loss composition: the effects of exercise following obesity surgery as measured by bioelectrical impedance analysis. Obes Surg. 2005;15:183–6.

Mohamed K, Copeland GP, Boot D a, Casserley HC, Shackleford IM, Sherry PG, et al. An assessment of the POSSUM system in orthopaedic surgery. J Bone Joint Surg Br. 2002;84:735–9.

Moonesinghe SR, Grocott MPW, Bennett-Guerrero E, Bergamaschi R, Gottumukkala V, Hopkins TJ, et al. American Society for Enhanced Recovery (ASER) and Perioperative Quality Initiative (POQI) joint consensus statement on measurement to maintain and improve quality of enhanced recovery pathways for elective colorectal surgery. Perioper Med. 2017;6:6. https://doi.org/10.1186/s13741-017-0062-7.

Moonesinghe SR, Harris S, Mythen MG, Rowan KM, Haddad FS, Emberton M, et al. Survival after postoperative morbidity: a longitudinal observational cohort study. Br J Anaesth. 2014;113:977–84.

Moonesinghe SR, Mythen MG, Das P, Rowan KM, Grocott MPW. Risk stratification tools for predicting morbidity and mortality in adult patients undergoing major surgery: qualitative systematic review. Anesthesiology. 2013;119:959–81. https://doi.org/10.1097/ALN.0b013e3182a4e94d.

Myers NA. Comparative vascular audit using the POSSUM scoring system. Ann R Coll Surg Engl. 1993;75:449.

Pinho S, Carvalho M, Soares M, Pinho D, Cavaleiro C, Machado HS. Obesity surgery mortality risk score: can we go beyond mortality prediction? J Anesth Clin Res. 2015;6:1–4.

Pinto A, Faiz O, Davis R, Almoudaris A, Vincent C. Surgical complications and their impact on patients' psychosocial well-being: a systematic review and meta-analysis. BMJ Open. 2016;6 http://bmjopen.bmj.com/content/6/2/e007224.abstract

Prytherch DR, Ridler BMF, Beard JD, Earnshaw JJ. A model for national outcome audit in vascular surgery. Eur J Vasc Endovasc Surg. 2001;21:477–83.

Saklad M. Grading of patients for surgical procedures. Anesthesiology. 1941;24:281–4.

Sanni A, Perez S, Medbery R, Urrego HD, McCready C, Toro JP, et al. Postoperative complications in bariatric surgery using age and BMI stratification: a study using ACS-NSQIP data. Surg Endosc Other Interv Tech. 2014;28:3302–9.

Swets JA. Measuring the accuracy of diagnostic systems. Science. 1988;240:1285–93. https://doi.org/10.1126/science.3287615.

Tekkis PP, Kocher HM, Bentley AJ, Cullen PT, South LM, Trotter GA, et al. Operative mortality rates among surgeons: comparison of POSSUM and p-POSSUM scoring systems in gastrointestinal surgery. Dis Colon rectum. 2000;43:1528–32.

The State of Food and Agriculture. (2013). Rome. http://www.fao.org/docrep/018/i3300e/i3300e.pdf.

Turner PL, Saager L, Dalton J, Abd-Elsayed A, Roberman D, Melara P, et al. A nomogram for predicting surgical complications in bariatric surgery patients. Obes Surg. 2011;21:655–62.

Van De Laar AWJM. Algorithm for weight loss after gastric bypass surgery considering body mass index, gender, and age from the Bariatric Outcome Longitudinal Database (BOLD). Surg Obes Relat Dis. 2014;10:55–61.

W.H.O. 2018 Obesity and overweight. Fact sheet. http://www.who.int/mediacentre/factsheets/fs311/en/.

Welbourn R, Small P, Finlay I, Sareela A, Somers S, Mahawar K. The National Bariatric Surgery Registry. 2014.

West MA, Loughney L, Lythgoe D, Barben CP, Sripadam R, Kemp GJ, et al. Effect of prehabilitation on objectively measured physical fitness after neoadjuvant treatment in preoperative rectal cancer patients: a blinded interventional pilot study. Br J Anaesth. 2015;114:244–51.

14

Total joint Perioperative Surgical Home

Darren R Raphael[1*], Maxime Cannesson[1], Ran Schwarzkopf[2], Leslie M Garson[1], Shermeen B Vakharia[1], Ranjan Gupta[2] and Zeev N Kain[1]

Abstract

Background: The numbers of people requiring total arthroplasty is expected to increase substantially over the next two decades. However, increasing costs and new payment models in the USA have created a sustainability gap. *Ad hoc* interventions have reported marginal cost reduction, but it has become clear that sustainability lies only in complete restructuring of care delivery. The Perioperative Surgical Home (PSH) model, a patient-centered and physician-led multidisciplinary system of coordinated care, was implemented at UC Irvine Health in 2012 for patients undergoing primary elective total knee arthroplasty (TKA) or total hip arthroplasty (THA). This observational study examines the costs associated with this initiative.

Methods: The direct cost of materials and services (excluding professional fees and implants) for a random index sample following the Total Joint-PSH pathway was used to calculate *per diem* cost. Cost of orthopedic implants was calculated based on audit-verified direct cost data. Operating room and post-anesthesia care unit time-based costs were calculated for each case and analyzed for variation. Benchmark cost data were obtained from literature search. Data are presented as mean ± SD (coefficient of variation) where possible.

Results: Total *per diem* cost was $10,042 ± 1,305 (13%) for TKA and $9,952 ± 1,294 (13%) for THA. Literature-reported benchmark *per diem* cost was $17,588 for TKA and $16,267 for THA. Implant cost was $7,482 ± 4,050 (54%) for TKA and $9869 ± 1,549 (16%) for THA. Total hospital cost was $17,894 ± 4,270 (24%) for TKA and $20,281 ± 2,057 (10%) for THA. In-room to incision time cost was $1,263 ± 100 (8%) for TKA and $1,341 ± 145 (11%) for THA. Surgery time cost was $1,558 ± 290 (19%) for TKA and $1,930 ± 374 (19%) for THA. Post-anesthesia care unit time cost was $507 ± 187 (36%) for TKA and $557 ± 302 (54%) for THA.

Conclusions: Direct hospital costs were driven substantially below USA benchmark levels using the Total Joint-PSH pathway. The incremental benefit of each step in the coordinated care pathway is manifested as a lower average length of stay. We identified excessive variation in the cost of implants and post-anesthesia care.

Keywords: Perioperative surgical home, Perioperative practice model, Perioperative care pathway, Total arthroplasty, Cost analysis, Cost variation

Background

Total knee arthroplasty (TKA) and total hip arthroplasty (THA) show high cost–utility, cost-effectiveness, and cost–benefit over other interventions [1-3]. However, the cost of care delivery in the USA has increased to the point that total arthroplasty (TA) is now the largest expenditure per procedure in Centers for Medicare and Medicaid Services (CMS)-provided interventions [4]. Coupled with declining reimbursement, hospitals have struggled to maintain profitability for these procedures. The passage of the Affordable Care Act and implementation of performance-based bundled payments threatens to exacerbate this sustainability gap if significant cost-control measures are not implemented. Furthermore, as the 'baby boomer' generation ages and obesity continues to rise in the general population, the demand for primary TKA and THA in the USA is expected to increase substantially over the next two decades [5,6].

* Correspondence: raphaeld@uci.edu
[1]Department of Anesthesiology and Perioperative Care, University of California, 333 The City Boulevard West, Suite 2150, Orange, Irvine, California 92868, USA
Full list of author information is available at the end of the article

It is well established that costs for TA during the initial hospital stay are mostly driven by three major factors: implant cost, hospital length of stay (LOS), and operating room (OR) cost [4,7-9]. Implant cost has increased sharply over the past two decades, with many new and more complex options brought to market. Implant cost minimization strategies may be found in the literature, including implant standardization, group purchasing, gain sharing, price ceilings, and the creation of a national joint database to track outcomes and inform purchasing decisions. LOS reduction efforts have examined modern surgical techniques and multimodal pain management, and described post-operative clinical pathways that employ early mobilization and rehabilitation as well as reduction of post-operative complications. OR cost reduction has focused mainly on surgical techniques and operational efficiency. These *ad hoc* interventions have been shown to reduce costs marginally in USA hospitals, but none has addressed the broader issue of a fragmented and inefficient perioperative system. The transition to performance-based bundled payments in the USA has illustrated the need for the adoption of perioperative practice models similar to those that have been in place in Europe for over a decade with proven financial benefits.

We submit that sustainable cost reduction lies only in a complete restructuring of how TA care is delivered. The Perioperative Surgical Home (PSH) is a recently proposed perioperative practice model in the USA. The goal of the PSH is to improve clinical outcomes while providing better perioperative service to patients at lower cost [10,11]. This model has been described as a 'patient-centered and physician-led multidisciplinary and team-based system of coordinated care that guides the patient throughout the entire surgical experience.' The first PSH program was implemented at UC Irvine Health in 2012 for all elective TKA and THA [12,13]. The intent of the program is to support the orthopedic surgeon, ensure adherence to mutually agreed-upon protocols, and manage medical issues that arise during the episode of care. The surgeon's role as ultimate decision-maker is maintained. A major aim of the Total Joint-PSH protocol is to reduce variation in care delivery, which will in turn reduce cost and improve outcomes [4,12-15]. This observational study examines the cost and cost variation associated with the Total Joint-PSH, and compares to reported benchmarks.

Methods

We performed an observational cost analysis for patients undergoing primary unilateral elective THA or TKA under the Total Joint-PSH model at UC Irvine Health between October 1, 2012 and September 30, 2013. Institutional review board approval was obtained with the purpose of analyzing and reporting our results, and patient

Table 1 Components of *per diem* cost

Time-based	Non time-based
Operating room time	Equipment
Post-anesthesia care unit time	Materials
	Laboratory
	Pharmacy
	Physical therapy
	Room and board

consent was waived (IRB HS#2012-9273). The implementation of the Total Joint-PSH program at our institution has been described in detail elsewhere [12,13].

Implementing the Total Joint-PSH program

The Total Joint-PSH program was created prior to reestablishment of an arthroplasty center at UC Irvine Health in 2012. The lack of an existing program allowed all stakeholders (including orthopedic surgeons, anesthesiologists, acute pain physicians, nurses, rehabilitation specialists, and hospital administrators) to have a voice in its design and implementation. All team members were trained in Lean Six Sigma (LSS), and agreed to adhere to the concepts of standardization and reduced variability. The goal of this process was to integrate four distinct perioperative phases: pre-operative, intra-operative, post-operative and post-discharge. A value stream map (flow diagram documenting in high detail every step of the process) was created for each perioperative phase. The pre-operative process incorporates expectation management, early discharge planning, protocol-driven health risk assessment, and medical optimization. Standardized anesthetic, nursing, and surgical care protocols, as well as Goal Directed Fluid Therapy (GDFT) underpin the intra-operative component. Post-operative management provides for multimodal analgesia, a targeted recovery plan, early ambulation, nutrition management, and prompt rescue from complications. Post-discharge care begins in

Table 2 Demographics of the included patients[a]

	TKA (n = 129)	THA (n = 77)
Age	65 ± 10.53	64 ± 13.82
BMI	30.7 ± 5.7	28.5 ± 7.2
Spinal anesthesia	61%	57%
General anesthesia	39%	43%
ASA grading		
I	0%	1%
II	15%	21%
III	79%	73%
IV	6%	5%

ASA, American Society of Anesthesiologists Physical Status; BMI, body mass index; THA, total hip arthroplasty; TKA, total knee arthroplasty.
[a]Data are expressed as mean ± SD.

Table 3 Summary of costs[a]

Costs	TKA	THA
Per diem cost (LOS = 3 days)	$10,042 ± 1305 (13%)	$9,952 ± 1294 (13%)
Orthopedic materials and implants	$7,482 ± 4050 (54%)	$9,869 ± 1549 (16%)
Total cost	$17,524 ± 4255 (24%)	$19,821 ± 2018 (10%)

LOS, length of stay; THA, total hip arthroplasty; TKA, total knee arthroplasty.
[a]Data are expressed as mean ± SD (coefficient of variation).

the hospital with coordinated transition to an appropriate rehabilitation setting. Once the perioperative pathways were fully vetted, the Total Joint-PSH program was officially launched on October 1, 2012.

Cost analysis

Per diem cost analysis

The direct cost of materials and services (excluding professional fees and implants) provided during each hospital day of care were obtained from the UC Irvine Health financial decision support office. Data were provided for a randomly chosen index sample (n = 29 or 14%) of patients who had undergone unilateral primary arthroplasty following the Total Joint-PSH pathway. Data from this sample were used to determine average per diem cost for each day of admission. Components of per diem cost are presented in Table 1. Per diem cost for post-operative day (POD) 0 included costs incurred during pre-operative health risk assessment and optimization in the operating room (OR) and in the post-anesthesia care unit (PACU). The cost of pre-operative orthopedic clinic professional visits was not included. Costs incurred during POD 1 to 3 included room and board as well as all activities related to recovery and discharge planning. The previously reported average LOS for the Total Joint-PSH was 2.7 ± 0.64 days for TKA and 2.6 ± 0.67 for THA [12], thus a conservative value of 3 days LOS was used to calculate total per diem cost.

Specialized orthopedic materials and implant cost analysis

All specialized orthopedic materials and implants used in the OR were recorded by nursing staff intra-operatively, and verified by the revenue audit department. Data from all patients (n = 206) undergoing elective primary unilateral TKA and THA were used to examine the cost of orthopedic materials and implants. The average cost of orthopedic materials and implants was calculated using the acquisition cost.

Total cost analysis

Total cost for primary TKA and THA performed as part of the Total Joint-PSH program was calculated as the sum of the total per diem cost, orthopedic materials cost, and implant cost. Total cost for was calculated for all cases.

Determination of OR and PACU cost per minute

The cost of OR time was calculated in the following manner. Aggregate direct cost data for the index patient sample was obtained from the decision support office. OR-related costs (excluding implants) were identified. Materials typically used during the first 30 minutes of OR time were also identified. Two average total costs were calculated, one for the first 30 minutes and one for costs incurred thereafter. Total OR time was obtained by database query of the intra-operative electronic medical record (EMR) (Surgical Information Systems, LLC, Alpharetta, GA, USA). Using these data, a cost per minute was calculated for the first 30 minutes and for subsequent OR time. An analogous process was performed to obtain cost per minute values for PACU time.

OR and PACU time variation and cost analysis

Total OR and PACU times were determined by database query of the intra-operative and post-operative EMR for all patients undergoing elective unilateral primary TKA and THA. In-room to incision time and surgical time

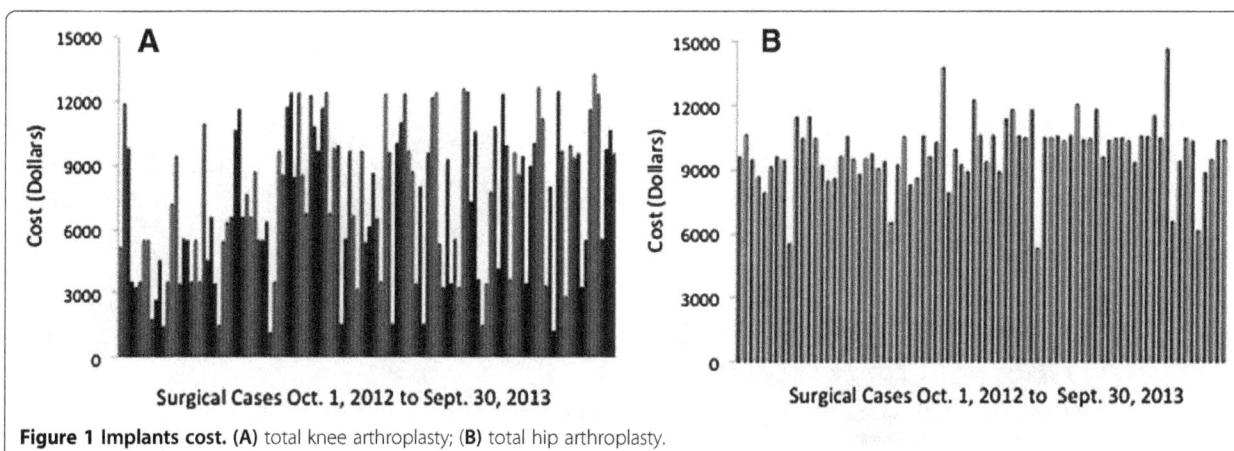

Figure 1 Implants cost. (A) total knee arthroplasty; **(B)** total hip arthroplasty.

Table 4 Summary of OR time costs[a]

	TKA	THA
In-room to incision time cost	$1,263 ± 100 (8%)	$1,341 ± 145 (11%)
Surgery time cost	$1,558 ± 290 (19%)	$1,930 ± 374 (19%)
PACU time cost	$507 ± 187 (36%)	$557 ± 302 (54%)
Total OR & PACU time cost	$3,329 ± 350 (11%)	$3,828 ± 559 (16%)

OR, operating room; PACU, post-anesthesia care unit; THA, total hip arthroplasty; TKA, total knee arthroplasty.
[a]Data are expressed as mean ± SD (coefficient of variation).

were also obtained. Using the calculated cost per minute values, a time-based cost was determined for the components of each case.

Data analysis

Variation in cost was assessed using coefficient of variation (defined as SD/mean). Data are presented as mean ± SD (coefficient of variation). All statistics were performed using SPSS software version 11.0 (SPSS Inc., Chicago, IL, USA).

Results

In total, 206 (n = 129 for TKA and n = 77 for THA) sequential patients undergoing unilateral primary TA were enrolled in the Total Joint-PSH protocol. Demographics are presented in Table 2.

Total cost analysis

A summary of costs (*per diem* cost, orthopedic materials and implants cost, and total calculated cost) is presented in Table 3. Individual cost of implants for all cases is presented in Figure 1.

Time-based cost analysis

A summary of OR time costs is presented in Table 4. Individual case costs (in-room to incision time cost, surgery time cost, PACU time cost, and total OR and PACU time cost) for TKA and THA are presented in Figure 2 and Figure 3, respectively.

Discussion

Our analysis shows a low total cost for unilateral primary TKA and THA in the setting of the first Total Joint-PSH. Prior to implementation of the Total Joint-PSH program, our institution had no active arthroplasty program. This study is observational in nature, and no comparison with prior costs was made. We sought instead to benchmark our cost data against figures reported in the literature. A recent retrospective study of

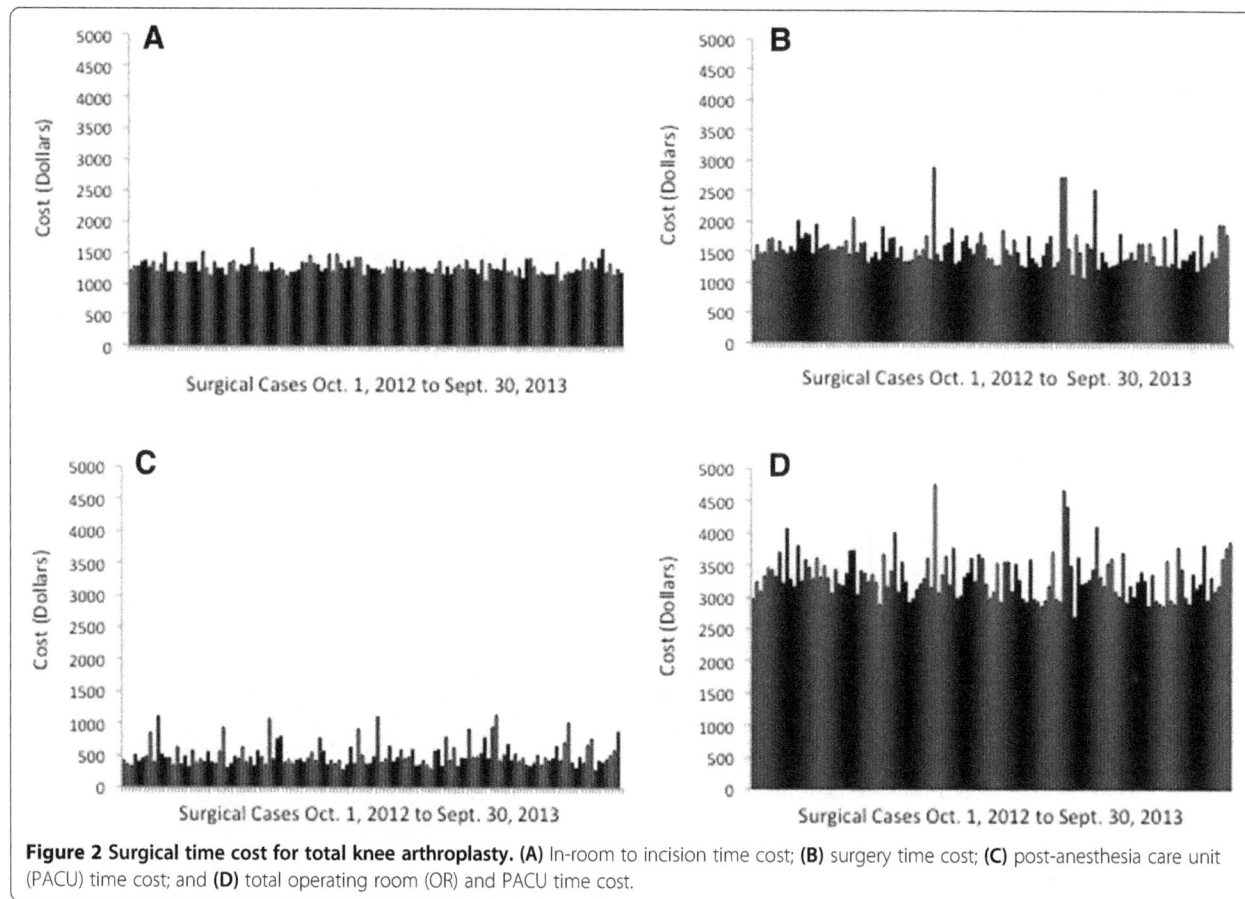

Figure 2 Surgical time cost for total knee arthroplasty. (A) In-room to incision time cost; **(B)** surgery time cost; **(C)** post-anesthesia care unit (PACU) time cost; and **(D)** total operating room (OR) and PACU time cost.

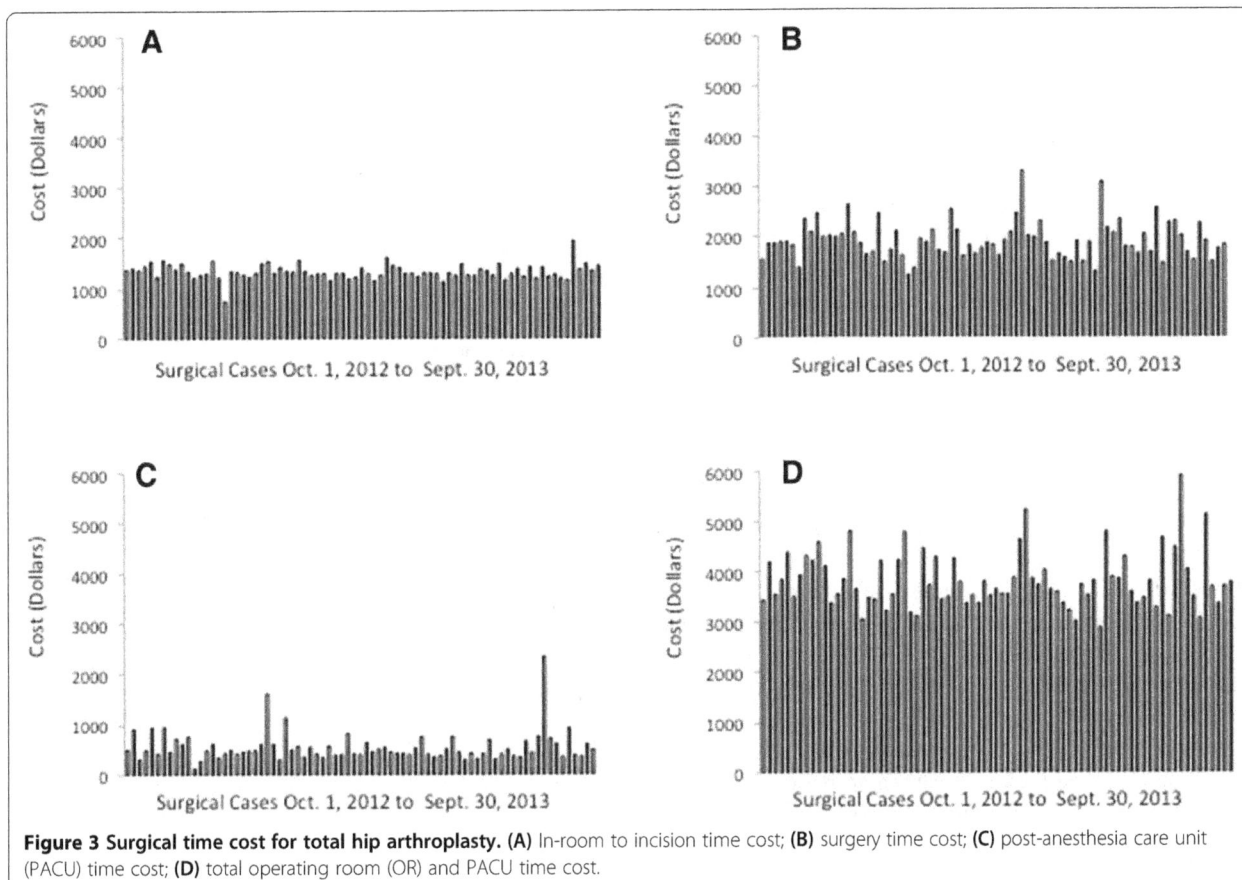

Figure 3 Surgical time cost for total hip arthroplasty. (A) In-room to incision time cost; **(B)** surgery time cost; **(C)** post-anesthesia care unit (PACU) time cost; **(D)** total operating room (OR) and PACU time cost.

primary total joint arthroplasty (TJA) found an average hospital cost (episode cost excluding implants) of $17,588 for TKA and $16,267 for THA. Hospital episode cost for the Total Joint-PSH patient at our institution ($10,042 ± 1305 for TKA and $9,952 ± 1294 for THA) was found to be significantly below this benchmark (Table 5). The reduced LOS in our institution (4 versus 3 days) is a major factor in this comparative cost reduction. We contend that the incremental benefit of each step in the Total Joint-PSH coordinated care pathway is manifested as a low average LOS (rapid recovery). Cost savings attributed to reduced LOS must be considered in the context of equivalent outcomes, as complications can contribute substantially to the overall cost of arthroplasty. We have previously reported low complication and re-admission rates for patients in the Total Joint-

PSH compared with published data [12], but the contribution of complications to overall cost of care was not considered in this analysis.

The second largest cost driver was identified as cost of implants $7,482 ± 4,050 (TKA) and $9,869 ± 1,549 (THA). Implant cost was recently examined in the literature, and found to range from $1,797 to $12,093 (TKA) and $2,392 to $12,361 (THA) [9]. Implant cost at our institution was within this benchmark range. However, the cost of implants was the largest source of cost variation in the Total Joint-PSH, at 54% (TKA) and 16% (THA). Variation in implant cost is appropriate as a reflection of patient demographics and underlying conditions, particularly in the setting of a tertiary care academic center. However, a component of this variation can be attributed to other factors. UC Irvine Health is currently engaged in an initiative to reduce implant cost variability and overall implant cost.

Operating room and PACU cost was determined using a time-based cost analysis. It has been argued that reduction in OR time does not result in cost savings unless enough time is saved to add an additional case during regular operating hours. This reasoning presumes all OR costs are fixed; however, a number of OR resources (such as staffing) are variable direct costs that can be reallocated if OR time is reduced. Determination of the

Table 5 Benchmark cost comparison: average hospital cost excluding implants[a]

	Total Joint-PSH	Benchmark [16]
TKA	$10,042 ± 1,305	$17,588
THA	$9952 ± 1,294	$16,267

PSH, perioperative surgical home; THA, total hip arthroplasty; TKA, total knee arthroplasty.
[a]Data are expressed as mean ± SD.

time-based cost can help to identify areas for OR cost savings and illustrate the importance of operational efficiency. We examined variation in terms of cost rather than time because our model assigns a higher cost to the initial 30 minutes of OR and PACU times. In our analysis, variation in OR time cost for the Total Joint-PSH was found to be low. Cost associated with in-room to incision time varied by 8% (TKA) and 11% (THA). We attribute this low variation to a well-defined, time-limited decision tree for conversion of difficult neuraxial to general anesthesia. Cost associated with surgery time varied by 19% (TKA and THA). Relatively low variation in these parameters enables predictable optimization of OR scheduling. Excessive variation of 36% (TKA) and 54% (THA) was found in the PACU time cost analysis. The data showed several outliers, which upon initial investigation were attributable to limited availability of beds in the orthopedic ward at the desired time of PACU discharge. This finding has alerted the Total Joint-PSH team to the need for further study and an LSS analysis of this process step.

Minimizing direct hospital costs without improvement in care or outcomes may simply shift cost to the post-discharge arena. The cost of orthopedic rehabilitation hospital care, home-based care, emergency room visits, complications, and readmissions must be closely tracked. A recent study of TJA costs found that post-discharge payments accounted for an average of 36% of total episode of care payments [16]. The current observational cost analysis of the Total Joint-PSH cohort did not consider post-discharge care, and some component of cost shifting may exist. We recognize this as a challenging and pressing area of future study.

The PSH is a care delivery model that has been endorsed by the American Society of Anesthesiologists (ASA), with the goal of improving clinical outcomes while providing better perioperative service at lower cost. Future studies will be geared toward comparing the PSH with other models of care.

Conclusions

We found that direct hospital costs can be driven substantially below benchmark levels using the Total Joint-PSH pathway, and suggest that implementation of a PSH model of care could help institutions to better control process costs and identify unwarranted costs. In the case of the Total Joint-PSH, we have identified an opportunity to decrease variation in the cost of implants and the cost of PACU time.

Abbreviations

ASA: American Society of Anesthesiologists; BMI: Body mass index; CMS: Centers for Medicaid and Medicare; EMR: Electronic medical record; GDFT: Goal directed fluid therapy; LOS: Length of Stay; LSS: Lean Six Sigma; OR: Operating room; PACU: Post-anesthesia care unit; POD: Post-operative day; PSH: Perioperative Surgical Home; TA: Total arthroplasty; THA: Total hip arthroplasty; TJA: total joint arthroplasty; TKA: Total knee arthroplasty.

Competing interests

RS performs consulting work for Smith & Nephew, owns stock in Gauss Surgical and Pristine and does research for Pricria; LMG owns stock warrants in Pristine; and SBV has received a fellowship grant from The Center for Healthcare Quality and Innovation for Urology Surgical Home. The other authors have no competing interests to declare.

Authors' contributions

DR participated in study design, was responsible for data acquisition, performed statistical analysis and figure design, and authored the manuscript; MC participated in study design, performed statistical analysis and figure design, and co-authored the manuscript; RS participated in study design, contributed to data analysis, and co-authored the manuscript; LG participated in study design, contributed to data acquisition, and co-authored the manuscript;. SV participated in study design and co-authored the manuscript; MC participated in study design and co-authored the manuscript; and ZK participated in study design, contributed to data analysis and co-authored the manuscript. All authors read and approved the final manuscript.

Acknowledgements

We thank Morris Frieling for providing cost data and Kwang Pak for assistance with data analysis.

Author details

[1]Department of Anesthesiology and Perioperative Care, University of California, 333 The City Boulevard West, Suite 2150, Orange, Irvine, California 92868, USA. [2]Department of Orthopedic Surgery, University of California, 101 The City Drive South Pavilion III, Building 29A Orange, Irvine, California 92868, USA.

References

1. Chang RW, Pellisier JM, Hazen GB: A cost-effectiveness analysis of total hip arthroplasty for osteoarthritis of the hip. JAMA 1996, 275:858–865.
2. Bozic KJ, Saleh KJ, Rosenberg AG, Rubash HE: Economic evaluation in total hip arthroplasty: analysis and review of the literature. J Arthroplasty 2004, 19:180–189.
3. Kumar S, Williams AC, Sandy JR: How do we evaluate the economics of health care? Eur J Orthod 2006, 28:513–519.
4. Bosco JA, Alvarado CM, Slover JD, Iorio R, Hutzler LH: Decreasing total joint implant costs and physician specific cost variation through negotiation. J Arthroplasty 2014, 29:678–680.
5. Rana AJ, Iorio R, Healy WL: Hospital economics of primary THA decreasing reimbursement and increasing cost, 1990 to 2008. Clin Orthop Relat Res 2011, 469:355–361.
6. Lovald ST, Ong KL, Malkani AL, Lau EC, Schmier JK, Kurtz SM, Manley MT: Complications, mortality, and costs for outpatient and short-stay total knee arthroplasty patients in comparison to standard-stay patients. J Arthroplasty 2014, 29:510–515.
7. Healy WL, Iorio R, Richards JA, Lucchesi C: Opportunities for control of hospital costs for total joint arthroplasty after initial cost containment. J Arthroplasty 1998, 13:504–507.
8. Healy WL, Ayers ME, Iorio R, Patch DA, Appleby D, Pfeifer BA: Impact of a clinical pathway and implant standardization on total hip arthroplasty: a clinical and economic study of short-term patient outcome. J Arthroplasty 1998, 13:266–276.
9. Robinson JC, Pozen A, Tseng S, Bozic KJ: Variability in costs associated with total hip and knee replacement implants. J Bone Joint Surg Am 2012, 94:1693–1698.
10. Schweitzer M, Fahy B, Leib M, Rosenquist R, Merrick S: The Perioperative Surgical Home Model. Am Soc Anesthesiol News Lett 2013, 77(6):58–59.
11. Oravetz P, Kelchlin A: Driving value through clinical practice variation reduction. In Presented at 2013 Healthcare Systems Process Improvement Conference. New Orleans: 2013 [http://www.iienet2.org/uploadedFiles/SHSNew/Feature%201%20Paper%20Ochsner%20Joint%20Improvement.pdf]

12. Garson L, Schwartzkopf R, Vakharia S, Alexander B, Stead S, Cannesson M, Kain ZN: Implementation of a total joint replacement-focused perioperative surgical home: a management case report. *Anesth Analg* 2014, **118**(5):1081–1089.
13. Kain ZN, Vakharia S, Garson L, Engwall S, Schwarzkopf R, Gupta R, Cannesson M: The Perioperative Surgical Home as a future perioperative practice model. *Anesth Analg* 2014, **118**(5):1126–1130.
14. Vetter TR, Boudreaux AM, Jones KA, Hunter JM, Pittet JF: The Perioperative Surgical Home: how anesthesiology can achieve and leverage the triple aim in healthcare. *Anesth Analg* 2014, **118**(5):1131–1136.
15. Vetter TR, Goeddel LA, Boudreaux AM, Hunt TR, Jones KA, Pittet JF: The Perioperative Surgical Home: how can it make the case so everyone wins? *BMC Anesthesiol* 2013, **13**:615.
16. Kozma CM, Slaton T, Paris A, Edgell ET: Cost and utilization of healthcare services for hip and knee replacement. *J Med Econ* 2013, **16**(7):888–896.

Perioperative corticosteroid administration

C. Groleau[1], S. N. Morin[2], L. Vautour[3], A. Amar-Zifkin[4] and A. Bessissow[2*]

Abstract

Background: Perioperative administration of corticosteroid is common and variable. Guidelines for perioperative corticosteroid administration before non-cardiac non-transplant surgery in patients with current or previous corticosteroid use to reduce the risk of adrenal insufficiency are lacking. Perioperative use of corticosteroid may be associated with serious adverse events, namely hyperglycemia, infection, and poor wound healing.

Objective: To determine whether perioperative administration of corticosteroids, compared to placebo or no intervention, reduces the incidence of adrenal insufficiency in adult patients undergoing non-cardiac surgery who were or are exposed to corticosteroids.

Methods: We searched MEDLINE via Ovid and PubMed, EMBASE via Ovid, and the Cochrane Central Register of Controlled Trials, all from 1995 to January 2017.

Selection criteria: We included randomized controlled trials (RCTs), cohort studies, case-studies, and systematic reviews involving adults undergoing non-cardiac non-transplant surgery and reporting the incidence of postoperative adrenal insufficiency.

Data collection and analysis: Two authors independently assessed studies' quality and extracted data. A descriptive and bias assessment analysis was performed.

Results: Two RCTs (total of 37 patients), five cohort studies (total of 462 patients), and four systematic reviews were included. Neither RCT showed a significant difference in the outcome. This result was like that of the five cohort studies. The quality of the evidence was low.

Conclusion: The current use of perioperative corticosteroid supplementation to prevent adrenal insufficiency is not supported by evidence. Given the significant studies' limitations, it is not possible to conclude that perioperative administration of corticosteroids, compared to placebo, reduces the incidence of adrenal insufficiency.

Background

It is increasingly common to encounter patients undergoing surgery who are on chronic corticosteroids or who have received large amounts of corticosteroids (Ergina et al. 1993). When evaluating the risk of adrenal insufficiency, it becomes a challenge for physicians to decide whether additional corticosteroid administration is required perioperatively.

Administration of stress-dose corticosteroids perioperatively for patients on long-term corticosteroid therapy began following the publication of two case reports in the 1950s. This happened despite the uncertainty regarding whether the patients in the case reports actually died of Addisonian crisis (Fraser et al. 1952; Lewis et al. 1953). Four decades later, a literature review demonstrated only three cases out of 57 in which death or hypotension could clearly be attributed to perioperative adrenal crisis in patients on long-term corticosteroid therapy (Salem et

* Correspondence: amal.bessissow@mcgill.ca
[2]Department of Medicine, Division of General Internal Medicine, McGill University Health Centre, Montreal, Canada
Full list of author information is available at the end of the article

al. 1994). More recently, studies have raised concern that supplementing corticosteroids in the perioperative period may lead to poorer postoperative outcomes as it may be associated with hyperglycemia, infectious complications, venous thromboembolism (VTE), poor surgical site healing, and increased length of stay (LOS) (Mathis et al. 2004; Nguyen et al. 2014; Gribsholt et al. 2015; Toner et al. 2017).

Because clinical guidelines are lacking, physicians face the challenge of balancing the risk of adrenal insufficiency in the perioperative period with the risk of postoperative complications related to corticosteroids. Therefore, we conducted a systematic review to answer the following question: In adult patients undergoing non-cardiac non-transplant surgery and who were or are exposed to corticosteroids, does the perioperative administration of corticosteroids, compared to placebo or no intervention, reduce the incidence of adrenal insufficiency?

Methods
Study design and participants
We included French or English language randomized controlled trials (RCTs), cohort studies (retrospective and prospective), case studies, and systematic reviews (SRs). We included articles involving humans aged ≥ 18 years old undergoing any type of surgery except cardiac surgery and transplant surgery. We excluded articles involving participants with primary adrenal insufficiency. We included articles evaluating the effect of corticosteroid administered preoperatively, regardless of the timing of administration and the duration of the corticosteroid and if corticosteroid were administered pre and post operatively. We included articles that compare corticosteroid administration to placebo, to standard of care/conventional management, or to no intervention. Articles reporting outcomes related to adrenal crisis such as hypotension, refractory hypotension, syncope, were included. Appendix 1 presents the study inclusion criteria in Table 1.

Information sources and search methods
We searched MEDLINE via Ovid, supplemented with a PubMed search for unindexed or in-process articles, EMBASE via Ovid, and the Cochrane Central Register of Controlled Trials. All databases were searched from 1995 to January 2017. We hand-searched the reference lists of all relevant articles. Refer to Additional file 1 for literature search strategies, Additional file 2 for screening forms, and Appendix 2 for methods of study selection, data collection process, and bias assessment methods.

Synthesis of results
Studies review revealed a wide variability in population characteristics, types of surgery, intervention, and outcomes. Since studies' characteristics were not conducive to quantitative analysis, we performed a descriptive analysis. Each study selected was summarized and assessed for risk of bias (refer to Appendix 4 and Additional file 3).

Results
Study selection
Our search strategy identified 995 unique references (refer to Appendix 3 for study flow diagram). Following independent assessment of the abstracts and titles by two authors (AB, CG), we identified 48 articles for full-text assessment. Of these, 37 did not fulfill inclusion criteria. Following discussions, the two authors were in full agreement in the selection of the studies.

Study characteristics and results
Eleven studies met selection criteria: two RCTs, five cohort studies, and four SRs. The results are discussed herein and summarized in Additional file 4. Refer to Appendix 4 for risk of bias assessment of RCTs. Refer to Additional file 3 for the risk of bias assessment of cohort studies.

Randomized controlled trials
Glowniak and Loriaux (1997) published the first RCT on the subject. Eighteen patients who had been taking prednisone (mean dose of 14 mg daily) over the past 2 months and with confirmed secondary adrenal insufficiency by Cortrosyn stimulation tests were randomized to continue their usual prednisone dose and either received 100 mg of hydrocortisone (HC) before entering the operating room (OR) followed by 25 mg every 6 h for 48 h then a taper or a placebo regimen of normal saline (NS). Most subjects ($N = 16$) underwent elective moderate risk surgeries such as abdominal surgeries or total knee arthroplasty. One patient in the placebo group had a significant episode of hypotension during the operation that improved following fluid administration. One patient in the corticosteroid-treated group had acute symptomatic hypotension 2 h after surgery from excess opioid administration. During the postoperative period, the blood pressure (BP), pulse rates, and postoperative complications such as fever or infection did not differ significantly between the two groups. The results of this study are limited by the small sample size. The authors note that their study could have been larger but they chose to exclude patients with a normal Cortrosyn stimulation test as well as patients undergoing surgeries they believed were

not physiologically very stressful such as transurethral biopsies of the prostate.

The second RCT, by Thomason et al. (1999), studied 20 organ transplanted patients undergoing gingival over-growth surgery under local anesthesia. All patients were on corticosteroids for ≥ 6 months prior to OR; the average daily prednisone at time of surgery was 7.9 mg. As each patient had overgrowth requiring two surgeries, each patient acted as their own control. Immediately before surgery, patients received either intravenous HC 100 mg or placebo in random, double-blind order. There was no significant difference in BP throughout surgery and postoperatively, and in ACTH measurements on com-pletion of surgery. The main limitation of this study is its small number of participants. The applicability of the study's findings is also limited by the studied surgi-cal procedure. Lastly, dental procedure under local anesthesia would generally not be considered as physio-logically stressful.

Cohort studies

Aytac et al. (2013) retrospectively analyzed patients with ulcerative colitis (UC) exposed to corticosteroids in the previous year who had undergone a restorative procto-colectomy and categorized them into two groups based on whether they received stress-dose corticosteroids. Among patient on corticosteroids up to the surgery, doses were similar among patients. Neither the mean nor median doses were reported. One hundred milli-grams of HC were administered intravenously immedi-ately before surgery, then 100 mg dose was administered every 8 h for the first 24 h and then tapered off. Pa-tients who were on corticosteroids until surgery re-ceived their regular corticosteroid regimen during the perioperative period. Eighty-nine patients received stress-dose corticosteroids and 146 patients did not. Stress-dose corticosteroids were more frequently ad-ministered to patients who were receiving chronic cor-ticosteroids until the time of surgery (37.1 vs 10.3%; $p < 0.001$). Sinus tachycardia developed more frequently in patients who received stress-dose corticosteroids during surgery (21.5 vs 17.8%; $p = 0.03$). One patient in the stress-dose corticosteroid group died on post-operative day 25 because of an anastomotic leak. There was no significant difference in bradycardia, BP and in postoperative complications including surgical site infection, anastomotic leak, hemorrhage, VTE, and LOS. This study was limited by its retrospective design, no matching of patients, and small number of adverse events. Also, the use of stress-dose corticoste-roids was not determined by uniform criteria as the physicians planned corticosteroids regimen at their discretion.

The following year, Lamore et al. (2014) retrospectively examined inflammatory bowel disease (IBD) patients exposed to corticosteroids within the previous year, undergoing colorectal surgery. Patients were divided into three groups at the time of surgery: [1] > 1 week of prior corticosteroid exposure, not receiving maintenance therapy ($n = 15$); [2] currently receiving budesonide ($n = 10$); and [3] currently receiving oral prednisone ($n = 24$). They received intraoperative corticosteroids, as follows: 8 patients (53%) in group 1, 7 (70%) in group 2, and 20 (83%) in group 3. Despite this being a IBD referral center, there was significant variability in postoperative GC dosing practices, particularly in patients who were receiving prednisone at the time of admission. The median intra-operative HC dose was 100 mg (range, 50–267 mg); the median total postoperative dose for the first 5 days after surgery was 485 mg (range, 50–890 mg). No patients had postoperative hemodynamic instability requiring intervention. No statistically significant difference in surgical site infection and 30-day re-admission rates were detected. This study was limited by its retrospective design, no matching of patients, very small sample size, and lesser number of events. Given the small sample size, they were unable to establish a statisti-cally significant difference in patient outcomes with and without perioperative corticosteroid exposure. The study also only evaluated in-hospital tapers, thus these findings likely underestimate the perioperative corticosteroid exposure.

Zaghiyan et al. (2011) retrospectively studied 49 consecu-tive corticosteroid-treated patients with IBD undergoing major colorectal surgery. Patients off corticosteroids at the time of surgery but previously treated with ≥ 5 mg of oral prednisone daily for > 1 week within the previous year were also included. Preoperative median maximum corticosteroid dose was prednisone 25 mg daily (range 5–60 mg), and the mean time from last corticosteroid dose to surgery was 4 months. Patients received either high-dose steroid (HSD group) consisting of HC 100 mg IV prior to OR then 100 mg IV every 8 h for 24 h followed by a taper, or no corticosteroids. The regimen choice was at the discre-tion of the surgeon. Aside from a higher incidence of tachycardia in the HDS group (82 vs 42%, $p = 0.04$), there was no significant difference in hemodynamic instability. One patient in the no corticosteroids group required a single dose of intraoperative vasopressor after aggressive beta-blockade. There was no significant difference in postoperative complications. This study was limited by its small sample size and by limitations in chart docu-mentation as to the precise preoperative corticosteroid doses and duration between corticosteroid therapy and surgery.

A year later, the same authors published a prospective cohort study of 32 consecutive corticosteroid-treated IBD patients undergoing major colorectal surgery (Zaghiyan et al. 2012a). Patients who were on corticosteroids preoperatively received a low-dose corticosteroid regimen (LDS). This consisted of one third of the IV HC equivalent of the daily preoperative corticosteroid dose (IVED) prior to OR, then one-third IVED every 8 h for the first 24 h, followed by one quarter IVED every 8 h. Patients who had previously been treated with corticosteroids but who were not on corticosteroid therapy at the time of operation were given no perioperative corticosteroids. Patient selection for this regimen was at the discretion of the surgeon. Five patients (23%) developed intra-operative or postoperative hypotension, all in the group not taking corticosteroids at the time of surgery. In all cases, hypotension resolved either spontaneously or with fluid bolus which allowed the authors to conclude that in steroid-treated IBD patients undergoing major colorectal surgery, the use of low-dose perioperative corticosteroids seems safe. This study was limited by its small sample size and by limitations in chart documentation as to the precise preoperative corticosteroid doses and duration between corticosteroid therapy and surgery. In addition, it is difficult to comment on the clinical importance of hemodynamic instability, fever, and hypothermia and surgical outcomes without a comparison group of patients treated with high-dose corticosteroids.

Subsequently, the same team published a retrospective study of 97 IBD patients on corticosteroids or who had previously been on corticosteroids undergoing major colorectal surgery (Zaghiyan et al. 2012b). Patients received one of two perioperative corticosteroid dosing regimens: HDS or LDS regimen as described in their previous studies (Zaghiyan et al. 2011, 2012a). Patients off corticosteroids at the time of surgery who were assigned to the LDS treatment group received no perioperative corticosteroids. In patients on corticosteroids at the time of surgery ($n = 48$), there was a significantly higher incidence of overall hemodynamic instability in the LDS group (16/16, 100%) compared with the HDS group (23/32, 72%) ($p = 0.02$). However, these differences in hemodynamic instability appeared to be clinically insignificant, as in 36 of the 39 patients' hemodynamic instability resolved with no intervention, fluid bolus, or blood transfusion. Three patients in the LDS group were treated with vasopressors. This study was limited by its small sample size and small number of events. It had a high risk of selection bias as the LDS algorithm was gradually implemented over time and was dependent on surgeon preference. At the beginning of the study period, LDS were administered to low-risk patients at the attending surgeons' discretion, with time it was then implemented for patients on higher dose of corticosteroids.

Systematic reviews

A total of four SRs met our inclusion criteria. de Lange and Kars (2008) included studies analyzing the need for perioperative corticosteroid supplementation, whether these studies included a stress-dose corticosteroid regimen or not. The same year, Marik and Varon (2008) undertook a SR, including RCTs comparing stress doses of corticosteroids with placebo and cohort studies that followed patients after surgery in which perioperative stress doses of corticosteroids were not administered. Yong et al. published a Cochrane SR including only two RCTs in 2009 and then an updated review in 2012 comparing use of supplemental perioperative corticosteroids to placebo in adults on maintenance doses of corticosteroids (Yong et al. 2009, 2012). The latter review was withdrawn from publication in 2013 due to questionable eligibility criteria and interpretation of summarized evidence. In all four SRs, authors highlighted that available evidence on this topic is limited by studies with small sample sizes and flawed methodology. de Lange and Kars and Marik and Varon concluded that in patients receiving long-term adrenally suppressive doses of corticosteroids, the combination of the patient's baseline exogenous corticosteroid plus endogenous corticosteroid production is possibly adequate to meet the demands of the physiologic stress of surgery. As for Yonge et al., given the poor level of evidence available, they decided not to support nor to refute the use of perioperative corticosteroids in patients with adrenal insufficiency. To note that all four SRs included the RCTs, we identified Glowniak and Loriaux (1997) and Thomason et al. (1999), which are reviewed in the "Randomized controlled trials" section.

Discussion
Summary of evidence
Though the prevalence of patients at risk of adrenal insufficiency in the perioperative period is increasing, there remains a paucity of studies on the subject (Benard-Laribiere et al. 2017; Fardet et al. 2011). Only two small RCTs (total of 37 patients) and five cohort studies (total of 462 patients) were identified for review. Neither RCT showed a significant difference in outcomes when stress-dose corticosteroids were administered compared to no perioperative corticosteroid use. This was supported by the findings of five cohort studies. The cohort studies done by Zaghiyan and colleagues in IBD patients suggest a possible benefit from receiving less corticosteroids, with HSD group reporting more tachycardia (Zaghiyan et al. 2011) and more blood loss than the LDS group (Zaghiyan et al. 2012b). Furthermore, though not included in our search due to our eligibility criteria, these results are supported

by five additional cohort studies in which patients received their usual daily dose of corticosteroids without the addition of stress-dose corticosteroids; none of the patients included demonstrated biochemical evidence of adrenal insufficiency (Mathis et al. 2004; Shapiro et al. 1990; Bromberg et al. 1991, 1995; Friedman et al. 1995).

Limitations

There have been very few studies done on the topic in the last decade, and no new RCT. As detailed above, all studies lack quality and need to be interpreted with caution. Importantly, there was significant heterogeneity within the studies in regard to both patients' previous exposure to corticosteroids, in the stress-dose regimen itself as well as in the type of surgery. The inclusion of gingival surgery and orthopedic surgeries is debatable, as previous studies had suggested that orthopedic surgery results in less increase in cortisol levels than, for instance, abdominal surgery (Naito et al. 1991; McIntosh et al. 1981; Jasani et al. 1968). Also, most studies did not report the use of a corticosteroid taper, which could have influenced the occurrence of postoperative complications. The anesthetic agents were also not reported, and this may have an impact on hemodynamics as etomidate, a commonly used agent, inhibits the 11β-hydroxylase enzyme that converts 11β-deoxycortisol into cortisol and predictably reduces cortisol synthesis for up to 48 h after a single intubating dose of this hypnotic agent (Jackson Jr 2005; Vinclair et al. 2008).

Conclusion

Based on the findings of this systematic review, it is not possible to conclude that the perioperative administration of corticosteroids, compared to placebo or standard of care, reduces the incidence of clinical adrenal insufficiency. Nonetheless, the above trials suggest that the demands of physiologic stress are met by a combination of increased endogenous adrenal function plus exogenous baseline doses of corticosteroids. Based on the very limited evidence available, it seems that stress-dose corticosteroid therapy in the perioperative period may therefore not be required as administration of the patient's daily maintenance dose of corticosteroid could be sufficient in most cases. This review allows us to conclude however that the current widespread practice of perioperative supra-physiological corticosteroid supplementation in patients who have been on steroids prior to surgery is not supported by the literature. Additionally, high doses of corticosteroids are associated with important postoperative complications that should not be ignored. This further reinforces the need for a high-quality randomized control trial on perioperative corticosteroid administration.

Appendix 1

Table 1 Study inclusion criteria

Inclusion criteria
Study designs: RCT, cohort studies, case-studies, SR
Articles in English or French

Population:
   Human participants not known to have adrenal insufficiency
   Age ≥ 18 years old
   Noncardiac nontransplant surgery

Intervention: corticosteroid administration before and after surgery
Comparator: standard of care, placebo, or no intervention
Outcomes: adrenal crisis, hypotension or syncope

RCT randomized controlled trials, *SR* systematic review

Appendix 2
Search methods
Study selection

Two authors (AB, CG) independently assessed the titles and abstracts of all articles identified by the above search. Any disagreements were resolved by consensus. Potentially relevant studies were subsequently retrieved in full text.

Data collection process

Two authors (AB, CG) independently extracted the data using a data extraction form. Any disagreements were resolved by consensus. Extracted data included study design, year of publication, surgery type, participant eligibility criteria, corticosteroid regimen used as intervention, comparative arm, sample size, primary and secondary outcomes, and results for the particular study. Studies that were found on full-text assessment not to meet inclusion criteria were subsequently excluded. Reasons for exclusion were recorded.

Risk of bias of individual studies

All studies meeting the inclusion criteria except for the systematic reviews were assessed for risk of bias within the individual study. Randomized controlled trials were assessed via Cochrane risk of bias tool described in the Handbook for Systematic Reviews of interventions version 5.1.0, Chapter 8 (The Cochrane Collaboration 2011). Overall risk of bias was assessed considering the risk of selection bias, performance bias, detection bias, attrition bias, and reporting bias. Each potential bias was characterized as having low, high, or unclear risk of bias. Observational studies were assessed using the agency for Healthcare Research and Quality analytic framework (Viswanathan et al. 2013). This tool was developed to consider source of confounding and risk of biases in observational studies used in systematic reviews.

Appendix 3

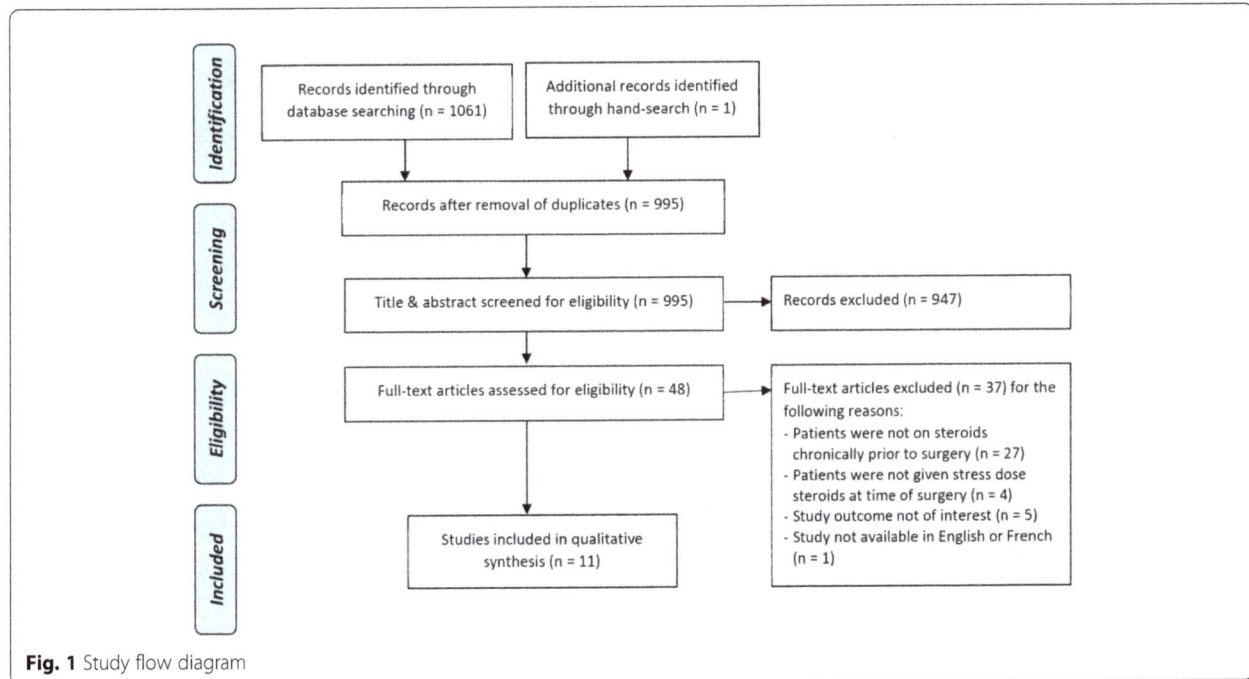

Fig. 1 Study flow diagram

Appendix 4
Risk of bias for RCTs
Risk of bias

Both studies were described by their authors as RCT; however, no information on the randomization process and on the method of concealment were described. Both studies stated patients were blinded by using a corresponding placebo. Glowniak et al. mention the surgical teams were blinded; however, the blinding of other parties is not described. No information was provided on personnel blinding in the Thomason et al.'s study. Detection and attrition bias were considered low risk in both studies as there were no differences between groups in how outcomes were determined and there were no noted withdrawals from the studies. Selective reporting bias was deemed unclear risk as the protocols of either study could not be obtained for comparison.

Additional files

Additional file 1: Literature search strategies. (DOCX 51 kb)

Additional file 2: Screening forms. (DOCX 44 kb)

Additional file 3: Risk of bias for cohort studies. Table S1. Risk of bias, confounding and precision summary: review authors' judgements about each risk of bias for each included cohort study. (Aytac et al. 2013; Lamore et al. 2014; Zaghiyan et al. 2011, 2012a, 2012b). (DOCX 51 kb)

Additional file 4: Summary of included studies. Table S2. Studies investigating the use of supplemental perioperative corticosteroids. (Glowniak and Loriaux 1997; Thomason et al. 1999; Aytac et al. 2013; Lamore et al. 2014; Zaghiyan et al. 2011, 2012a, 2012b; de Lange and Kars 2008; Marik and Varon 2008; Yong et al. 2012, 2009). (DOCX 67 kb)

Abbreviations

ACTH: Adrenocorticotropic hormone; BP: Blood pressure; CC: Case control; CD: Crohn's disease; HC: Hydrocortisone; HDS: High dose steroids; HR: Heart rate; IBD: Inflammatory bowel disease; ICU: Intensive care unit; IV: Intravenous; IVED: Intravenous hydrocortisone equivalent of the daily preoperative steroid dose; IVF: Intravenous fluids; LDS: Low dose steroids; LOS: Length of stay; NA: Not applicable; ND: Not determined; NR: Not reported; NS: Normal saline; OR: Operation room; POD: Postoperative day; RA: Rheumatoid arthritis; RCT: Randomized controlled trial; RYGB: Roux-en-Y gastric bypass surgery; SBP: Systolic blood pressure; SR: Systematic review; UC: Ulcerative colitis; VTE: Venous thromboembolism

Fig. 2 Risk of bias summary for included randomized controlled study. Green: low risk of bias; yellow: unclear risk of bias; red: high risk of bias

Authors' contributions
CG and AB contributed to the conception and design, data collection, data analysis, and manuscript writing. AA-Z contributed to the conception and design. SNM and LV contributed to the conception and design and manuscript writing. All authors read and approved the final manuscript.

Competing interests
The authors declare that they have no competing interests.

Author details
[1]Hematology Residency Program, McGill University, Montreal, Canada. [2]Department of Medicine, Division of General Internal Medicine, McGill University Health Centre, Montreal, Canada. [3]Department of Medicine, Division of Endocrinology, McGill University Health Centre, Montreal, Canada. [4]Medical library, McGill University Health Centre, Montreal, Canada.

References
Aytac E, Londono JM, Erem HH, Vogel JD, Costedio MM. Impact of stress dose steroids on the outcomes of restorative proctocolectomy in patients with ulcerative colitis. Dis Colon Rectum. 2013;56(11):1253–8.

Benard-Laribiere A, Pariente A, Pambrun E, Begaud B, Fardet L, Noize P. Prevalence and prescription patterns of oral glucocorticoids in adults: a retrospective cross-sectional and cohort analysis in France. BMJ Open. 2017; 7(7):e015905.

Bromberg JS, Alfrey EJ, Barker CF, Chavin KD, Dafoe DC, Holland T, et al. Adrenal suppression and steroid supplementation in renal transplant recipients. Transplantation. 1991;51(2):385–90.

Bromberg JS, Baliga P, Cofer JB, Rajagopalan PR, Friedman RJ. Stress steroids are not required for patients receiving a renal allograft and undergoing operation. J Am Coll Surg. 1995;180(5):532–6.

de Lange DW, Kars M. Perioperative glucocorticosteroid supplementation is not supported by evidence. Eur J Intern Med. 2008;19(6):461–7.

Ergina PL, Gold SL, Meakins JL. Perioperative care of the elderly patient. World J Surg. 1993;17(2):192–8.

Fardet L, Petersen I, Nazareth I. Prevalence of long-term oral glucocorticoid prescriptions in the UK over the past 20 years. Rheumatology (Oxford). 2011; 50(11):1982–90.

Fraser CG, Preuss FS, Bigford WD. Adrenal atrophy and irreversible shock associated with cortisone therapy. J Am Med Assoc. 1952;149(17):1542–3.

Friedman RJ, Schiff CF, Bromberg JS. Use of supplemental steroids in patients having orthopaedic operations. J Bone Joint Surg Am. 1995;77(12):1801–6.

Glowniak JV, Loriaux DLA. Double-blind study of perioperative steroid requirements in secondary adrenal insufficiency. Surgery. 1997;121(2):123–9.

Gribsholt SB, Svensson E, Thomsen RW, Richelsen B, Sorensen HT. Preoperative glucocorticoid use and risk of postoperative bleeding and infection after gastric bypass surgery for the treatment of obesity. Surg Obes Relat Dis. 2015;11(6):1212–7.

Jackson WL Jr. Should we use etomidate as an induction agent for endotracheal intubation in patients with septic shock?: a critical appraisal. Chest. 2005; 127(3):1031–8.

Jasani MKFP, Boyle JA, Reid AM, Diver MJ, Buchanan WW. Studies of the rise in plasma 11-hydroxycorticosteroids (11-OHCS) in corticosteroid-treated patients with rheumatoid arthritis during surgery: correlations with the functional integrity of the hypothalamo-pituitary adrenal axis. Q J Med. 1968; 37:(407).

Lamore RF 3rd, Hechenbleikner EM, Ha C, Salvatori R, Harris LH, Marohn MR, et al. Perioperative glucocorticoid prescribing habits in patients with inflammatory bowel disease: a call for standardization. JAMA Surg. 2014;149(5):459–66.

Lewis L, Robinson RF, Yee J, Hacker LA, Eisen G. Fatal adrenal cortical insufficiency precipitated by surgery during prolonged continuous cortisone treatment. Ann Intern Med. 1953;39(1):116–26.

Marik PE, Varon J. Requirement of perioperative stress doses of corticosteroids: a systematic review of the literature. Arch Surg. 2008;143(12):1222–6.

Mathis AS, Shah NK, Mulgaonkar S. Stress dose steroids in renal transplant patients undergoing lymphocele surgery. Transplant Proc. 2004;36(10):3042–5.

McIntosh TK, Lothrop DA, Lee A, Jackson BT, Nabseth D, Egdahl RH. Circadian rhythm of cortisol is altered in postsurgical patients. J Clin Endocrinol Metab. 1981;53(1):117–22.

Naito Y, Fukata J, Tamai S, Seo N, Nakai Y, Mori K, et al. Biphasic changes in hypothalamo-pituitary-adrenal function during the early recovery period after major abdominal surgery. J Clin Endocrinol Metab. 1991;73(1):111–7.

Nguyen GC, Elnahas A, Jackson TD. The impact of preoperative steroid use on short-term outcomes following surgery for inflammatory bowel disease. J Crohns Colitis. 2014;8(12):1661–7.

Salem M, Tainsh RE Jr, Bromberg J, Loriaux DL, Chernow B. Perioperative glucocorticoid coverage. A reassessment 42 years after emergence of a problem. Ann Surg. 1994;219(4):416–25.

Shapiro R, Carroll PB, Tzakis AG, Cemaj S, Lopatin WB, Nakazato P. Adrenal reserve in renal transplant recipients with cyclosporine, azathioprine, and prednisone immunosuppression. Transplantation. 1990;49(5):1011–3.

The Cochrane Collaboration. In: Higgins J, Green S, editors. Cochrane handbook for systematic reviews of interventions. Version 5.1.0 ed; 2011.

Thomason JM, Girdler NM, Kendall-Taylor P, Wastell H, Weddel A, Seymour RA. An investigation into the need for supplementary steroids in organ transplant patients undergoing gingival surgery. A double-blind, split-mouth, cross-over study. J Clin Periodontol. 1999;26(9):577–82.

Toner AJ, Ganeshanathan V, Chan MT, Ho KM, Corcoran TB. Safety of perioperative glucocorticoids in elective noncardiac surgery: a systematic review and meta-analysis. Anesthesiology. 2017;126(2):234–48.

Vinclair M, Broux C, Faure P, Brun J, Genty C, Jacquot C, et al. Duration of adrenal inhibition following a single dose of etomidate in critically ill patients. Intensive Care Med. 2008;34(4):714–9.

Viswanathan M, Berkman ND, Dryden DM, Hartling L. AHRQ methods for effective health care. Assessing risk of bias and confounding in observational studies of interventions or exposures: further development of the RTI item bank. Rockville: Agency for Healthcare Research and Quality (US); 2013.

Yong SL, Coulthard P, Wrzosek A. Supplemental perioperative steroids for surgical patients with adrenal insufficiency. Cochrane Database Syst Rev. 2012;12: CD005367.

Yong SL, Marik P, Esposito M, Coulthard P. Supplemental perioperative steroids for surgical patients with adrenal insufficiency. Cochrane Database Syst Rev. 2009;(4):CD005367. https://doi.org/10.1002/14651858.CD005367.pub2.

Zaghiyan K, Melmed G, Murrell Z, Fleshner P. Are high-dose perioperative steroids necessary in patients undergoing colorectal surgery treated with steroid therapy within the past 12 months? Am Surg. 2011;77(10):1295–9.

Zaghiyan K, Melmed G, Murrell Z, Fleshner P. Safety and feasibility of using low-dose perioperative intravenous steroids in inflammatory bowel disease patients undergoing major colorectal surgery: a pilot study. Surgery. 2012a; 152(2):158–63.

Zaghiyan KN, Murrell Z, Melmed GY, Fleshner PR. High-dose perioperative corticosteroids in steroid-treated patients undergoing major colorectal surgery: necessary or overkill? Am J Surg. 2012b;204(4):481–6.

16

Self-reported mobility as a preoperative risk assessment tool in older surgical patients compared to the American College of Surgeons National Surgical Quality Improvement Program

Sunghye Kim[1,2], Rebecca Neiberg[3], W. Jack Rejeski[4], Anthony P. Marsh[4], Stephen B. Kritchevsky[2], Xiaoyan I. Leng[3] and Leanne Groban[2,5*]

Abstract

Background: The American College of Surgeons National Surgical Quality Improvement Program (NSQIP®) developed a surgical risk calculator using data from 1.4 million patients and including 1557 unique Current Procedural Terminology (CPT) codes. Although this calculator demonstrated excellent performance in predicting postoperative mortality, morbidity, and six surgical complications, it was not developed specifically for use in older surgical patients who have worse surgical outcomes and additional unique risk factors compared to younger adults. We aimed to test the ability of a simple self-reported mobility tool to predict postoperative outcomes in the older surgical population compared to the NSQIP.

Methods: We used data from a prospective cohort study that enrolled 197 older surgical patients (≥ 69 years) undergoing various elective surgeries and assessed 30-day surgical outcomes. Statistical models included data from the Mobility Assessment Tool-short form (MAT-sf) alone, covariates alone, and MAT-sf data and covariates. We used leave-one-out (LOO) cross-validation of the models within our cohort and compared their performance for predicting postoperative outcomes against the NSQIP calculator based on receiver operating characteristic area under the curve (ROC AUC).

Results: Patients with poor self-reported mobility experienced higher rates of postoperative complications and nursing home placement. There was no difference in performance between any of our models and the NSQIP calculator ($p > 0.1$), with AUC between 0.604 and 0.697 for predicting postoperative complications and 0.653 and 0.760 for predicting nursing home placement. All models also predicted a length of stay (LOS) similar to the actual LOS.

Conclusion: Mobility assessment alone using MAT-sf can predict postoperative complications, nursing home placement, and LOS for older surgical patients, with accuracy comparable to that of the NSQIP calculator. The simplicity of this noninvasive risk assessment tool makes it an attractive alternative to the NSQIP calculator that requires 20 patient predictors and the planned procedure, or CPT code to predict the chance that patients will have 15 different adverse outcomes following surgery.

Keywords: Preoperative, Risk calculator, NSQIP, Mobility

* Correspondence: lgroban@wakehealth.edu
[2]Sticht Center for Healthy Aging and Alzheimer's Prevention, Wake Forest School of Medicine, Medical Center Boulevard, Winston-Salem, NC 27157, USA
[5]Department of Anesthesiology, Wake Forest School of Medicine, Medical Center Boulevard, Winston-Salem, NC 27157-1009, USA
Full list of author information is available at the end of the article

Background

The American College of Surgeons National Surgical Quality Improvement Program (NSQIP®) surgical risk calculator (American College of Physicians n.d.), released in 2013 (Bilimoria et al. 2013), was developed using data from more than 1.4 million patients, encompassing 1557 unique Current Procedural Terminology (CPT) codes. Patient-related preoperative variables include age, sex, functional status, American Society of Anesthesiologists (ASA) classification, steroid use for chronic conditions, ascites within 30 days prior to surgery, systemic sepsis within 48 h prior to surgery, ventilator dependency, disseminated cancer, diabetes (DM), hypertension (HTN), congestive heart failure 30 days prior to surgery, dyspnea, current smoker within 1 year, history of severe chronic obstructive pulmonary disease (COPD), dialysis, acute renal failure, and body mass index (BMI). The calculator also takes into account the type of surgery, based on specific CPT codes and emergency status (American College of Physicians n.d.). Although the NSQIP surgical risk calculator demonstrated excellent performance in predicting postoperative mortality (c-statistic = 0.944), morbidity (c-statistic = 0.816), and six surgical complications (c-statistics > 0.8), it was not developed specifically for use in the older patient population, which is rapidly growing in the USA and is known to have worse surgical outcomes than younger patients (Sukharamwala et al. 2012; Raats et al. 2015; Bentrem et al. 2009). Specifically, the NSQIP surgical risk calculator does not include factors such as frailty and mobility that are known to be important predictors of surgical outcomes in older patients (Kim et al. 2016; Makary et al. 2010).

The NSQIP and the American Geriatric Society published a best practice guideline for optimal preoperative assessment of older surgical patients (Chow et al. 2012). The guideline recommends assessment of patients' gait and mobility impairment and fall risk, using tests such as the Timed Up and Go test to assess surgical risk in older patients. While the NSQIP surgical risk calculator does include patients' functional status as a categorical variable with three options (independent, partially dependent, and totally dependent), this variable does not capture the various degrees of functional limitation that older patients experience. Furthermore, the NSQIP surgical risk calculator does not take into account patients' mobility status.

In a prospective study of older surgical patients, we assessed preoperative self-reported mobility using a novel tool, the Mobility Assessment Tool-short form (MAT-sf), and found it to be a good predictor for postoperative complications, hospital length of stay (LOS), and nursing home placement (Kim et al. 2016). Here, we used data from that study to develop a simplified preoperative risk assessment model that includes measures of self-reported mobility to predict postoperative outcomes in older

patients. The aim of this study was to compare the performance of these simple surgical risk calculators to the NSQIP surgical risk calculator in predicting postoperative outcomes among older patients.

Methods

Study design

We previously conducted a prospective cohort study of older patients (≥ 69 years) who were undergoing elective, noncardiac surgery from July 2012 to February 2014 (Kim et al. 2016). Eligible patients were asked to provide written informed consent (IRB approval number 000193921; 4/23/2012) before undergoing standardized assessments. Preoperative risk factors, including comorbidity, BMI, and ASA Physical Status Classification, were obtained at enrollment. Self-reported mobility was assessed using the MAT-sf, administered by trained study personnel. The MAT-sf is a 10-item, computer-based assessment of mobility using animated video clips (Rejeski et al. 2013). The 10 items ask patients to report on their ability to perform a broad range of functions, including walking on level ground, slow jogging, walking outdoors on uneven terrain, walking up a ramp with and without use of a handrail, stepping over hurdles, ascending and descending stairs with and without use of a handrail, and climbing stairs while carrying bags (Rejeski et al. 2010a). Each item is accompanied by an animated video clip together with the responses for that question (number of minutes, number of times, yes/no). The MAT-sf was validated by two separate stepwise regression analyses, one for the Short Physical Performance Battery (SPPB) and a second for the 400-m walk. In these analyses, the Pepper Assessment Tool for Disability (PAT-D) mobility score was entered first followed by the MAT-sf scores. In both analyses, the entry of the MAT-sf contributed over and above the PAT-D mobility subscale to the explanation of performance-based function; for the SPPB, the change in R^2 was an additional 9.8% and for the 400-m walk it was 16.7%. The zero order correlations of the MAT-sf to the SPPB and 400-m walk gait speed were 0.59 ($p < 0.001$) and 0.58 ($p < 0.001$), respectively. It is also of interest to point out the standardized β weight for the MAT-sf was substantially larger than the PAT-D mobility subscale in both analyses (Rejeski et al. 2013; Rejeski et al. 2010b).

Postoperative outcomes were assessed by medical record review, including postoperative complications within 30 days of the operation, LOS, and nursing home placement. The NSQIP definition of postoperative complications was used and included surgical site infection (superficial, deep, and organ space), wound disruption, pneumonia, unplanned intubation, thromboembolism, on ventilator > 48 h, urinary tract infection, progressive renal insufficiency, acute renal failure, cerebrovascular accident, cardiac arrest, myocardial infarction, and sepsis (Khuri et al. 1998).

Statistical analysis

Sex differences in MAT-sf scores were compared using Student's *t* test. Percentages of postoperative complications and nursing home placement among patients by sex-specific mobility tertile (best, mid, and worst tertiles of MAT-sf score) were compared using chi-square tests. Length of stay was compared across MAT-sf tertiles using the Wilcoxon rank sum test.

To compare our risk models to the ASC NSQIP surgical risk calculator, we first calculated predicted surgical outcomes using risk factors obtained at enrollment by the NSQIP calculator (American College of Physicians n.d.). Next, logistic regression models were used to estimate probabilities of postoperative complications and nursing home placement and a Poisson regression model was used to estimate LOS for each participant. Three sets of models were created including (1) MAT-sf scores alone; (2) covariates alone: age, sex, BMI, ASA status, DM, HTN, and surgical risk; and (3) both the covariates and MAT-sf scores. Since the NSQIP surgical risk calculator estimates of LOS and probability of postoperative complications and nursing home placement are predictions, and we already knew these outcomes for our cohort, we utilized the leave-one-out (LOO) cross-validation method when fitting our models to obtain model-based predictions for the observation left out. Finally, the receiver operating characteristic (ROC) areas under the curve (AUCs) were calculated for estimated probabilities of postoperative complications and nursing home placement from both the NSQIP surgical risk calculator and our models. Estimates of AUC standard errors and confidence intervals for all models and the NSQIP surgical risk calculator were obtained, and comparisons of AUCs were done through a nonparametric approach using the SAS ROC macro (SAS Institute, Cary, NC) (DeLong et al. 1988). For LOS, the estimates between each of the models and the actual LOS were compared in a mixed model ANOVA accounting for correlation between measurements on the same patient. The Spearman's rank correlation was also used to test associations between the MAT-sf and the NSQIP-calculated length of stay, any complications, and probability of nursing home placement.

Results

Patient cohort

For this study, we utilized data from a total of 197 patients undergoing elective, noncardiac surgery who were enrolled in a prospective trial (Kim et al. 2016). The mean (± SD) age was 75.2 years (± 5.0), 51% of the patients were female, and the cohort was predominantly white (Table 1). After surgery, 30 (15.2%) of the patients had postoperative complications within 30 days of the operation, while 27 (13.7%) were placed to nursing homes. The median (interquartile range [IQR]) LOS

Table 1 Characteristics of patient cohort (*n* = 197)

Age, mean (SD)	75.2 (5.0)
Female, *n* (%)	101 (51)
Race, *n* (%)	
White	179 (91)
African American	15 (8)
Other	3 (1.5)
Body mass index, kg/m², mean (SD)	27.8 (5.6)
ASA physical status, *n* (%)	
I	0 (0)
II	47 (24)
III	136 (69)
IV	14 (7)
Surgical risk, *n* (%)	
Low	35 (18)
Intermediate-to-high	162 (82)
Mobility Assessment Tool-short form score, median (IQR)	53.1 (46.4–61.6)

ASA American Society of Anesthesiologists, *IQR* interquartile range, *SD* standard deviation

was 3.0 (2.0–4.0) days and the mean ± SD was 3.6 ± 4.2 days.

Mobility measured by MAT-sf

As we have reported previously, the median MAT-sf score was 53.1 (IQR 46.4–61.6). Men had higher MAT-sf scores (58.3 [IQR 48.3–65.5]) than women (49.9 [IQR 42.2–55.5]), *p* < 0.001. Patients in lower sex-specific MAT-sf tertiles had higher rates of postoperative complications (*p* = 0.014) and nursing home placement (*p* = 0.009), as well as longer LOS (*p* < 0.0001; Fig. 1).

Comparison of new models and NSQIP surgical risk score

We developed and cross-validated models using MAT-sf only, covariates only (age, gender, BMI, ASA status, DM, HTN, and surgical risk), and MAT-sf plus covariates to predict postoperative outcomes. Table 2 summarizes the ROC AUC of each cross-validated model and the NSQIP surgical risk score for the outcomes of postoperative complications and nursing home placement. There was no significant difference in AUC between any of the new models and the NSQIP surgical risk score for either postoperative complications or nursing home placement. Figure 2 illustrates the AUC of the MAT-sf only model and the NSQIP surgical risk score for postoperative complications (AUC 0.643 [95% CI 0.538–0.748] and 0.697 [0.580–0.813], respectively, *p* = 0.54). Figure 3 illustrates the AUC of the MAT-sf only model and the NSQIP surgical risk score for nursing home placement (AUC 0.723 [0.632–0.813] and 0.760 [0.640–0.880], respectively, *p* = 0.58). Table 3 lists the estimated LOS

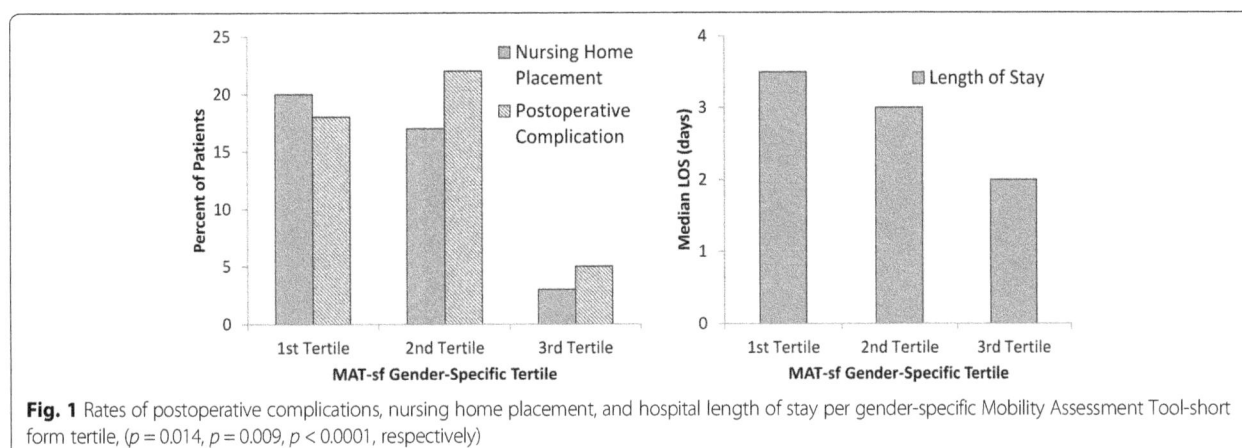

Fig. 1 Rates of postoperative complications, nursing home placement, and hospital length of stay per gender-specific Mobility Assessment Tool-short form tertile, ($p = 0.014$, $p = 0.009$, $p < 0.0001$, respectively)

based on our three models and the NSQIP surgical risk score. There were no significant differences between the actual LOS in the cohort and LOS estimated using our three models or the NSQIP surgical risk score. The correlations between the MAT-sf and NSQIP-calculated length of stay, any complications, and probability of nursing home placement are shown in Table 4. There was a significant association between these two scoring systems for postoperative outcomes.

Discussion

We set out to develop a surgical risk calculator that was simple and specific to the older surgical patient population. We developed three models using data from our prospective cohort of 197 older surgical patients and cross-validated the models to provide robust probabilities of risk. The model using only the MAT-sf score had similar ability for predicting postoperative complications and nursing home placement as the NSQIP surgical risk calculator. Thus, the MAT-sf score provides a simple, easy to use tool to predict surgical outcomes in older patients. The model performed as well as the NSQIP surgical risk calculator in predicting LOS.

The NSQIP risk calculator was developed using data from more than 1.4 million patients and has demonstrated excellent performance in predicting postoperative outcomes (American College of Physicians n.d.; Bilimoria et al. 2013). However, the NSQIP calculator was not specifically developed for use in an older patient population, in which unique factors, such as mobility, are important predictors of surgical outcomes. There have been efforts to develop simpler tools to predict postoperative outcomes in the older patient population. A few studies have used mobility as a marker of postoperative outcomes. Robinson et al. tested the Timed Up and Go test as a predictive tool among 272 older patients (98 patients undergoing colorectal surgery and 174 patients undergoing cardiac surgery). The Timed Up and Go test measures the time it takes for an individual to rise from a chair, ambulate 10 ft, turn around a cone marker, return to the chair, and sit back down. In patients undergoing either colorectal or cardiac surgery, the study reported the ROC AUC for predicting postoperative complications using the Timed Up and Go test as 0.775 and 0.684, respectively, compared to 0.554 and 0.552 for standard-of-care surgical risk calculators (Robinson et al. 2013). The MAT-sf tool had similar

Table 2 Comparisons of cross-validated models and NSQIP® surgical risk score for predicting postoperative outcomes in older patients

Outcomes	Model	ROC AUC (95% CI)	Estimate of difference (95% CI)*	p value*
Postoperative complications	MAT-sf only	0.643 (0.538–0.748)	− 0.054 (− 0.227, 0.120)	0.54
	Covariates only†	0.604 (0.496–0.711)	− 0.093 (− 0.232, 0.046)	0.19
	MAT-sf + covariates†	0.641 (0.529–0.753)	− 0.056 (− 0.203, 0.092)	0.46
	ACS NSQIP surgical risk score	0.697 (0.580–0.813)		
Nursing home placement	MAT-sf only	0.723 (0.632–0.813)	− 0.037 (− 0.167,0.094)	0.58
	Covariates only†	0.653 (0.543–0.762)	− 0.107 (− 0.238,0.024)	0.11
	MAT-sf + covariates†	0.708 (0.596–0.821)	− 0.051 (− 0.184, 0.081)	0.45
	NSQIP surgical risk score	0.760 (0.640–0.880)		

NSQIP® National Surgical Quality Improvement Program, *AUC* area under the curve, *MAT-sf* Mobility Assessment Test-short form, *ROC* receiver operator characteristic
*Comparing each model to NSQIP surgical risk score
†Covariates include age, gender, body mass index, ASA status, diabetes mellitus, hypertension, and surgical risk

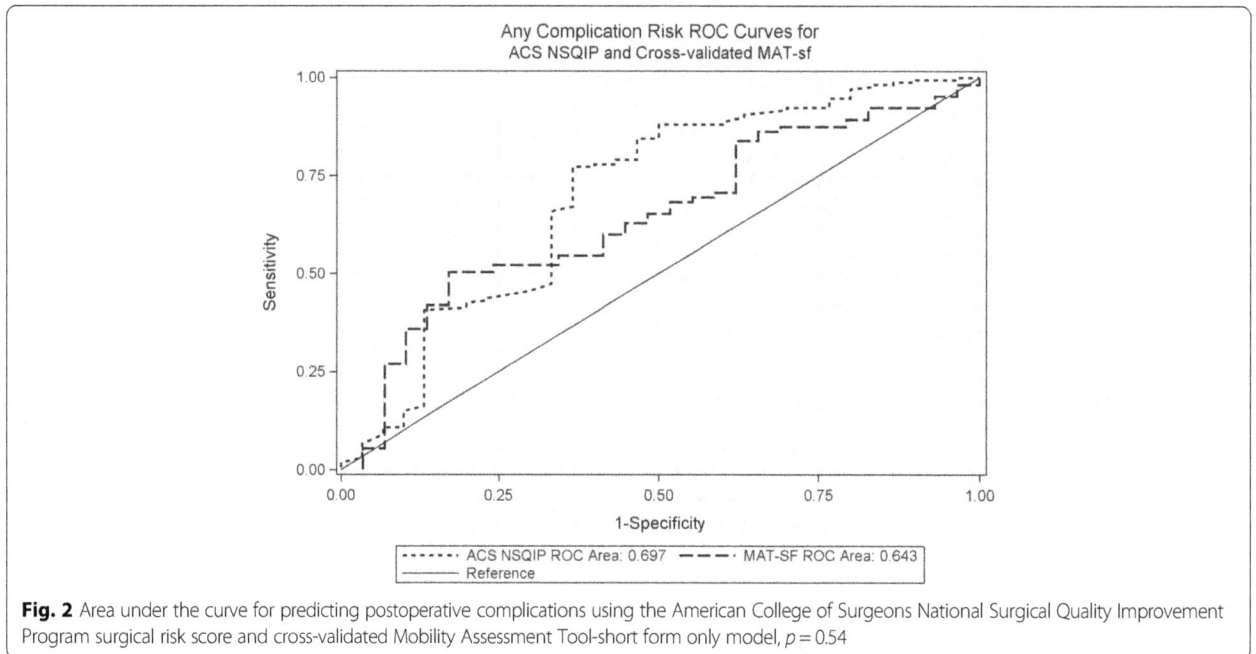

Fig. 2 Area under the curve for predicting postoperative complications using the American College of Surgeons National Surgical Quality Improvement Program surgical risk score and cross-validated Mobility Assessment Tool-short form only model, $p = 0.54$

ROC AUCs for postoperative complications as those reported for the Timed Up and Go test, and we did not see any difference between the MAT-sf tool and the NSQIP surgical risk calculator. One important distinction between these two simple perioperative risk score measures is that the Timed Up and Go is a performance test of physical function whereas the MAT-sf is a self-report measure. Consequently, the Timed Up and Go might not be as feasible due to space and patient limitations. Since the study by Robinson et al. limited the enrollment criteria

to patients who were undergoing colorectal or cardiac surgery and analyzed them separately, the risk associated with each type of surgery could be controlled. By contrast, our study enrolled any older patients who were undergoing elective surgery (Table 5). Given the relatively small sample size of our study, we could not control for the risk associated with each type of surgery. In the models that used the covariates alone or covariates plus MAT-sf, we controlled for the surgical risk in terms of low vs. intermediate-to-high risk using the definitions from

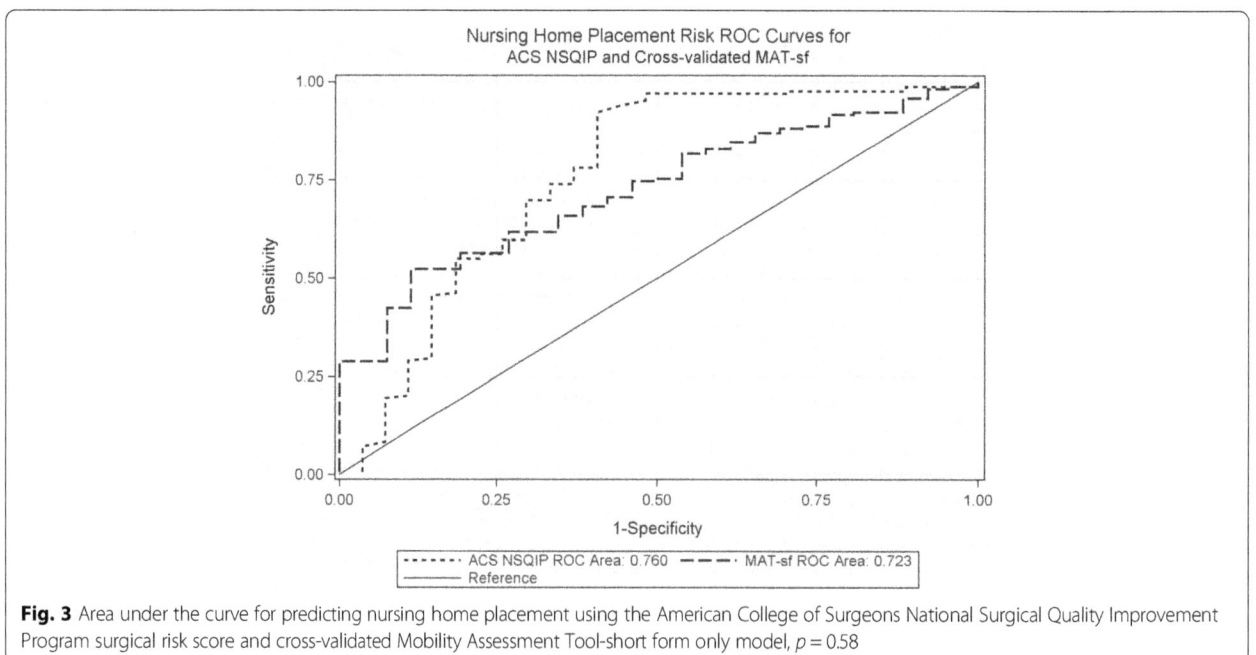

Fig. 3 Area under the curve for predicting nursing home placement using the American College of Surgeons National Surgical Quality Improvement Program surgical risk score and cross-validated Mobility Assessment Tool-short form only model, $p = 0.58$

Table 3 Comparison of actual and model-based estimates of postoperative hospital length of stay in older patients

Model	Predicted LOS (mean ± SD)	Difference from actual LOS (95% CI)	p value*
Mobility Assessment Tool-short form only	3.55 ± 0.76	− 0.04 (− 0.61–0.54)	0.90
Covariates only†	3.59 ± 1.54	− 0.00 (− 0.41–0.42)	0.99
Mobility Assessment Tool-short form + covariates†	3.55 ± 1.59	− 0.03(− 0.59–0.53)	0.92
NSQIP surgical risk score	3.36 ± 2.40	− 0.22(− 0.78–0.33)	0.43
Actual LOS	3.58 ± 4.15	−	

LOS length of stay, NSQIP* National Surgical Quality Improvement Program, SD standard deviation
*Comparing estimated length of stay from each model and NSQIP surgical risk score to actual length of stay
†Covariates include age, gender, body mass index, ASA status, diabetes mellitus, hypertension, and surgical risk

American College of Cardiology/American Heart Association guidelines (Fleisher et al. 2014).

Reddy and colleagues examined the ability of a stair climbing activity to predict surgical outcomes in 264 patients ≥ 19 years of age who were undergoing elective abdominal surgery. They reported that stair climbing predicted morbidity better than the NSQIP surgical risk calculator (AUC = 0.81 vs. 0.62, $p < 0.0001$). However, the stair climbing task caused physiologic stress, especially in those patients who were slower climbers, causing a 16.6 and 21.8% increase in heart rate and mean arterial pressure, respectively, compared to 7.4 and 7.9% for faster climbers (Reddy et al. 2016). Although this study demonstrated excellent power of stair climbing time as a tool to predict postoperative outcomes, it is an even more intensive test than the Timed Up and Go test, with higher risk (including falls and cardiac events with physiologic stress). Also, the time and space constraints, as well as personnel requirements, clearly limit the feasibility of the stair climbing test in clinical practice.

What is noteworthy is that our models were not different from the NSQIP surgical risk calculator in predicting postoperative hospital LOS. Indeed, the biggest factor that determines postoperative hospital LOS is the type of surgery; for example, patients who undergo laparoscopic cholecystectomy will have a much shorter LOS than patients who undergo open hemicolectomy. The NSQIP surgical risk calculator was developed using 1557 unique CPT codes and

allows input of a single procedure CPT code. Even though our models did not include the surgical risk in the model (e.g., MAT-sf only model) or reflect the risks fully (only two degrees of surgical risks [low vs. intermediate-to-high]), the predictions for LOS using the simple MAT-sf model were remarkably similar to the universal calculator. Adequately incorporating procedure complexity and risk into future studies that use the simple MAT-sf could solidify its efficacy in forecasting surgical outcomes.

Table 5 Summary of surgical procedures by sex

Surgery	Male	Female	Total
Orthopedic surgery	42	72	114
Hip	13	26	
Knee	9	18	
Spine	18	21	
Other	2	7	
Urology	25	4	29
Kidney	5	2	
Prostate	10	0	
Other	10	2	
Intraperitoneal	13	7	20
Colorectal	5	4	
Hernia	3	1	
Other	5	2	
Otolaryngology	5	8	13
Thyroid	0	3	
Other	5	5	
Vascular	6	3	9
Carotid endarterectomy	4	1	
Other	2	2	
Gynecology	0	4	4
Hysterectomy	0	2	
Other	0	2	
Neurosurgery	2	1	3
Pituitary	1	1	
Other	1	0	
Other	3	2	5

Table 4 Spearman's correlation between MAT-sf and NSQIP calculator predicted outcomes

Spearman correlation coefficients
Prob > |r| under H0: Rho = 0

	MAT-sf	LOS	Any complications	Nursing home placement
MAT-sf	1.00000	− 0.33034 < 0.0001	− 0.16252 0.0229	− 0.44940 < 0.0001
Length of stay	− 0.33034 < 0.0001	1.00000	0.69552 < 0.0001	0.67603 < 0.0001
Any complications	− 0.16252 0.0229	0.69552 < 0.0001	1.00000	0.25218 0.0004
Nursing home placement	− 0.44940 < 0.0001	0.67603 < 0.0001	0.25218 0.0004	1.00000

MAT-sf Mobility Assessment Test-short form, LOS length of stay

The limitations of the study include its single-center design and use of a majority white patient cohort, features of the study design that compromise the external validity of the findings. We were unable to include the full list of measures included in the NSQIP calculator due to our small sample size and lack of variability in some measures such as cancer and chronic heart failure, among others. Since this issue could have accounted for the similarities observed between the universal calculator and the MAT-sf models, the results must be interpreted with caution. Nonetheless, we expect that our estimation of postoperative risks and LOS with the MAT-sf tool may have been better if we had a larger sample with increased variability. Although we used the LOO cross-validation method, our findings still need to be tested in a separate cohort. Lastly, the models were developed from relatively small number of older patients ($n = 197$), which may not accurately reflect surgical risk.

Conclusion

The MAT-sf can predict postoperative outcomes (complications, LOS, and nursing home placement) in older surgical patients with predictive performance comparable to the NSQIP surgical risk calculator. Given the simplicity and noninvasive nature of the MAT-sf tool, it can be easily adopted into clinical practice for preoperative risk assessment. Future studies in a larger cohort of patients undergoing a single type of surgery are warranted to validate this new method to predict postoperative outcomes.

Abbreviations

ASA: American Society of Anesthesiologists; AUC: Area under the curve; BMI: Body mass index; COPD: Chronic obstructive pulmonary disease; CPT: Current Procedural Terminology; DM: Diabetes mellitus; HTN: Hypertension; IQR: Interquartile range; LOO: Leave one out; LOS: Length of stay; MAT-sf: Mobility Assessment Tool-short form; NSQIP®: National Surgical Quality Improvement Program; ROC: Receiver operating characteristic

Funding

This study was funded in part by the Anesthesia Patient Safety Foundation (LG), the Translational Science Center at Wake Forest University (LG), the Grants for Early Medical/Surgical Specialists' Transition to Aging Research (GEMSSTAR, R03 AG050919) (SKim), and the Claude D. Pepper Center Older Americans Independence Center (P30 AG21332) (SKritchevsky), Wake Forest School of Medicine, Winston-Salem, NC.

Authors' contributions

SKim and LG were responsible for the study conception and design. SKim, RN, LG, and XIL contributed to the data acquisition, analysis, production of figures, and data interpretation. The manuscript was drafted by SKim, RN, XIL, and LG. Critical revision was performed by APM, WJR, SKritchevsky, and LG. All authors read and approved the final manuscript.

Competing interests

The authors declare that they have no competing interests.

Author details

[1]Department of Internal Medicine, Section of General Internal Medicine, Wake Forest School of Medicine, Medical Center Boulevard, Winston-Salem, NC 27157, USA. [2]Sticht Center for Healthy Aging and Alzheimer's Prevention, Wake Forest School of Medicine, Medical Center Boulevard, Winston-Salem, NC 27157, USA. [3]Division of Public Health Sciences, Department of Biostatistical Sciences, Wake Forest School of Medicine, 525 Vine, Winston-Salem, NC 27101, USA. [4]Department of Health and Exercise Science, Wake Forest University, PO Box 7868, Winston-Salem, NC 27109, USA. [5]Department of Anesthesiology, Wake Forest School of Medicine, Medical Center Boulevard, Winston-Salem, NC 27157-1009, USA.

References

American College of Physicians. n.d. ACS NSQIP surgical risk calculator. https://riskcalculator.facs.org/RiskCalculator/. Accessed 16 June 2017.

Bentrem DJ, Cohen ME, Hynes DM, Ko CY, Bilimoria KY. Identification of specific quality improvement opportunities for the elderly undergoing gastrointestinal surgery. Arch Surg. 2009;144:1013–20.

Bilimoria KY, Liu Y, Paruch JL, Zhou L, Kmiecik TE, Ko CY, et al. Development and evaluation of the universal ACS NSQIP surgical risk calculator: a decision aid and informed consent tool for patients and surgeons. J Am Coll Surg. 2013; 217:833–42.

Chow WB, Rosenthal RA, Merkow RP, Ko CY, Esnaola NF. American College of Surgeons National Surgical Quality Improvement Program; American Geriatrics Society. Optimal preoperative assessment of the geriatric surgical patient: a best practices guideline from the American College of Surgeons National Surgical Quality Improvement Program and the American Geriatrics Society. J Am Coll Surg. 2012;215:453–66.

DeLong ER, DeLong DM, Clarke-Pearson DL. Comparing the areas under two or more correlated receiver operating characteristic curves: a nonparametric approach. Biometrics. 1988;44:837–45.

Fleisher LA, Fleischmann KE, Auerbach AD, Barnason SA, Beckman JA, Bozkurt B, et al. 2014 ACC/AHA guideline on perioperative cardiovascular evaluation and management of patients undergoing noncardiac surgery: a report of the American College of Cardiology/American Heart Association Task Force on practice guidelines. J Am Coll Cardiol. 2014;64:e77–137.

Khuri SF, Daley J, Henderson W, Hur K, Demakis J, Aust JB, et al. The Department of Veterans Affairs' NSQIP: the first national, validated, outcome-based, risk-adjusted, and peer-controlled program for the measurement and enhancement of the quality of surgical care. National VA Surgical Quality Improvement Program. Ann Surg. 1998;228:491–507.

Kim S, Marsh AP, Rustowicz L, Roach C, Leng XI, Kritchevsky SB, et al. Self-reported mobility in older patients predicts early postoperative outcomes after elective noncardiac surgery. Anesthesiology. 2016;124:815–25.

Makary MA, Segev DL, Pronovost PJ, Syin D, Bandeen-Roche K, Patel P, et al. Frailty as a predictor of surgical outcomes in older patients. J Am Coll Surg. 2010;210:901–8.

Raats JW, van Eijsden WA, Crolla RM, Steyerberg EW, van der Laan L. Risk factors and outcomes for postoperative delirium after major surgery in elderly patients. PLoS One. 2015;10:e0136071.

Reddy S, Contreras CM, Singletary B, Bradford TM, Waldrop MG, Mims AH, et al. Timed stair climbing is the single strongest predictor of perioperative complications in patients undergoing abdominal surgery. J Am Coll Surg. 2016;222:559–66.

Rejeski WJ, Ip EH, Marsh AP, Barnard RT. Development and validation of a video-animated tool for assessing mobility. J Gerontol A Biol Sci Med Sci. 2010b;65: 664–71.

Rejeski WJ, Marsh AP, Anton S, Chen SH, Church T, Gill TM, et al. The MAT-sf: clinical relevance and validity. J Gerontol A Biol Sci Med Sci. 2013;68:1567–74.

Rejeski WJ, Marsh AP, Chmelo E, Rejeski JJ. Obesity, intentional weight loss and physical disability in older adults. Obes Rev. 2010a;11:671–85.

Robinson TN, Wu DS, Sauaia A, Dunn CL, Stevens-Lapsley JE, Moss M, Stiegmann GV, et al. Slower walking speed forecasts increased postoperative morbidity and 1-year mortality across surgical specialties. Ann Surg. 2013;258:582–8.

Sukharamwala P, Thoens J, Szuchmacher M, Smith J, DeVito P. Advanced age is a risk factor for post-operative complications and mortality after a pancreaticoduodenectomy: a meta-analysis and systematic review. HPB (Oxford). 2012;14:649–57.

17

Exploring the experience of an enhanced recovery programme for gynaecological cancer patients

Stephanie Archer[1,2*], Jane Montague[1] and Anish Bali[3]

Abstract

Background: Perioperative enhanced recovery programmes (ERPs), identified as initiatives that improve care and save money, have been adopted by NHS Improvement and are currently being rolled out across many surgical departments within the NHS. To date, five papers have specifically explored patients' experiences of ERPs; none, however, has explored the gynaecological cancer patient experience.

Methods: In total, 14 women (mean age, 66 years) participated in an audio-recorded face-to-face or telephone interview in which they discussed their experience of taking part in an ERP. The resulting data were transcribed verbatim and analysed using interpretative phenomenological analysis.

Results: Two main themes emerged from the analysis. The first, 'Taking part in the programme', highlights two important aspects of the ERP: being given an opportunity to receive information and, following this, to build knowledge about the programme. The theme also explores the challenges associated with the programme, particularly around getting mobile and complying with its demands - the women report experiencing a constant battle between intuition and instruction. The second theme, 'Home', focuses on the role home plays in motivating the patients to aim for an early discharge from hospital. Patients describe their need to return to a suitable home and the need for support from others. They also discuss the importance of the follow-up phone call.

Conclusion: Overall, the patients in this study positively assessed the individual aspects of the ERP, in particular, information resources, the availability of the physiotherapist and the delivery of follow-up phone calls. These findings highlight the importance of developing and maintaining individual aspects of ERPs over time, to ensure their sensitivity and responsiveness to patient needs.

Keywords: Enhanced recovery programmes, Gynaecological cancer, Patient experience

Background

Initiatives such as Lord Darzi's High Quality Care for All [1], the Strategy for Cancer: Improving Outcomes [2] and the Quality, Innovation, Productivity and Prevention Challenge [3] have all highlighted the need for the NHS to deliver more services but without compromising quality. Enhanced recovery programmes (ERPs) have been identified as initiatives that are beneficial both for improving care and for saving money; as a result these have been implemented in hospital trusts across the country [4]. The aim of ERPs is to 'improve the quality of patients' care, through improving their clinical outcomes and experience, and to reduce the length of elective care inpatient pathways across the NHS by utilising good practice principles of the enhanced recovery model of care' [5].

'Enhanced' or 'fast track' recovery combines several perioperative interventions to reduce the length of inpatient stay in hospital and to promote early recovery after surgery [6]. Other benefits of ERPs are increased utilisation of beds (that is, available beds having a higher turnover of patients) and reduced healthcare expenditure [7]. The fundamental aspects of ERPs focus on pain control, reduction of surgical stress, enhanced nutrition, heat loss

* Correspondence: stephanie.archer@imperial.ac.uk
[1]Psychology Department, Faculty of Education, Health & Science, University of Derby, Kedleston Road, Derby DE22 1GB, UK
[2]Centre for Patient Safety and Service Quality, Imperial College London, Medical School Building, St Mary's Campus, Norfolk Place, London W2 1PG, UK
Full list of author information is available at the end of the article

and mobilisation as key factors in patient recovery [8]. These aspects are just a selection of those that have been built into ERPs over the past 15 years [9] and, although originally developed for colorectal surgery, ERPs are now widely used for surgical procedures in both cancer and non-cancer populations.

There are currently only five papers that specifically explore patients' experiences of ERP; three papers looking at patients with colorectal cancer, and two papers exploring patients' experiences of hysterectomy [10-14]. Research by Wagner et al. [13,14], explored the patient experiences of ERPs in terms of hysterectomy, although this purposely left out the gynaecological cancer patients 'because the supplementary diagnosis can have an impact on the women's experiences of the admission to hospital' [14]. It is important, therefore, to look at the ERP experiences of cancer patients outside of the colorectal discipline to ascertain the programme's efficacy.

The study reported here explores the experience of a group of women taking part in an ERP at an East Midlands regional cancer centre while having surgery for gynaecological cancer. This qualitative study gives insight into the lived experience of an ERP for this group of women. It provides an in-depth, and previously unexplored, view of the ERP from the gynaecological cancer patients' perspective.

Methods
Participant recruitment
Participants recruited for the study had taken part in the ERP between October 2010 and April 2011 and had undergone elective open surgery for gynaecological cancer. The clinical team identified qualifying patients through hospital records and contact details supplied by the ERP project lead. In total, 34 patients were identified with 33 of these being asked to take part in the study. The 34th patient had returned home to a country outside of the UK and her contact details were not available.

Patients were sent an information sheet, an invitation to participate and a reply slip on which they could indicate whether they were consenting to take part in the evaluation. Those who agreed to take part could choose a face-to-face or a telephone interview. In total, 25 women responded to the invitation; 11 of the respondents opted not to take part in the evaluation. Of the 14 who agreed, four patients chose to be interviewed by telephone and 10 chose face-to-face interviews.

Participant characteristics and demographics
All patients taking part in the evaluation had undergone a full open hysterectomy, +/- bilateral salpingo-oopherectomy, +/- omentectomy, +/- pelvic lymph node dissection at an East Midlands regional cancer centre. Patients were all living in the East Midlands at the time

of the operation and spoke fluent English; the sample comprised of women from various ethnic origins. The age range of the patients was 53 to 80 years (mean age, 66 years).

Data collection
A semi-structured interview method was utilised, allowing for all participants to be asked similar questions within a flexible framework [15,16]. All interviews were conducted in a place suitable for the women (which was chosen by them) and were recorded on a digital voice recorder. Participants dictated the flow of the interview, covering topics in an order with which they felt most comfortable. Questions focused on the women's experiences of participating in the ERP as well as any other aspects of their hospital care they felt to be important. If further clarification or exploration of a topic was required, the researcher 'revisited' these topics before the close of the interview.

The study conformed to British Psychological Society ethical standards [17]; the protocol was approved by the University of Derby Psychology Ethics Committee and was approved as a current audit by the NHS hospital audit team at the Royal Derby Hospital. Participants gave written informed consent, and pseudonyms were used to protect their anonymity. Patients were also debriefed after their participation in the study and directed to suitable support agencies where necessary.

Analytic procedure
The choice of a qualitative methodology for this study was informed by researchers such as Starks & Brown Trinidad [18], who state that 'qualitative research methods enable health sciences researchers to delve into questions of meaning, examine institutional and social practices and processes, identify barriers and facilitators to change and discover the reasons for the success or failure of interventions'. Analysis was conducted using an interpretative phenomenological analysis (IPA) approach, a methodology frequently used in health services research [15,19-22]. IPA was developed to 'explore the participant's view of the world' and to adopt, as far as possible, an 'insider perspective' [23] and is informed by phenomenology and hermeneutics [24].

In line with the IPA methodology, interviews were transcribed verbatim, and initially coded by reading and re-reading the transcript and making notes, drawing on observations made during the interviews and transcription. Transcripts were then coded line by line: describing, summarising and attending to linguistic elements such as pronoun and metaphor use [15]. Emergent themes were developed from these codes and clustered with related themes.

Results

Two emergent themes are explored in this paper: 'Taking part in the programme' and 'Home', both of which focus on the role of ERP in the medical setting. The theme of home is further split into two subthemes: 'Going home' and 'The follow-up phone call'.

Taking part in the programme

Overall, the introductory information provided to these women about enhanced recovery was reported as informative both for them and for significant others. Patients described available information as increasing their knowledge; leading to a greater understanding of why they were being asked to comply with each part of the programme.

"So you know everything went so smoothly and when he said you are going to go into that fast-track programme, I thought well that's absolutely splendid... I was absolutely thrilled to bits, you know, and I must admit I had all the details, the information that was given to me was terrific, I felt perfectly confident and happy about everything... and I took it home anyhow and studied it, because I thought if I am fast-tracking I want to be part of this" (Betty 42-88).

Existing health psychology literature recognises that seeking and using information (or not) can be indicative of, or linked to, coping style [25-27]. Those patients who use a problem focused coping strategy are suggested to benefit from the ERP's enhanced information as it helps them to understand their experience [28-30]. This was reflected in this group's reported experiences, which suggested that they were more likely to use problem focused than emotion focused coping strategies in dealing with their illness. Enabling patients to actively participate in their own care through being informed maintains a sense of autonomy which in turn prompts their motivation to adhere to a care programme [31].

Patients cited getting active as an important part of the programme, and receiving information and gaining knowledge enabled them to achieve this more quickly. It seemed that knowing what was expected of them and why helped them regain the control that is often reported as lost when undergoing surgery [32,33]. For this group, being active was the key to going home; once this was achieved then their return home was assured. The route to being active, however, was not straightforward and a number of barriers were identified, such as getting out of bed:

"The fact that I knew what I was going to have to do when I came round. I knew I was going to have to get up, and I knew that I had to get up and walk. The preparation is good" (Lynn 564-567).

In some ways the ERP, with its emphasis on getting up and active rather than resting and recuperating, contradicts the traditional post-surgery behaviour that this group of women would be more familiar with. A number of them had undergone gynaecological surgery in the past and most had had contact with someone else who had undergone a similar experience; being asked to get up almost immediately seemed, therefore, to be counterintuitive.

"I think there is a fright in moving because, well I had a big scar that does right across my abdomen... but it was this horrible feeling that you are going to burst it or something, because it's always there I suppose in your mind that are the clips going to hold? But you know, you have to have confidence in all of these things. They have done it thousands of times before, so it's very rare that you would have a big problem as long as you do, you move how they tell you" (Lynn 205-216).

Although patients included in an ERP are told that they will be expected to get out of bed, this does not transfer into intention, and subsequently, behaviour. There are several reasons why patients do not want to get out of bed and mobilise, such as discomfort or pain or because they believe that they cannot, or even that they should not, be getting out of bed so soon.

"I think there were about three things and I was doing them all the time, to keep everything going. I knew I had got to get off the bed as much as I could, but you really don't want to. You don't want to" (Sharon 347-349).

The role of the physiotherapist is integral to getting patients out of bed; they successfully get patients out of bed and encourage them to be mobile [34,35]. Postoperatively, in particular, the visit from the physiotherapist forms a key part of the start of the mobility aspect of the programme. By giving the patient permission to mobilise, the physiotherapist can build confidence that no harm will result.

"Well I think they took the, the drip thing out and then the physios were round quite early, and they got me out of bed, and then I'd still got the catheter in - that was the thing that bothered me the most before I went in, was having a catheter... so the physios came round and sort of helped me out of bed, and made sure I did it the right way. But I'd been practising at home, but it's not quite the same is it when you get there. And she took me for a walk along the corridor, and went through things again, what I should be doing" (Jane 418-430).

Once they are out of bed, patients report that being mobile is not as difficult as they expected. This enables them to move towards completing 'everyday' tasks such as getting dressed, brushing their teeth and bathing. This return to 'normal activities' is important post-surgery; it helps patients take some control of their own care and builds confidence. The women in the current study reported a belief that these are the first steps on the road to being able to return home and their rapid resumption of physical activity suggests a much less stressful post-surgery experience than might usually be the case.

Home

Going home

On Day Two of the ERP, patients are up and out of bed, can eat normally, have been to the toilet and have had a shower; they feel that they are ready to go home and they believe that this is possible. Patients in this sample felt that they had completed their 'end of the bargain' so should be given the reward of going home. Home seems to be the desirable place for discharge for most patients and all patients in this sample were being discharged to their own home. Previous research highlights that patients on ERPs who are not discharged to their home (so to a nursing home or to hospital) do not have as reduced a length of stay as those who are. It seems, then, that a return to 'own home' is a motivator for early discharge [36].

"Yes, yes definitely, because I knew that I would be going home quicker and you feel better at home, you feel more relaxed at home, and I just felt better going home, sooner be at home" (Liz 310-313).

Similarly, recovery is discussed as being easier to achieve in more familiar surroundings.

"The all round business of being able to get and move more easily at home, I mean there is no doubt that I began to recover the minute I got home" (Betty 368-370).

It appears, then, that in terms of this sample, home has a special significance which seems to be more than just 'not wanting to be in hospital'. Home is personal and symbolises a certain level of normality in their lives, especially after diagnosis. This desire to return home more quickly was not as apparent in all cases, however, and if the patient did not feel fully recovered, home was a less attractive option.

"No, I was panicking at that point because I felt so rough when I woke up on the Friday morning and I said to him [consultant], "well I don't know if I want to [go home] because I didn't feel well this morning", and he said "well I'm happy, I know you are going to be cared for at home, quite well, I've met your

husband, I know you will be cared for. If you're up to it, you can go home..." and I said "can I stay because I really don't feel too good"" (Sharon 455- 460).

Overall, then, this group of patients report a lack of pleasure in being in the hospital environment when they feel 'well' and express a strong desire to go home. On the other hand, they feel that the hospital environment is beneficial for their recovery, when they feel that they are not yet recovered. This may be because they do not want to leave hospital when they are unwell, or because they do not want to return to the home environment feeling ill.

Home is related to normality and the illness (in this case surgery for cancer) has disrupted that normality for them. After surgery, familiar activities become more difficult. Home, therefore, can be viewed as restrictive: what was once easily performed in a familiar environment is now difficult (for example, climbing the stairs). Traditionally, hospital has allowed patients to experience those negative aspects of illness (in this case recovery from surgery) in an external environment, thus leaving the home intact and devoid of the experience of illness. This idea is challenged by ERPs: patients return home earlier in their recovery journey, while everyday tasks are still difficult, thus blurring the boundaries between hospital and home. The early return home also necessitates a different level of support, at least for a while.

"I had our mum in law, my mum in law live with me for a while so we had got a stair lift, so that was very handy because I would have never took the stairs because we are in an Edwardian house with very steep stairways, so I wouldn't have got up and down" (Lily 311-316).

Previous research has found that having a partner was positively associated with engagement in activities such as reading, washing oneself, ambulating and exercising in the days following surgery [37]. The analysis reported here reveals that significant others (generally husbands in this sample) are required to fulfil a number of functions including carer, enforcer of rules and companion. In some circumstances this marks a pronounced change or reversal of roles within the household with significant others receiving little or no preparation regarding their involvement in, and the practicalities associated with, having to care for someone in the early stages of recovery.

"And the consultant explained again that if everything was OK he'd check again on the circumstances at home, and that James would be at home for a while, he said that if he was happy to have me home, then there would be no reason why I couldn't go home" (Sheila 111-116).

Patients often feel that they can do more than they are 'supposed to' resulting in partners or family members policing them to prevent them from doing things that they should not.

"I know they say no lifting for 6 weeks afterwards, you could almost, I almost felt as if I could get, if I didn't have my husband around saying don't do that, I'll lift that and all the rest of it, I did feel extremely well" (Rachel 276-287).

The idea, from this sample, that they can do more than asked is reinforced by their completion of the tasks set by the hospital and the consequent reward of discharge. Once discharged, though, patients struggle to reconcile intuition and instruction; they generally feel well and are able to attempt or complete many 'everyday' tasks around the home, without always needing the support from their significant other. They become the 'recovering patients' in comparison to the 'active patients' that they have been in hospital. Furthermore, they are not just 'recovering from the operation' but are moving to 'recovering from cancer'.

The follow-up telephone call
In the role of 'recovering patient' at home following the ERP it is important to maintain and continue communication with the hospital. The analysis conducted for this study revealed, however, that there was a clear breakdown of communication once these patients returned home. Many feel as if they are alone and are reluctant to call for assistance from the hospital even if it is to ask for advice. ERP patients are instructed to call the hospital if they have any questions or queries once they get home. This avenue of communication is one of the reasons that ERPs work: though the care is transferred from the hospital to the home this communication channel eases the transition from one to the other [5]. The current analysis suggests otherwise: little communication is reported and patients feel uncomfortable contacting the hospital, even if there is a problem.

"Yes, yeah, because I think that even though they say that if you've got any problems you can ring us, well I know, I don't know other people but, but me personally you know, I, I know that I tend to leave things a bit too long maybe, and I don't like to bother people, and I probably wouldn't have phoned unless I was really, really worried. (Jane 573-580).

The project lead for the ERP explored here initiated the use of follow-up phone calls to ease the transition from one environment to the other. This initiative met with some success and is supported by research conducted in other areas [38,39]. The analysis clearly highlights that patients value the follow-up phone call and believe that this is beneficial in their transition to being at home.

"It was nice to know that she was going to ring when I got out of the hospital, because I thought I've got the weekend now, and, am I going to be alright, I mean I don't want to be a nuisance, although the ward had reassured me to ring if there was a problem. But I didn't want to sort of be a nuisance as such, and I was a bit worried that what would happen just in case they were any problems, but it was nice to know Katy was going to call on Monday" (Sheila 1010-1024).

The use of telecommunication is not new, but is a resource that is becoming increasingly beneficial for those in the medical profession. The ability to be able to contact patients outside of the hospital environment is of benefit to both the patient and the hospital, as it means that valuable bed days are saved for the hospital and that patients are reassured that they are not expected to manage on their own. The follow-up phone call provides an opportunity through which information can be reinforced, which may increase compliance whilst ensuring that patients are both physically and emotionally comfortable [40]. It also means that both sides are given the opportunity to give and receive important information.

"Yes, yes the enhanced recovery people actually phoned up to the ward to see how I was doing, and when I got home... they wanted to see how I was doing. They had pre warned me that they were going to be keeping an eye on me which was nice really" (Lily 328-335).

Of course, one challenge is that the calls *must* happen: patients must have that contact with the hospital if they are expecting it, in the same way as if a visit from a doctor was promised at the hospital; deviation from the expected can lead to a negative experience for patients, as they may well be relying on the follow-up phone call from the hospital to discuss any difficulties or to ask any questions that they may have after discharge. Not implementing the follow-up call may result in other healthcare providers having to see patients in clinic or in the home (GP practices or district nurses) when a follow-up phone call may have dealt with the question in a more timely and efficient manner.

Discussion
Main findings
Prior to surgery, the receipt of information about the coming days is particularly important for patients and their significant others. It allows them to understand why they are being asked to comply with the programme and helps set their expectations about what is required

from them after surgery. This information moderates the relationship between instruction and intuition, which is an ongoing battle for patients taking part in ERPs. Patients find that initiating physical movement (getting out of bed) most difficult; physiotherapists have an important role to play in patients' mobility as they, in part, give patients both permission and confidence to mobile within a structured environment.

Patients who see a physiotherapist at the preoperative appointment are shown how to get off the bed, and are given information to support this. This process was highlighted in the patients' accounts of their experience as being important for them, so is something that should be encouraged, particularly as it may improve patients' self-efficacy in getting out of bed and starting to mobilise [41-43]. It is known that self-efficacy represents a personal resource factor that may facilitate coping both during and after surgery [44]. Bandura described that one of the ways to improve self-efficacy is though vicarious experience (watching someone else who is comparable with the patient) [43]. In light of this, it may be worthwhile having a resource available for patients to watch or use that shows patients how to correctly get out of bed (modelled by an appropriate actor), in something as simple as a video that could be distributed on CD, online or shown in clinic [45].

ERPs allow patients to go home sooner, and for many this is the place that they desire to be (albeit when they are confident to return home). However, home is not as 'easy' as before the operation. Early discharge with reduced mobility alters the role of home and the interaction that patients have with this place. Additionally, early discharge challenges the roles of those who are associated with home (primarily spouses or other close family members). Information about what patients should and should not do after their operation is detailed in the literature given to them at the preoperative stage and is followed by confirmation on discharge. As long ago as 1999, however, researchers found that physicians overestimate patients' understandings of the post-discharge treatment plan, and suggested that steps should be taken to improve communication about post-discharge treatment [46]. More recently, research has found that husbands who were asked to watch videotaped information designed to assist patients in their recovery after surgery were more successful in helping their wives achieve this, thus suggesting that information specifically written for significant others may be of benefit [47].

The implementation of follow-up phone calls assists with the transition from the hospital to the home environment. The analysis highlights that patients are unlikely to contact the hospital themselves. Therefore, the follow-up phone calls must happen in order to prevent unnecessary readmission and use of primary care resources. An intervention that would encourage patients to call the ward when necessary would be beneficial. This may include some sort of prompt sheet in the discharge material that details the type of problems to look out for (that is, with wounds or bowel movements). This would be beneficial for both patients and significant others as it would raise awareness of some of the issues that are associated with this type of surgery and which ones are problematic and require hospital intervention. In addition to this, it may be beneficial for those completing the discharge to emphasise the availability of contact with the ward to the significant other who is staying with the patient on their return home. The significant other often becomes the main carer and is on occasion faced with the decision about whether to seek medical assistance [11]. The availability of communication with a healthcare professional on the ward may well reduce some of the worry or stress associated with caring for a patient at home who is on day two of recovery from surgery.

Strengths and limitations

This is the first study looking at the experiences of taking part in an ERP for women undergoing surgery for gynaecological cancer. The analysis of the interview data gives a previously unseen view of ERPs from the patient experience and has highlighted a number of areas for consideration when designing perioperative care for gynaecological cancer patients. However, there are a number of limitations. Patients included in the analysis were recruited from a larger sample of women. All patients on the ERP within a given time frame were asked to take part, and out of 33 patients, only 14 chose to participate. This self-selecting sample may have been the patients who have 'something to say' about the programme and chose this evaluation as an avenue for discussion. Further to this, the interviews were conducted after a considerable period of time for some patients (up to 8 months after the operation). For future research it may be beneficial to interview patients closer to the time of surgery. However, for this study it was difficult to interview participants who were still on active treatment, as they did not have time to participate, and in some cases, did not feel ready to explore their experiences of surgery.

This sample also consisted of older women. With a mean age of 66 years, there was little reflection of the breadth of ages of patients with gynaecological cancer. Younger patients were invited to take part but declined the offer. It would be interesting to compare the experience of younger patients (that is, those with cervical cancer) with that of the older generation to explore any impact of age on the perception of the programme and their expectations. In addition to this, all patients in this sample were returning to their own home rather than an alternative place of discharge such as a nursing home or a long-term hospital bed. Research suggests that patients who return to a destination other than home experience longer lengths of stay than those who return home [36]. As the current analysis had such a large focus on home and the role of home in enhanced recovery, additional research with a diverse patient group is required to effectively explore other possible experiences.

Conclusion

ERPs are highly valued by the patients taking part in them. For patients, ERPs are more than just a reduction in length of stay. Patients value the individual aspects of the ERP, in particular, information resources, the availability of physiotherapists and the delivery of follow-up phone calls. This highlights the need to develop and maintain the individual aspects of ERPs over time to ensure that ongoing developments in the programme are sensitive and responsive to patient needs. Ongoing research into the patient experiences of ERP are required to ensure that quality care is being delivered to patients, and that the patient experience is considered alongside length of stay data in terms of determining the efficacy of ERPs.

Competing interests

There are no competing interests for any of the authors of this paper.

Authors' contributions

SA, JM and AB were all involved in the planning of the research, the analysis of the data and the preparation of the manuscript. All authors approved the final version of the manuscript.

Acknowledgements

We would like to acknowledge the contribution of Claire Hill, who was the project lead for the ERP; Claire contributed to the recruitment of patients in the audit. Additionally, we would like to acknowledge Dr. Heidi Sowter for her preliminary comments on the paper. Our thanks go to the Gynaecological Cancer Fund, which is part of the Derby Hospital Charity for the funding supplied to support this project.

Author details

[1]Psychology Department, Faculty of Education, Health & Science, University of Derby, Kedleston Road, Derby DE22 1GB, UK. [2]Centre for Patient Safety and Service Quality, Imperial College London, Medical School Building, St Mary's Campus, Norfolk Place, London W2 1PG, UK. [3]Gynaecology/Oncology, Maternity and Gynaecology Level 2, Women and Children's Services, Royal Derby Hospital, Uttoxeter Road, Derby DE22 3NE, UK.

References

1. Department of Health: *High quality care for all: NHS next stage review Final Report*. London: Department of Health; 2008.
2. Department of Health: *Improving Outcomes: A Strategy for Cancer*. London: Department of Health; 2011.
3. Department of Health: *The NHS Quality, Innovation, Productivity and Preventions Challenge: an introduction for clinicians*. London: Department of Health; 2010.
4. NHS Improvement: *Enhanced Recovery Partnership Programme - Fulfilling the potential: A better journey for patients and a better deal for the NHS*. Leicester: NHS Improvement; 2012.
5. Department of Health: *Enhanced Recovery Partnership Programme – Report March 2011*. London: Department of Health; 2011.
6. Wilmore DW, Kehlet H: Recent advances: management of patients in fast track surgery. *Br Med J* 2001, **332**:473–476.
7. Delaney CP, Fazio VW, Senagore B, Robinson AL, Halverson A, Remzi FH: 'Fast Track' postoperative management protocol for patients with high co-morbidity undergoing complex abdominal and pelvic colorectal surgery. *Br J Surg* 2001, **88**:1533–1538.
8. Kehlet H: Multimodal approach to control postoperative pathophysiology and rehabilitation. *Br J Anaesth* 1997, **78**:606–617.
9. Fearon KCH, Ljungqvist O, Von Mayenfeldt M, Revhaug A, Dejong CHC, Lassen K, Nygren J, Hausel J, Soop M, Andersen J, Kehlet H: Enhanced recovery after surgery: a consensus review of clinical care for patients undergoing colonic resection. *Clin Nutr* 2005, **24**:466–477.
10. Blazeby JM, Soulsby M, Winstone K, King PM, Bulley S, Kennedy RH: A qualitative evaluation of patients' experiences of an enhanced recovery programme for colorectal cancer. *Color Dis* 2010, **12**:e236–e242.
11. Norlyk A, Harder I: After colonic surgery: the lived experience of participating in a fast track programme. *Int J Qual Stud Health Well-being* 2009, **4**:170–180.
12. Norlyk A, Harder I: Recovering at home: participating in a fast track colon cancer surgery programme. *Nurs Inq* 2011, **18**:165–173.
13. Wagner L, Carlslund AM, Moller C, Ottesen B: Patient and staff (doctors and nurses) experiences of abdominal hysterectomy in accelerated recovery programme. *Dan Med Bull* 2004, **51**:418–421.
14. Wagner L, Carlslund AM, Sorensen M, Ottesen B: Women's experiences with short admission in abdominal hysterectomy and their patterns of behaviour. *Scand J Caring Sci* 2005, **19**:330–336.
15. Smith JA, Flowers P, Larkin M: *Interpretative Phenomenological Analysis: Theory, Method & Research*. London: Sage; 2009.
16. Dearnley C: A reflection on the use of semi-structured interviews. *Nurse Res* 2005, **13**:19–28.
17. British Psychological Society: *Codes of Ethics and Conduct*. Leicester: The British Psychological Society; 2009.
18. Starks H, Brown Trinidad S: Choose your method: a comparison of phenomenology, discourse analysis, and grounded theory. *Qual Health Res* 2007, **17**:1372–1380.
19. McDonough MH, Sabiston CM, Crocker PRE: An interpretative phenomenological examination of psychosocial changes among breast cancer survivors in their first season of dragon boating. *J Appl Sport Psychol* 2008, **20**:425–440.
20. Earle EA, Davies H, Greenfield D, Ross R, Eiser C: Follow-up care for young people who have been treated for cancer: a focus groups analysis. *Eur J Cancer* 2005, **41**:2882–2886.
21. Hannan J, Gibson F: Advanced cancer in children: how parents decide on final dying place for their child. *Indian J Palliat* 2005, **11**:284–291.
22. Phillips E, Elander J, Montague J: Managing multiple goals during fertility treatment: an interpretative phenomenological analysis. *J Health Psychol* 2014, **19**:531–543.
23. Smith JA: Beyond the divide between cognition and discourse: using interpretative phenomenological analysis in health psychology. *Psychol Health* 1996, **11**:261–271.
24. Smith JA, Osborn M: Interpretative phenomenological analysis. In *Qualitative psychology: a practical guide to research methods*. Edited by Smith JA. London: Sage; 2003:53–80.
25. Eheman CR, Berkowitz Z, Lee J, Mohile S, Purnell J, Rodreguez EM, Roscoe J, Johnson D, Kirshner J, Morrow G: Information-seeking styles among cancer patients before and after treatment by demographics and use of information sources. *J Health Commun Int Perspect* 2009, **14**:487–502.
26. van Der Molem B: Relating information needs to the cancer experience: 1. Information as a key coping strategy. *Eur J Cancer Care (Engl)* 1999, **8**:238–238.
27. Mills ME, Sullivan K: The importance of information giving for patients newly diagnosed with cancer: a review of the literature. *J Clin Nurs* 1999, **8**:631–642.
28. Lambert SDN, Loiselle CGN, Macdonald ME: An in-depth exploration of information-seeking behavior among individuals with cancer: Part 2: Understanding patterns of information disinterest and avoidance. *Cancer Nurs* 2009, **32**:26–36.
29. Walker JA: What is the effect of preoperative information on patient satisfaction? *Br J Nurs* 2007, **16**:27–32.
30. Suhonen R, Leino-Kilpi H: Adult surgical patients and the information provided to them by nurses: a literature review. *Patient Educ Couns* 2006, **61**:5–15.
31. Williams G, Freedman Z, Deci E: Supporting autonomy to motivate patients with diabetes for glucose control. *Diabetes Care* 1998, **21**:1644–1651.

32. Heike IM, Mahler HIM, Kulik JA: **Preferences for health care involvement, perceived control and surgical recovery: a prospective study.** *Soc Sci Med* 1990, **31**:743–751.

33. Taylor SE: **Hospital patient behaviour: reactance, helplessness or control?** *J Soc Issues* 1979, **35**:156–184.

34. Stockton K, Mengersen K: **Effect of multiple physiotherapy sessions on functional outcomes in the initial postoperative period after primary total hip replacement: a randomized controlled trial.** *Arch Phys Med Rehabil* 2009, **90**:1652–1657.

35. Wainwright T, Middleton R: **An orthopaedic enhanced recovery pathway.** *Curr Anaesth Crit Care* 2010, **21**:114–120.

36. Brasel KJ, Lim HJ, Nirula R, Weigelt JA: **Length of stay: an appropriate quality measure?** *Arch Surg* 2007, **142**:461–466.

37. Schroder K, Schwarzer R, Konertz W: **Coping as a mediator in recovery from cardiac surgery.** *Psychol Health* 1998, **13**:83–97.

38. Mistiaen P, Poot E: *Telephone follow up, initiated by a hospital-based health professional, for post-discharge problems in patients discharged from hospital to home (Review).* Oxford: The Cochrane Collaboration, John Wiley & Sons, Ltd; 2008.

39. Dudas V, Bookwalter T, Kerr KM, Pantilat SZ: **The impact of follow-up phone calls to patients after hospitalisation.** *Am J Med* 2001, **111**:S26–S30.

40. Cox K, Wilson E: **Follow up for people with cancer: nurse led services and telephone interventions.** *J Adv Nurs* 2003, **43**:51–61.

41. Sirur R, Richardson J, Wishart L, Hanna S: **The role of theory in increasing adherence to prescribed practice.** *Physiotherapy* 2009, **61**:68–77.

42. Cheal B, Clemson L: **Older people enhancing self-efficacy in fall-risk situations.** *Aust Occup Ther J* 2001, **48**:80–91.

43. Bandura A: **Self-efficacy mechanism in human agency.** *Am Psychol* 1982, **37**:122–147.

44. Knoll N, Rieckmann N, Schwarzer R: **Coping as a mediator between personality and stress outcomes: a longitudinal study with cataract surgery patients.** *Eur J Personal* 2005, **19**:1–19.

45. Lee LL, Arthur A, Avis M: **Using self-efficacy theory to develop interventions that help older people overcome psychological barriers to physical activity: a discussion paper.** *Int J Nurs Stud* 2008, **45**:1690–1699.

46. Calkins DR, Davis RB, Reiley P, Phillips RS, Pineo KLC, Delbanco TL, Iezzoni LI: **Patient-Physician communication at hospital discharge and patients understanding of the post-discharge treatment plan.** *Arch Intern Med* 1999, **157**:1026–1030.

47. Mahler HIM, Kulik JA: **Effects of a videotape information intervention for spouses on spouse distress and patient recovery from surgery.** *Health Psychol* 2002, **21**:427–437.

18

Design and methodology of SNAP-1: a Sprint National Anaesthesia Project to measure patient reported outcome after anaesthesia

Suneetha Ramani Moonesinghe[1,2]*, Eleanor Mary Kate Walker[1,2], Madeline Bell[2] and the SNAP-1 investigator group

Abstract

Background: Patient satisfaction is an important metric of health-care quality. Accidental awareness under general anaesthesia (AAGA) is a serious complication of anaesthesia care which may go unrecognised in the immediate perioperative period but leads to long-term psychological harm for affected patients. The SNAP-1 study aimed to measure patient satisfaction with anaesthesia care and the incidence of AAGA, reported on direct questioning within 24 h of surgery, in a large multicentre cohort. A secondary aim of SNAP-1 was to test the effectiveness of a new network of Quality Audit and Research Coordinators in NHS anaesthetic departments, to achieve widespread study participation and high patient recruitment rates. This manuscript describes the study methodology.

Methods: SNAP-1 was a prospective observational cohort study. The study protocol was approved by the National Research Ethics Service. All UK NHS hospitals with anaesthetic departments were invited to participate. Adult patients undergoing any type of non-obstetric surgery were recruited in participating hospitals on 13th and 14th May 2014. Demographic data were collected by anaesthetists providing perioperative care. Patients were then approached within 24 h of surgery to complete two questionnaires—the Bauer patient satisfaction questionnaire (to measure patient reported outcome) and the modified Brice questionnaire (to detect possible accidental awareness). Completion of postoperative questionnaires was taken as evidence of implied consent. Results were recorded on a standard patient case report form, and local investigators entered anonymised data into an electronic database for later analysis by the core research team.

Results: Preliminary analyses indicate that over 15,000 patients were recruited across the UK, making SNAP-1 the largest NIHR portfolio-adopted study in anaesthesia to date. Both descriptive and analytic epidemiological analyses will be used to answer specific questions about the patient perception of anaesthesia care overall and in surgical sub-specialties and to determine the incidence of AAGA.

Conclusions: The SNAP-1 study recruited a large number of UK hospitals and thousands of perioperative patients using newly established networks in the UK anaesthetic profession. The results will provide benchmarking information to aid interpretation of patient satisfaction data and also determine the incidence of AAGA reported on a single postoperative visit.

Keywords: Patient-reported outcome, Patient satisfaction, Anesthesia awareness, Epidemiology, Cohort study

* Correspondence: rmoonesinghe@gmail.com
[1]UCL/UCLH Surgical Outcomes Research Centre, University College Hospital NIHR Biomedical Research Centre, London NW1 2BU, UK
[2]National Institute for Academic Anaesthesia's Health Services Research Centre, Royal College of Anaesthetists, Churchill House 35 Red Lion Square, London WC1R 4SG, UK

Background

Patient feedback metrics are viewed as important assessments of the quality of health care. Broadly, the patient's viewpoint can be sought in three domains. First, they can provide feedback on interactions with health-care professionals and specifically communications skills: colloquially, this might be referred to as the "bedside manner" test; and in the UK, this is a mandatory assessment for clinical doctors as part of the revalidation process. Second, patients can provide feedback on their *experience* of health care; such questionnaires would usually seek the patient viewpoint on a diverse range of issues such as cleanliness of the care environment, efficiency of treatment and services and the courtesy and trustworthiness of staff. Finally, patients may provide their views on the efficacy of their treatment, using patient-reported outcome measures (PROMs). The National Health Service (NHS) has a mandated programme of patient-reported outcome measures for a number of surgical procedures which are aimed at alleviating symptoms and improving health-related quality of life, such as hip and knee joint replacement and varicose vein repairs.

In perioperative anaesthesia practice, the patient perspective on their care can be sought through the administration of patient satisfaction measures. Patient satisfaction has been previously described as a construct which comprises a cognitive evaluation and an emotional response to the care received [1]. It is important to use an appropriately designed questionnaire to measure patient satisfaction, so that reliable and valid results are obtained. A systematic review has recently been published which qualitatively assessed the psychometric development and validation of published patient satisfaction questionnaires relating to anaesthesia practice [2]. This study concluded that the Bauer questionnaire [3] was amongst the best for use in the perioperative setting, both in terms of the rigour with which it was developed and the acceptability of the questionnaire to patients.

While it is of clear importance to measure patient experience and satisfaction, in anaesthetic practice, an important adverse outcome which is not commonly searched for or reported in routine practice is accidental awareness under general anaesthesia (AAGA). Estimates of the incidence of AAGA vary from 1–2 per 1,000 patients in clinical trials, [4-6] to considerably lower (approximately 1 in 15,000 or 20,000 general anaesthetics) in observational studies and surveys [7-9]. As with patient satisfaction, of paramount importance in being able to estimate the incidence of AAGA is the type of questionnaire or interview administered to patients. Traditionally, the Brice questionnaire and protocol has been adopted to elicit reports of AAGA—a series of five open-ended questions which are administered to the patient three times within 30 days of surgery [10]. A modified Brice questionnaire, which used

closed questions with multiple choice answers, was subsequently adopted for a large randomised control trial evaluating the efficacy of a protocoled use of Bi-spectral Index monitoring in the prevention of AAGA [6].

While most anaesthetists will be aware of the availability both of patient satisfaction questionnaires and Brice methods, clinical experience tells us that they are infrequently used in routine practice in the United Kingdom (UK). Reasons for this may include a lack of familiarity with validated measures and a lack of benchmarking data to aid interpretation of patient satisfaction data. Furthermore, there are only limited data evaluating the reported incidence of AAGA where patients have been approached using a Brice-style questionnaire in a real-world setting. Therefore, the first UK Sprint National Anaesthesia Project (SNAP-1) aimed to prospectively measure patient reported outcome after anaesthesia in a large multicentre cohort. This paper describes the methods and analysis plan for the SNAP-1 study.

Methods

Aims and objectives

The aims of SNAP-1 are to report the descriptive and analytic epidemiology of the delivery and patient-reported outcomes of anaesthesia in the UK. Objectives are as follows:

1. To describe conduct of perioperative anaesthesia in the UK, including personnel, technology support and pharmacological management and postoperative resource utilisation;
2. To describe the characteristics of the patient population undergoing surgery involving an anaesthetist;
3. To measure patient satisfaction after anaesthesia using a validated survey on a national scale;
4. To determine the relationship between individual patient predicted risk using validated scoring systems and patient-reported postoperative outcome
5. To record the reported incidence of AAGA in routine UK practice using a modified Brice questionnaire administered within 24 h of surgery;
6. To determine associations between patient characteristics, procedural factors and adverse patient-reported outcomes

In addition to these main aims and objectives, a secondary aim of SNAP-1 is to determine the effectiveness of the Quality Audit and Research Coordinator (QuARC) network, at achieving local engagement and coordination with a national research project. The QuARC network was established by the National Institute for Academic Anaesthesia's Health Services Research Centre (NIAA HSRC); all UK anaesthetic departments were asked to nominate a consultant anaesthetist as the QuARC, with the aim of liaising between the clinical department and the NIAA HSRC in national survey, audit, quality improvement and research projects. A particular aim of SNAP-1 was also to engage trainee anaesthetists in research. Previous surveys have shown that many trainees are unable to access opportunities to participate in research, despite a desire to do so; [11,12] therefore, SNAP-1 was proposed as an opportunity to address this gap.

Study design and ethics

SNAP-1 was a multicentre observational study. Ethics approval was granted by the UK National Research Ethics Service (West Midlands Committee; REC reference 14/WM/0043). The study was approved as a research study, with implied consent being provided by patients upon completion of the questionnaires.

Recruitment, inclusion and exclusion criteria

All adult (≥18 years) patients in participating hospitals undergoing any type of surgery or procedure under anaesthesia (local, regional or general) or sedation administered by an anaesthetist were eligible for inclusion. The following patient groups were excluded:

- Age less than 18 years
- Patients unable to understand spoken or written English
- Obstetric patients
- Patients too unwell or confused to be able to complete the questionnaire
- Patients who refused consent

The recruitment dates for SNAP-1 were 13 and 14 May 2014. All eligible patients having procedures involving an anaesthetist in participating on those dates were given a participant information sheet (Additional file 1) before their procedure, explaining that they would be approached postoperatively to complete the study questionnaires. No specific consent form was required as the ethics approval stated that completion of the follow-up questionnaires could be taken as implied consent: this was explained to patients in the participant information sheet. The target recruitment rate for the study was 7,500 patients.

Dataset

The dataset comprised three questionnaires: a demographic questionnaire (completed by the perioperative anaesthetist at the time of surgery; Additional file 2), the Bauer patient satisfaction questionnaire and a modified Brice questionnaire (MBQ) (Additional file 3). The MBQ was adapted from that used in the BAG-RECALL study [6]. Demographic data were collected on all patients in

participating centres who met inclusion criteria on the study days. The variables within the demographic questionnaire included patient factors, personnel factors and process factors. The patient risk variables were based on simple previously validated preoperative predictors of objective adverse postoperative outcomes. Patients were subsequently approached to complete the follow-up questionnaires (see Additional file 3) either on the day of surgery before hospital discharge (for ambulatory surgery patients) or within 24 h of surgery (for those undergoing inpatient surgery). Both the date of the procedure and the date of survey completion were noted for each patient. Data were collected on paper case report forms (CRFs) and subsequently transcribed by local investigators into electronic CRFs via a secure web-based data entry portal. A unique identifier for each case was generated through the creation of each new eCRF.

Data management

The paper CRFs include fields for patient identifiers (name, date of birth and hospital number). These CRFs are securely stored at each participating site in accordance with the principles of information governance and good clinical practice. The electronic CRFs did not contain fields for patient identifiable information: therefore, each local investigator was required to keep a recruitment log to enable later identification of patients if required. Thus, no patient identifiable data was transferred outside the local hospital environment either electronically or on paper.

Post-study investigator questionnaire

In order to assess the impact of this study on engagement with research amongst UK anaesthetists, a post-study questionnaire was issued to all registered investigators (see Additional file 4).

Study coordination and funding

Investigators were sought from every anaesthetic department in the UK which provided perioperative services to adult non-obstetric patients. Site and investigator recruitment was facilitated through the Quality Audit and Research Coordinator (QuARC) network. Recruitment of trainee investigators was particularly encouraged. SNAP-1 was also adopted onto the National Institute for Health Research clinical research portfolio, thereby enabling Clinical Research Network support to be provided to participating hospitals.

Study management was led by a core group of investigators based at the UCL/UCLH Surgical Outcomes Research Centre and the NIAA's HSRC. The core group consisted of the Chief Investigator, a trainee lead investigator and a study administrator based at the NIAA HSRC. Study oversight was provided by the Executive

Management Board of the NIAA's HSRC. The study sponsor was the University College London Hospitals NHS Foundation Trust. The study was funded through a grant of £18,069 from the National Institute for Academic Anaesthesia and through salary support (for the Chief Investigator and trainee lead investigator) from the University College London Hospitals NHS Foundation Trust and its National Institute for Health Research Biomedical Research Centre.

Analysis plan

All results will be reported in accordance with the "Strengthening the Reporting of Observational Studies in Epidemiology" (STROBE) statement [13]. The main focus of analysis is to describe the epidemiology of the practice of anaesthesia and patient-reported outcome after anaesthesia in the overall cohort and, where feasible, in surgical sub-specialty groups and for specific surgical procedures.

Study recruitment and missing data

Study recruitment rates and missing data will be reported. The total number of sites that participated (broken down by country) will be presented in addition to the total number of patients recruited. The number of eligible patients who did not complete the questionnaires and the reasons reported for this will be stated. Comparison will be made of the demographics of patients who did and did not complete follow-up questionnaires. A description will be provided of any missing data points.

Descriptive epidemiology

The information collected from the patient demographic and perioperative questionnaire will be presented. The number of cases per specialty and type of procedure will be stated. Point estimates and ranges will be given for patient descriptors (for example, age, ASA grade, comorbidities and body mass index) in addition to detail of the use of long-term analgesics or benzodiazepines. The characteristics of surgery will be described by urgency, severity and length of operation. The personnel (i.e. seniority of the anaesthetist(s)) involved will be described as well as the type and site of anaesthesia induction. Anaesthetic technique and postoperative destination will be described and summarised both overall and for surgical sub-specialty groups.

The variables for three risk prediction/adjustment tools were included in the dataset: the population-based ASA grade; [14] the Surgical Risk Scale; [15] and the Surgical Outcome Risk Tool [16]. The latter two of these systems have been validated for the prediction of 30-day mortality after surgery. The predicted mortality based on these scoring systems will be presented for the overall patient population and for surgical sub-specialty groups. Data will be presented describing patterns of admission to high dependency or intensive care facilities compared with the predicted risk of 30-day mortality according to these systems, in order to assess compliance with national recommendations on postoperative care [17,18].

Bauer patient satisfaction questionnaire

For each of questions 1–10 (on anaesthesia-related discomfort), counts and percentages will be reported for each of the three potential responses. For questions 11–15 (which ask about satisfaction with anaesthesia care), counts and percentages of each of the four potential responses will be reported. Further analysis of the all these responses within different categories using chi-square testing with Bonferroni's correction to compare outcomes between categories, such as (for example):

- Ambulatory surgery—comparisons by specialty and operative procedure
- Inpatient surgery—comparisons by specialty and operative procedure
- Elective/expedited versus immediate/urgent

Within surgical categories, comparison will be made between the responses to the patient satisfaction questionnaires depending on whether the questionnaire was administered on the day of surgery or day 1 postoperatively.

Univariate analysis will be used to demonstrate associations between patient factors and adverse outcomes, defined as the worst category answer for each question. Logistic regression will be used to determine independent risk factors for the adverse outcomes. Analyses will be conducted for the overall population and for surgical and patient categories where the sample size allows. The decision on whether to conduct regression analyses in particular subgroups will be informed by consideration of the principles described by Vittinghoff and McCulloch, including consideration of whether continuous or binary variables are included, the number of events per outcome variables and the sample size itself [19].

Modified Brice questionnaire (MBQ)

Counts and percentages for the responses to each question will be presented. Comparison will be made between the patients' perception of the anaesthetic technique (general versus sedation or regional) and the actual anaesthetic technique.

The responses to the MBQ will be analysed to identify cases which may potentially represent AAGA. Both the responses to the closed multiple choice questions and free-text responses will be analysed for this purpose. If a case is found where any of these responses would be consistent with a potential case of AAGA, the lead local investigator for the site where the patient was anaesthetised will be informed and asked to follow up the case according to their local departmental guidelines. Local investigators will be asked to provide structured feedback to the core research team. Following review of information received from local investigators, the case will be classified as either proven awareness, not awareness, or unable to determine.

As the SNAP-1 study only asks patients about awareness once within 24 h of surgery, the results will be extrapolated to determine an estimate of the likely actual incidence of awareness, based on the results of previous studies which used three separate interviews (on approximately day 0, days 1–2 and day 30 postoperatively) and reported the incidence of awareness occurring on each day [20]. Depending on the event rate and sample size, regression analyses to determine independent risk factors for awareness may be undertaken.

Results and discussion
SNAP-1 follows similar methodology to previous studies of surgical [21] and anaesthesia-related epidemiology, [22] in adopting a "snapshot" approach to gather a large sample of data in a short time frame. However, these studies did not require patient consent or any interaction with patients outwith the usual practice of the anaesthesia or perioperative team. Thus, to our knowledge, this is the first such study in the UK to measure patient-reported outcome related to anaesthesia using this methodology. Preliminary analyses indicate that this is the highest recruiting NIHR portfolio-adopted consenting research study in anaesthesia to date.

SNAP-1 has introduced the concept of using a validated survey to measure patient satisfaction with anaesthesia to the majority of UK hospitals. It is hoped that individual departments will reflect on the resources that were required to facilitate the study and use this to inform future attempts to measure patient satisfaction for the purposes of quality improvement, research and revalidation. The post-study survey will assess the impact of the study on anaesthetists' willingness to engage with the measurement of patient satisfaction and the screening of patients for AAGA in routine practice.

Once analysed and reported, it is hoped that SNAP-1 results will inform the development of patient information leaflets for different types of surgery, which can be used to better inform patients about the likely short-term outcomes of their anaesthetic and surgical experience. Summary national data should provide benchmarking information for future local and national surveys of patient-reported outcome after anaesthesia.

The study has received little primary funding and may provide important data on the feasibility of conducting such large-scale studies on a limited budget. While the study methodology was simple and the intervention (the administration of a questionnaire) was not complex, the logistics of coordinating a study which required individual Research and Development department approval in all four UK-devolved nations was considerable. The post-study investigator questionnaire should improve our understanding of the baseline level of experience of "non-academic" anaesthetists with research and research methodology and the potential benefits (and pitfalls) of engaging with clinical research for both trainees and career-grade doctors. Additionally, it will provide information about the motivation for anaesthetists' participation in this study, including whether the promise of acknowledgment on study manuscripts was a significant incentive to take part. (see Additional file 5).

Conclusions
SNAP-1 should provide new and important data on patient-reported outcome after anaesthesia, the incidence of AAGA in a "real-world" clinical setting and the impact of participation in nationally coordinated patient-focussed research for clinical anaesthetists in the UK, particularly trainees.

Additional files

Additional file 1: Participant information sheet.
Additional file 2: Patient demographics questionnaire.
Additional file 3: Bauer and Brice questionnaires.
Additional file 4: Post-study investigators questionnaires.
Additional file 5: SNAP-1 investigator list (collaborators).

Abbreviations
AAGA: Accidental awareness under general anaesthesia; SNAP-1: Sprint national anaesthesia project; QuARC: Quality audit and research coordinator; MBQ: Modified brice questionnaire; BPS: Bauer patient satisfaction questionnaire; NIAA: National institute for academic anaesthesia; HSRC: Health services research centre; ASA: American society of anesthesiology physical status score.

Competing interests
The authors declare that they have no competing interests.

Authors' contributions
SRM led the study design and conduct and drafted the manuscript. EMKE contributed to the study design and conduct and with SRM drafted the manuscript. MH contributed to the study conduct. All authors approved the final version of the manuscript.

Acknowledgements
This study was funded by the National Institute for Academic Anaesthesia and the Royal College of Anaesthetists and supported by the National Institute for Health Research University College London Hospitals Biomedical Research Centre.
This manuscript has been written on behalf of the SNAP-1 investigators who contributed to the conduct of the study and are listed in Additional file 5.

References

1. Pascoe GC. Patient satisfaction in primary health care: a literature review and analysis. Eval Program Plann. 1983;6:185–210.

2. Barnett SF, Alagar RK, Grocott MP, Giannaris S, Dick JR, Moonesinghe SR. Patient-satisfaction measures in anesthesia: qualitative systematic review. Anesthesiology. 2013;119:452–78.

3. Bauer M, Bohrer H, Aichele G, Bach A, Martin E. Measuring patient satisfaction with anaesthesia: perioperative questionnaire versus standardised face-to-face interview. Acta Anaesthesiol Scand. 2001;45:65–72.

4. Myles PS, Leslie K, McNeil J, Forbes A, Chan MT. Bispectral index monitoring to prevent awareness during anaesthesia: the B-Aware randomised controlled trial. Lancet. 2004;363:1757–63.

5. Avidan MS, Zhang L, Burnside BA, Finkel KJ, Searleman AC, Selvidge JA, et al. Anesthesia awareness and the bispectral index. N Engl J Med. 2008;358:1097–108.

6. Avidan MS, Jacobsohn E, Glick D, Burnside BA, Zhang L, Villafranca A, et al. Prevention of intraoperative awareness in a high-risk surgical population. N Engl J Med. 2011;365:591–600.

7. Pandit JJ, Cook TM, Jonker WR, O'Sullivan E. A national survey of anaesthetists (NAP5 baseline) to estimate an annual incidence of accidental awareness during general anaesthesia in the UK. Br J Anaesth. 2013;110:501–9.

8. Pollard RJ, Coyle JP, Gilbert RL, Beck JE. Intraoperative awareness in a regional medical system: a review of 3 years' data. Anesthesiology. 2007;106:269–74.

9. Pandit JJ, Andrade J, Bogod DG, Hitchman JM, Jonker WR, Lucas N, et al. 5th National Audit Project (NAP5) on accidental awareness during general anaesthesia: summary of main findings and risk factors. Br J Anaes. 2014. doi:10.1093/bja/aeu313.

10. Brice DD, Hetherington RR, Utting JE. A simple study of awareness and dreaming during anaesthesia. Br J Anaesth. 1970;42:535–42.

11. Ross-Anderson D, Reddy S, Setty S, Moonesinghe SR. Ivory towers and academic utopia: research and audit training in anaesthesia. Bull R Coll Anaesth. 2009;58:8–10.

12. Mesbah A, Yeung J. Trainees and anaesthesia research: a survey of research activity during UK anaesthesia training. Bull R Coll Anaesth. 2014;85:32–4.

13. von Elm E, Altman DG, Egger M, Pocock SJ, Gotzsche PC, Vandenbroucke JP. The Strengthening the Reporting of Observational Studies in Epidemiology (STROBE) statement: guidelines for reporting observational studies. J Clin Epidemiol. 2008;61:344–9.

14. Saklad M. Grading of patients for surgical procedures. Anesthesiology. 1941;2:281–5.

15. Sutton R, Bann S, Brooks M, Sarin S. The surgical risk scale as an improved tool for risk-adjusted analysis in comparative surgical audit. Br J Surg. 2002;89:763–8.

16. Protopapa K, Simpson J, Smith N, Moonesinghe SR. Development and validation of the Surgical Outcome Risk Tool (SORT): a novel preoperative risk stratification tool. Br J Surg. in press.

17. Anderson ID. The higher risk general surgical patient: towards improved care for a forgotton group. Royal College of Surgeons and the Department of: Health; 2011.

18. Findlay GP, Goodwin APL, Protopapa K, Smith NCE, Mason M. Knowing the risk: a review of the perioperative care of surgical patients. National Confidential Enquiry into Patient Outcome and Death. 2011.

19. Vittinghoff E, McCulloch CE. Relaxing the rule of ten events per variable in logistic and Cox regression. Am J Epidemiol. 2007;165:710–8.

20. Sandin RH, Enlund G, Samuelsson P, Lennmarken C. Awareness during anaesthesia: a prospective case study. Lancet. 2000;355:707–11.

21. Pearse RM, Moreno RP, Bauer P, Pelosi P, Metnitz P, Spies C, et al. Mortality after surgery in Europe: a 7 day cohort study. Lancet. 2012;380:1059–65.

22. Sury MRJ, Palmer JHMG, Cook TM, Pandit JJ. The State of UK anaesthesia: a survey of National Health Service activity in 2013. Br J Anaes. 2014; doi:10.1093/bja/aeu292.

19

Perioperative clinical and economic outcomes associated with replacing first-generation high molecular weight hydroxyethyl starch (Hextend®) with low molecular weight hydroxyethyl starch (Voluven®) at a large medical center

Raquel R Bartz[1], William D White[1] and Tong J Gan[2*]

Abstract

Background: Several plasma volume expander alternatives exist to enhance intravascular volume status in patients undergoing surgery. The optimal intravascular volume expander in the perioperative setting is currently unknown. Low molecular weight hetastarch, Voluven® (130/0.4), may have a better safety profile than high molecular weight hetastarch, Hextend® (450/0.7). We examined the clinical and cost outcomes of converting from Hextend® to Voluven® in a large tertiary medical center.

Methods: Using a large electronic database, we retrospectively compared two different time periods (2009 and 2010) where the availability of semisynthetic colloids changed. Perioperative and postoperative outcomes including the use of red blood cells (RBC), platelets and coagulation factors, length of stay in the postoperative acute care unit (PACU), intensive care unit and hospital, as well as 30-day and 1-year mortality were compared. In addition, direct acquisition costs of all intraoperative and PACU colloids and crystalloid use were determined.

Results: A total of 4,888 adult subjects were compared of which 1,878 received Hextend® (pre-conversion) and 2,759 received Voluven® (post-conversion) during two separate 7-month periods within 1 year apart, with the remainder receiving Plasmanate. The patients were similar in terms of patient demographics, preoperative comorbidities, ASA status, emergency surgery, types of surgery, intraoperative, and PACU times. In unadjusted outcomes, patients in the Hextend® group received more lactated Ringer's than in the Voluven® group $(2,220 + 1,312$ vs. $1,946 \pm 1,097$ ml; $P < 0.0001$). The use of albumin (Plasmanate) was reduced from 10.5% of patients to 1.1% when Voluven® was substituted for Hextend®. Unadjusted outcomes were similar in each group including hospital LOS, percent change from baseline creatinine and receipt of intraoperative and PACU blood product administration. However, overall unadjusted total fluid costs were greater in the Voluven® compared to Hextend® group ($116.7 compared to $59.3; $P < 0.001$).

Conclusions: Conversion from Hextend® to Voluven® in the perioperative period resulted in decreased albumin use and was not associated with changes in clinical outcomes and short- and long-term mortality. The conversion was associated with decreases in crystalloid use and an increase in colloid use and hence IV fluid acquisition costs in the Voluven® group.

Keywords: Hetastarch, Perioperative fluid administration, Hextend®, Voluven®

* Correspondence: tong.gan@stonybrookmedicine.edu
[2]Department of Anesthesiology, Stony Brook University, HSC Level 4, Rm 060, Stony Brook, NY 11794-8480, USA
Full list of author information is available at the end of the article

Background

Both human and semisynthetic colloids have been successfully used to increase intravascular volume in the perioperative period [1-4]. However, recent trials of volume replacement in the intensive care unit (ICU) have questioned the safety and efficacy of both human and synthetic colloids with one trial suggesting no benefit of albumin over saline for resuscitation and others suggesting harm with the use of semisynthetic colloids in this patient population [5-8]. The issue of safety has not been directly resolved in the perioperative setting. And, in many institutions, semisynthetic colloids are still available for use in patients undergoing surgical procedures where a benefit in decreased costs associated with intraoperative volume replacement may exist.

One of these semisynthetic products, Voluven®, was recently introduced into the US market. It has a lower molecular weight (150 kD) and molar substitution (0.4) and therefore has a theoretical lower plasma accumulation and tissue storage [9,10]. Previous investigations of Voluven® suggest less impact on factor VIII and Von Willebrand factor concentrations with a sustained plasma volume expansion effect resulting in less disturbance of coagulation with subsequent reduced blood loss and blood transfusion when compared to older larger molecular weight (MW) hydroxyethyl starch (HES) solutions [11,12]. In addition, up to 50 ml/kg of Voluven® can be given (about 3,500 ml in a 70-kg adult) compared to a maximum of 1,500 ml (20 ml/kg) of high MW hydroxyethyl starch to adult patients [13,14]. Therefore, Voluven® has the potential to reduce the need for other more costly plasma volume expanders such as 5% albumin as well as the need for blood transfusion. However, because of recent recommendations against the use of these products in ICU patients by regulatory agencies, hospitals have to evaluate the rationale for maintaining their availability for use in the perioperative period.

Additionally, anesthesiologists in the US are limited to using isotonic crystalloids and human albumin-based products (albumin or Plasmanate) in patients requiring intravascular volume expansion. Because of these institutional shifts of colloid types, hospital formulary costs will change. Currently, there is paucity of data that have examined the impact to hospital costs related to the use of different intravascular volume expanders. Therefore, we investigated two different periods evaluating the clinical and direct acquisition cost impact of converting from Hextend® to Voluven® in a large tertiary medical center. By comparing cases in which some colloid was given during two different periods, we sought to determine what differences in overall perioperative volume use, overall fluid costs, and certain perioperative outcomes might be associated with the use of the two different colloids.

Methods

We conducted a retrospective comparison of two different time periods at a large academic medical center, Duke University Medical Center (DUMC). In March 2010, DUMC converted from Hextend® (hetastarch 6%, MW 670 kD, in balanced electrolyte solution) to Voluven® (hydroxyethyl tetrastarch 6% in sodium chloride 0.9%) as the semisynthetic colloid for use in the perioperative period. After Duke University Medical Center Institutional Review Board approval, de-identified data was obtained from an electronic anesthesia database which consists of physiologic and treatment characteristics used for perioperative care of the patient. Because de-identified clinical data was used, this study was determined to be exempt from patient consent. Two separate 7-month periods were investigated from 1 June 2009 to 30 December 2009 (Hextend®) and 1 June 2010 to 30 December 2010 (Voluven®). Anesthesia and surgical practice was otherwise similar in these two time periods; however, overall surgical volume increased due to increased operating room capacity in 2010. We avoided the 3-month interval before and after the conversion to ensure a period of stability in practice. Pre- and postoperative data were obtained by procedure ICD-9 codes, and our local institutional data warehouse known as the Decision Support Repositories was then linked to perioperative anesthesia records. Follow-up closed for both periods on 31 December 2012. All sequential cases greater than 18 years old, who received Hextend®, Voluven®, or albumin (Plasmanate®), were examined for inclusion. Cases in which <500 ml of Hextend® or Voluven® were recorded were not included in the analysis.

Patient demographics including gender, age, surgical comorbidities, type of surgery, duration of surgery, and type of anesthesia were obtained. Patient outcomes were compared between HES periods including volume of all crystalloids and colloids administered in the intraoperative and post-anesthesia care unit (PACU), the use of red blood cells (RBC) and platelets and coagulation factors. The length of stay in the PACU, hospital length of stay, intensive care unit length of stay, and 30-day and 1-year mortality were also compared. Fluid costs were calculated using the Red book acquisition costs of each product multiplied by the number of whole or partial units received intraoperatively or in the PACU. For 2013, these costs were Hextend® (500 ml) $37.80, Voluven® (500 ml) $61.06, Plasmanate (250 ml) $41.00, lactated Ringer's (1,000 ml) $2.04, and 0.9% normal saline (1,000 ml) $2.65.

Statistical analysis

Descriptive statistics including mean and standard deviation are presented for all measures, and mean values did not differ meaningfully form median. For the primary comparison of total fluid cost between periods, we used initial Wilcoxon rank-sum tests not subject to influence by extreme outliers, followed by multivariable regression analysis adjusting for BMI, duration of surgery, emergency status, regional or general anesthesia, and type of procedure. Unadjusted two-group tests were used to compare periods on other variables. For categorical demographic and outcome variables including gender, preoperative characteristics, type of anesthesia used, and death within 30 days and 1 year, the Pearson chi-square tests were used to determine P values, or the Pearson exact tests if counts were sparse. For comparisons of continuous measures and outcomes such as fluid volumes, length of stay, red blood cells used, and percent change creatinine, Wilcoxon rank-sum tests were used to determine P values. A P value <0.05 was considered statistically significant. All analyses were conducted on non-missing data; where data was incomplete, it was assumed to be consistent with non-missing data. SAS software version 9.3 (Cary, NC, USA) was used for statistical analysis.

Results

Our database query for our defined sample initially returned a set of 5,548 cases. We then excluded 95 whose fluid volumes were zero and 196 aged <18 years old. We further excluded 206 who received <500 ml of Voluven® alone and 163 receiving <500 ml of Hextend® alone. The final overall analysis sample thus included 4,888 cases including 175 who received Plasmanate/albumin alone.

From 1 June 2009 to 30 December 2009, 2,098 were in the group in which Hextend® was the primary synthetic colloid and from 1 June 2010 to 30 December 2010, 2,790 patients were in the group in which Voluven® was available. An increase in surgical capacity accounts for the increased number of patients in the 2010 period. Otherwise, the patient demographics were similar in terms of patient characteristics, preoperative comorbidities, and emergency surgery with inconsequential differences in proportions of ASA status and types of surgery (Tables 1 and 2). Fewer patients in the 2010 group (90.1% vs. 93%, $P < 0.001$) received general anesthesia (Table 2). Intraoperative time and PACU time were similar between periods; however, in unadjusted outcomes, mean volume of lactated Ringer's given differed significantly between periods; 2,252.9 ml in 2009 - Hextend® group vs. 1,958.9 in 2010 - Voluven® group; $P < 0.0001$. As expected, long-term follow-up also differed significantly between periods (Table 2). In 2009, 1,906 subjects received a mean of 767 ml (SD ± 301.8 ml) of Hextend®

Table 1 Patient characteristics

	2009 (n = 2,098)			2010 (n = 2,790)			P value
	Total N	Mean or n	SD or percentage	Total N	Mean or n	SD or percentage	
Age (yrs) (mean, SD)	2,098	58.1	15.4	2,790	58	15.6	0.8910
Female gender (n,%)	1,972	902	45.7	2,767	1,343	48.5	0.0574
Race (n,%)	1,966			2,762			0.7380
White		1,454	74		2,043	74	0.9933
Black		430	21.9		601	21.8	0.9266
Nat. Amer		23	1.2		26	0.9	0.4444
Asian		21	1.1		22	0.8	0.3322
Other		35	1.8		65	2.4	0.1621
Multiracial		3	0.2		5	0.2	1.0000
BMI (mean, SD)	1,884	29.6	7.3	2,639	29.5	7.3	0.9510
CAD preop (n,%)	1,383	721	52.1	1,839	1,016	55.2	0.0792
COPD preop (n,%)	1,383	83	6	1,839	116	6.3	0.7207
CABG preop (n,%)	1,383	9	0.7	1,839	12	0.7	0.9951
MI preop (n,%)	1,383	21	1.5	1,839	29	1.6	0.8942
Preop valve dz (n,%)	1,383	48	3.5	1,839	67	3.6	0.7938
Diabetes type I (n,%)	1,383	6	0.4	1,839	11	0.6	0.6274
Diabetes type II (n,%)	1,383	224	16.2	1,839	331	18	0.1799
Hypertension preop (n,%)	1,383	721	52.1	1,839	1,016	55.2	0.0792
Preop creatinine (mean, SD)	1,370	1	0.6	1,847	1.1	1.3	0.1725

yrs, years; Nat. Amer, Native American; BMI, body mass index; h/o, history of; CAD, coronary artery disease; COPD, chronic obstructive pulmonary disease; Preop valve dz, preoperative valve disease; CABG, coronary artery bypass graft; MI, myocardial infarction; DM, diabetes mellitus; preop, preoperative; SD, standard deviation.

Table 2 Procedural characteristics

	2009 (n = 2,098)			2010 (n = 2,790)			P value
	Total N	Mean or n	SD or percentage	Total N	Mean or n	SD or percentage	
Emergency surgery (n,%)	1,878	149	7.9	2,677	226	8.4	0.5390
ASA class (n,%)	1,880			2,682			0.0045
1		48	2.6		59	2.2	0.4376
2		636	33.8		785	29.3	0.0011
3		1,074	57.1		1,612	60.1	0.0443
4		120	6.4		222	8.3	0.0168
5		2	0.1		4	0.1	1.0000
Procedure category	1,977			2,774			<0.0001
Misc. diagnostic (n,%)		4	0.2		10	0.4	0.4202
Obstetrical (n,%)		21	1.1		37	1.3	0.4007
Cardiovascular (n,%)		153	7.7		301	10.9	0.0003
Digestive (n,%)		398	20.1		530	19.1	0.3795
Ear (n,%)		32	1.6		73	2.6	0.0192
Endocrine (n,%)		17	0.9		33	1.2	0.2723
Eye (n,%)		3	0.2		4	0.1	1.0000
Female genital (n,%)		104	5.3		127	4.6	0.2811
Heme/lymphatic (n,%)		35	1.8		47	1.7	0.8427
Integumentary (n,%)		62	3.1		102	3.7	0.3141
Male genital (n,%)		104	5.3		104	3.7	0.0121
Musculoskeletal (n,%)		689	34.9		857	30.9	0.0041
Nervous system (n,%)		30	1.5		114	4.1	<0.0001
Nose, mouth, pharynx (n,%)		0	0		9	0.3	0.0129
Thoracic (n,%)		123	6.2		137	4.9	0.0553
Urinary (n,%)		139	7		199	7.2	0.8502
Other (n,%)		63	3.2		90	3.2	0.9115
General anes used (n,%)	1,977	1,848	93.5	2,774	2,499	90.1	<0.0001
Regional anes used (n,%)	1,977	647	32.7	2,774	930	33.5	0.5642
Surg. time (mins) (mean, SD)	1,505	240.8	128.6	2,399	242	131.8	0.8516
Rec'd any RBC, FFP, cryo (n,%)	1,977	440	22.3	2,774	578	20.8	0.2398
Days of follow-up (mean, SD)	1,976	1,081.6	323.6	2,774	776.7	211.6	<0.0001

Anes, anesthesia; SD, standard deviation; Misc, miscellaneous; Rec'd, received; RBC, red blood cell; Surg., surgical; Mins, minutes; FFP, fresh frozen plasma; Cryo, cryoprecipitate.

in the intraoperative period and 51 cases received a mean of 578.4 ml (SD ± 215 ml) in the PACU. The mean amount of Hextend® given for the entire operative and PACU period was 773.1 ml (SD ± 306.9 ml) compared to 933.7 ml (SD ± 518.4 ml) of Voluven® in 2010. Whereas, 2,650 subjects in the 2010 cohort received a mean of 905.8 ml (SD ± 495.5 ml) of Voluven® in the operative period and 263 subjects received 645.3 ml (SD ± 260.7 ml) of Voluven® in the PACU. Considering the volume of hetastarch, the mean volume of Hextend® received per case in 2009 was significantly lower than the mean volume of Voluven® received per case in 2010 (P < 0.001). The number of patients who received albumin,

either alone or in combination with a perioperative product, decreased from 220 to 31 patients from the 2009 - Hextend® to 2010 - Voluven® period, although the mean volume of Plasmanate/albumin received per case did not change significantly between periods.

In unadjusted outcomes, we did not find a difference in blood product use in patients between periods; 22% of patients in 2009 and 21% in 2010 received a blood product which consisted of either a packed RBC, fresh frozen plasma, or cryoprecipitate (Table 3). Patient outcomes did not differ significantly between periods. Hospital length of stay, change in creatinine from baseline represented as percent change from baseline creatinine, and

Table 3 Fluid volumes given

	2009 (n = 2,098)			2010 (n = 2,790)			P value
	Total N	Mean or n	SD or percentage	Total N	Mean or n	SD or percentage	
Hextend intraop (ml) (mean, SD)	1,906	767	301.8				
Hextend given in PACU (ml) (mean, SD)	51	578.4	215				
Hextend entire case (ml) (mean, SD)	1,941	773.1	306.9				
Voluven given intraop (ml) (mean, SD)				2,650	905.8	495.5	
Voluven given in PACU (mean, SD)				263	645.3	260.7	
Voluven entire case (ml) (mean, SD)				2,772	933.7	518.4	
Plasmanate total (mean, SD)	220	467.4	346.9	31	460.5	267.8	0.5029
Lactated Ringer's intraop (mean, SD)	1,861	2,232.7	1,324.7	2,591	1,943.7	1,098.5	<0.0001
Lactated Ringer's PACU (mean, SD)	87	536.2	432.1	104	471.6	388.1	0.2710
Tot lac. Ringer's (ml) (mean, SD)	1,865	2,252.9	1,332.5	2,596	1,958.9	1,106.2	<0.0001
Normal saline intraop (mean, SD)	335	932.7	766.9	488	940	739.4	0.7984
Normal saline PACU (mean, SD)	12	175.3	158.1	45	194	205.7	0.8882
Tot N saline (ml) (Mean, SD)	344	914.5	767.4	524	892.1	744.5	0.5633
RBC's intraop (mean, SD)	388	1,166.7	1,406.3	505	1,058.3	1,084.5	0.4291
RBC's PACU (mean, SD)	72	597.9	313.6	82	557.6	227.9	0.8751
RBC's total (mean, SD)	433	1,144.9	1,342.3	564	1,028.7	1,039.8	0.1790
FFP intraop (mean, SD)	123	1,069.5	1,095.3	171	947.7	938.8	0.1482
FFP PACU (mean, SD)	10	407.2	150.6	8	485.9	160.6	0.4205
Tot FFP (ml) (mean, SD)	131	1,035.3	1,071.2	177	937.5	926.6	0.2260
Cryoprecipitate intraop (mean, SD)	10	161.6	68.5	30	149.5	94.3	0.3885
Cryoprecipitate total (mean, SD)	10	161.6	68.5	31	147.9	93.1	0.3502

Intraop, intra-operative; ml, milliliters; PACU, post-anesthesia care units; Tot, Total; ml, milliliters; Lac, lactated Ringer's; N, normal; RBC, red blood cell; FFP, fresh frozen plasma.

number of intraoperative and PACU RBC transfused were similar between periods (Tables 3 and 4). Similarly, postoperative mortality at 30-day and 1-year mortality was also similar (Table 4). However, surprising overall total fluid costs in the operating room and the PACU in 2013 dollars were significantly greater in the group in 2010 - Voluven® period compared to the 2009 - Hextend® period ($122.1 compared to $68.03; P <0.001) (Table 5). After adjusting for age, BMI, length of surgery, and type of anesthetic, Voluven® was still associated with increased fluid costs. The R^2 for this multivariable model was 0.379, and the difference between periods remained significant with P < 0.001. Age, COPD, history of hypertension, and preoperative creatinine were also tested but dropped as non-significant effects. Results of the confirmatory analyses comparing all pre- vs. post-conversion cases were very consistent with the primary results.

Discussion

In this study, we had expected that the switch from Hextend® to Voluven® would be associated with overall decreased fluid acquisition costs due to lower utilization of albumin, an improved profile on intravascular coagulation

and less need for other intravascular volume expanders as well as blood products. However, although patient demographics and outcomes were similar between trial periods, in both unadjusted and adjusted analyses, overall costs associated with the 2010 - Voluven® period were greater than the 2009 - Hextend® period. The lower cost of Plasmanate/albumin was more than offset by the considerably higher unit cost of Voluven® coupled with a higher volume of Voluven® given per case.

As many hospitals in the US are receiving bundled payments for surgical procedures, the overall hospital costs associated with surgery is becoming more important to define [15-17]. This is the first study to present the effects of a switch from Hextend® to Voluven® on fluid costs to the hospital during the perioperative period. Many surgical groups are using enhanced recovery after surgery (ERAS) protocols in colorectal and other surgeries which recommend giving a semisynthetic colloid as a plasma volume expander in the intraoperative goal-directed fluid therapy algorithm in an effort to reduce total crystalloid use [18]. The use of colloid in combination with crystalloid has been shown to decrease postoperative bowel dysfunction, including incidence of

Table 4 Health-care outcomes

	2009 (n = 2,098)			2010 (n = 2,790)			P value
	Total N	Mean or n	SD or percentage	Total N	Mean or n	SD or percentage	
Any PACU time (n,%)	1,977	1,498	75.8	2,774	2,053	74	0.1681
PACU time (hrs, incl. 0) (mean, SD)	1,977	3.2	3.3	2,774	3.2	3.3	0.0848
PACU hrs if > 0 (mean, SD)	1,498	4.3	3.2	2,053	4.3	3.2	0.2991
Any ICU stay (n,%)	1,971	339	17.2	2,774	629	22.7	<0.0001
ICU days	1,971			2,774			<0.0001
None (n,%)		1,632	83		2,145	77	<0.0001
1 day (n,%)		137	7		247	9	0.0150
2 to 3 days (n,%)		114	6		189	7	0.1530
4+ days (n,%)		88	4		193	7	0.0003
Total ICU days (incl. 0) (mean, SD)	1,971	0.9	4.8	2,774	1	4.2	<0.0001
ICU days if > 0 (mean, SD)	339	5.2	10.7	629	4.5	7.8	0.3676
Highest postop creatinine (mean, SD)	1,901	1.2	1	2,634	1.4	1.5	0.0884
Creatinine pre-post percentage change (mean, SD)	1,310	24.1	69	1,735	24.1	63.6	0.4533
LOS (days) (mean, SD)	1,977	7.3	9.2	2,774	7.3	9.6	0.8711
Death - 30 days (n,%)	1,977	32	1.6	2,774	49	1.8	0.6981
Death - 1 year (n,%)	1,977	164	8.3	2,774	238	8.6	0.7286

PACU, post-anesthesia care units; postop, postoperative; hrs, hours; SD, standard deviation; ICU, intensive care unit; creatinine pre-post, creatinine pre-surgery post-surgery; LOS, length of stay.

postoperative nausea and vomiting, use of rescue antiemetic, as well as pain and edema symptoms in major surgery [2]. Although our study showed an increased direct acquisition cost to the hospital in 2010 - Voluven® over 2009 - Hextend® period. A recent study at this institution suggests that goal-directed fluid therapy in which Voluven® was used as part of an ERAS algorithm resulted in a 1-L decrease in crystalloid use overall and earlier return to bowel function in patients undergoing bowel surgery as well as a 2-day reduction in hospital length of stay [19]. Whether the use of a plasma expander or other parts of the ERAS bundle contributed to this decreased length of stay needs further study. We did not target a specific

population in our study, and future studies should specifically focus on this area of investigation and question which part of the ERAS bundle leads to the most beneficial patient outcomes.

Several limitations to the current study need consideration. This is a single center study, and hence, the results may not be generalizable to other institutions or other countries given differences in fluid acquisition costs and availability depending on regulatory agencies. Also, given the retrospective nature of this study, unaccounted confounders may exist which may have skewed our results. However, because baseline demographics are similar as the types of surgeries, this is less likely to be a major issue.

Table 5 Direct fluid acquisition costs in the Hextend® and Voluven® groups

	2009 (n = 2,098)			2010 (n = 2,790)			P value
	Total N	Mean	SD	Total N	Mean	SD	
Hextend units cost	2,098	$55.13	$27.80	2,790	$0.00	$0.00	<0.0001
Voluven units cost	2,098	$0.00	$0.00	2,790	$116.01	$65.05	
Plasmanate units cost	2,098	$8.07	$29.85	2,790	$0.85	$9.21	<0.0001
LR units cost	1,977	$4.84	$2.93	2,774	$4.31	$2.52	<0.0001
NS units cost	1,977	$0.60	$1.49	2,774	$0.64	$1.53	0.196
Colloids (Hex/Vol + Plas) cost	2,098	$63.20	$33.53	2,790	$116.87	$64.80	<0.0001
All fluids units cost (observed)	1,977	$68.03	$33.22	2,774	$122.10	$65.85	<0.0001
All fluids units cost (imputed)	2,098	$68.65	$34.68	2,790	$121.82	$65.82	

Cost ($) statistics include all cases (none given = $0). ml, milliliters; LR, lactated Ringer's; NS, normal saline; SD, standard deviation.

Conclusions

In summary, after converting from Hextend® to Voluven® in a large tertiary medical institution, no differences were seen in short- and long-term mortality, renal outcome, blood and blood product utilization, ICU, or hospital length of stay. Although the number of cases receiving albumin decreased, total intraoperative and PACU intravascular volume fluid acquisition costs were greater.

Abbreviations

CI: confidence interval; ERAS: enhanced recovery after surgery; ICU: intensive care unit; kD: kilodalton; ml: milliliter; MW: molecular weight; PACU: post-anesthesia care unit; RBC: red blood cells; SD: standard deviation.

Competing interests

This study was supported in part by the Fresenius. RRB and WDW declare they have no competing interests. TJG had previously received grant support and honoraria from Fresenius.

Authors' contributions

RRB, WDW, and TJG helped conceive of the design of the analysis, interpreted the analysis, and contributed to the completion of the manuscript. All authors have read and approve of the final version of the manuscript.

Acknowledgements

This study was supported in part by a grant from the Fresenius.

Author details

[1]Department of Anesthesiology, Duke University Medical Center, Durham, NC, USA. [2]Department of Anesthesiology, Stony Brook University, HSC Level 4, Rm 060, Stony Brook, NY 11794-8480, USA.

References

1. Sander O, Reinhart K, Meier-Hellmann A. Equivalence of hydroxyethyl starch HES 130/0.4 and HES 200/0.5 for perioperative volume replacement in major gynaecological surgery. Acta Anaesthesiol Scand. 2003;47:1151–8.
2. Moretti EW, Robertson KM, El-Moalem H, Gan TJ. Intraoperative colloid administration reduces postoperative nausea and vomiting and improves postoperative outcomes compared with crystalloid administration. Anesth Analg. 2003;96:611–7.
3. Groeneveld AB, Navickis RJ, Wilkes MM. Update on the comparative safety of colloids: a systematic review of clinical studies. Ann Surg. 2011;253:470–83.
4. Gan TJ, Bennett-Guerrero E, Phillips-Bute B, Wakeling H, Moskowitz DM, Olufolabi Y, et al. Hextend®, a physiologically balanced plasma expander for large volume use in major surgery: a randomized phase III clinical trial. Hextend® study group. Anesth Analg. 1999;88:992–8.
5. Myburgh JA, Finfer S, Bellomo R, Billot L, Cass A, Gattas D, et al. Hydroxyethyl starch or saline for fluid resuscitation in intensive care. N Engl J Med. 2012;367:1901–11.
6. Perner A, Haase N, Guttormsen AB, Tenhunen J, Klemenzson G, Aneman A, et al. Hydroxyethyl starch 130/0.42 versus Ringer's acetate in severe sepsis. N Engl J Med. 2012;367:124–34.
7. Brunkhorst FM, Engel C, Bloos F, Meier-Hellmann A, Ragaller M, Weiler N, et al. Intensive insulin therapy and pentastarch resuscitation in severe sepsis. N Engl J Med. 2008;358:125–39.
8. Finfer S, Bellomo R, Boyce N, French J, Myburgh J, Norton R. A comparison of albumin and saline for fluid resuscitation in the intensive care unit. N Engl J Med. 2004;350:2247–56.
9. Hoffmann JN, Vollmar B, Laschke MW, Inthorn D, Schildberg FW, Menger MD. Hydroxyethyl starch (130 kD), but not crystalloid volume support, improves microcirculation during normotensive endotoxemia. Anesthesiology. 2002;97:460–70.
10. Leuschner J, Opitz J, Winkler A, Scharpf R, Bepperling F. Tissue storage of 14C-labelled hydroxyethyl starch (HES) 130/0.4 and HES 200/0.5 after repeated intravenous administration to rats. Drugs R D. 2003;4:331–8.
11. Langeron O, Doelberg M, Ang ET, Bonnet F, Capdevila X, Coriat P. Voluven®, a lower substituted novel hydroxyethyl starch (HES 130/0.4), causes fewer effects on coagulation in major orthopedic surgery than HES 200/0.5. Anesth Analg. 2001;92:855–62.
12. Entholzner EK, Mielke LL, Calatzis AN, Feyh J, Hipp R, Hargasser SR. Coagulation effects of a recently developed hydroxyethyl starch (HES 130/0.4) compared to hydroxyethyl starches with higher molecular weight. Acta Anaesthesiol Scand. 2000;44:1116–21.
13. Westphal M, James MF, Kozek-Langenecker S, Stocker R, Guidet B, Van Aken H. Hydroxyethyl starches: different products - different effects. Anesthesiology. 2009;111:187–202.
14. Ertmer C, Kohler G, Rehberg S, Morelli A, Lange M, Ellger B, et al. Renal effects of saline-based 10% pentastarch versus 6% tetrastarch infusion in ovine endotoxemic shock. Anesthesiology. 2010;112:936–47.
15. Miller DC, Gust C, Dimick JB, Birkmeyer N, Skinner J, Birkmeyer JD. Large variations in Medicare payments for surgery highlight savings potential from bundled payment programs. Health Aff (Millwood). 2011;30:2107–15.
16. Bozic KJ, Ward L, Vail TP, Maze M. Bundled payments in total joint arthroplasty: targeting opportunities for quality improvement and cost reduction. Clin Orthop Relat Res. 2014;472:188–93.
17. Birkmeyer JD, Gust C, Baser O, Dimick JB, Sutherland JM, Skinner JS. Medicare payments for common inpatient procedures: implications for episode-based payment bundling. Health Serv Res. 2010;45:1783–95.
18. Ramirez JM, Blasco JA, Roig JV, Maeso-Martinez S, Casal JE, Esteban F, et al. Enhanced recovery in colorectal surgery: a multicentre study. BMC Surg. 2011;11:9.
19. Miller TE, Thacker JK, White WD, Mantyh C, Migaly J, Jin J, et al. Reduced length of hospital stay in colorectal surgery after implementation of an enhanced recovery protocol. Anesth Analg. 2014;118:966–75.

20

Stroke volume variation to guide fluid therapy: is it suitable for high-risk surgical patients?

Ib Jammer[1,2]*, Mari Tuovila[3] and Atle Ulvik[2]

Abstract

Background: Perioperative goal-directed fluid therapy (GDFT) may improve outcome after high-risk surgery. Minimal invasive measurement of stroke volume variation (SVV) has been recommended to guide fluid therapy. We intended to study how perioperative GDFT with arterial-based continuous SVV monitoring influences postoperative complications in a high-risk surgical population.

Methods: From February 1st 2012, all ASA 3 and 4 patients undergoing abdominal surgery in two university hospitals were assessed for randomization into a control group or GDFT group. An arterial-line cardiac output monitor was used to measure SVV, and fluid was given after an algorithm in the intervention group. Restrictions of the method excluded patients undergoing laparoscopic surgery, patients with atrial fibrillation and patients with severe mitral/aortal stenosis. To detect a decrease in number of complication from 40 % in the control group to 20 % in the GDFT group, $n = 164$ patients were needed (power 80 %, alpha 0.05, two-sided test). To include the needed amount of patients, the study was estimated to last for 2 years.

Results: After 1 year, 30 patients were included and the study was halted due to slow inclusion rate. Of 732 high-risk patients scheduled for abdominal surgery, 391 were screened for randomization. Of those, $n = 249$ (64 %) were excluded because a laparoscopic technique was preferred and $n = 95$ (24 %) due to atrial fibrillation.

Conclusions: Our study was stopped due to a slow inclusion rate. Methodological restrictions of the arterial-line cardiac output monitor excluded the majority of patients. This leaves the question if this method is appropriate to guide fluid therapy in high-risk surgical patients.

Trial registration: ClinicalTrials.gov: NCT01473446.

Background

Maintaining adequate oxygen supply to body organs is one of the main goals during anaesthesia, and giving intravenous fluid is one way to achieve this goal. A Cochrane systematic review found that complication rate and length of hospital stay, but not mortality, were reduced when global blood flow is optimized perioperatively by means of fluid and or drugs [1].

Recent studies show the development and use of several minimal invasive methods to estimate cardiac output and guide fluid therapy [2]. Despite the unclear evidence in the literature and contradictory findings in clinical trials, the pressure on clinicians to use a goal-directed fluid therapy approach is high. In the UK, there is even a governmental financial incentive for hospitals to use Oesophageal Doppler for its patients [3] because the goal-directed approach may be cost effective [4].

High-risk patient may have the greatest benefit of a goal-directed fluid approach [5, 6]. Less capability to compensate hypo- and hypervolemia may increase the

* Correspondence: ib.jammer@helse-bergen.no
[1]Department of Clinical Medicine, University of Bergen, 5020 Bergen, Norway
[2]Department of Anaesthesia and Intensive Care, Haukeland University Hospital, 5021 Bergen, Norway
Full list of author information is available at the end of the article

rate of complications in a poorly optimized fluid balance [7, 8]. Benes et al. evaluate the effect of minimal invasive cardiac output-monitored fluid therapy exclusively in a high-risk abdominal surgery population [9]. Pearse describes the use of an arterial-line cardiac output monitoring in a high-risk surgery population [10]. Both studies where done on high-risk patients, using a strict definition of "high-risk". However, we could not find a consensus in the literature about the definition of "high-risk surgery". To simplify our approach to high-risk surgery, we defined therefore ASA 3 and 4 patients as high-risk patients. Then we intended to conduct a multicentre international prospective clinical trial to study what impact goal-directed fluid therapy based on continuous SVV (stroke volume variation) monitoring has on postoperative complications in this patient group.

Methods
Trial design
We planned a two-centre, assessor concealed, prospective randomized clinical trial conducted in Norway and Finland. The trial was approved by the institutional board in Norway (2011/947/REK Vest) and Finland (EETTMK:10/2012).

Participants
From 1 February 2012 to 31 January 2013, all high-risk patients defined by ASA score 3 and 4, older than 18 years scheduled for major abdominal surgery in two university hospitals were assessed for eligibility. Patients who were able to give consent when an investigator was available were screened for eligibility. Patient undergoing liver or oesophageal surgery where not screened because they follow a more restrictive fluid regimen. Exclusion criteria after screening were the following: atrial fibrillation, severe aortic or mitral stenosis, and laparoscopic surgery or declined participation. Patients were included consecutively. Informed consent was obtained from each randomized patient.

Interventions
Patients were randomized into two groups: a control group receiving traditional fluid therapy and a group with a goal-directed fluid therapy (GDFT) regimen guided by an arterial pressure-based cardiac output device (LiDCOrapid, LiDCO Ltd, London, UK) to measure SVV [11]. For more details of the study protocol, see Additional file 1.

Sample size calculation
The complication rate for lower gastrointestinal surgery in elective patients in one of the study hospitals was 40 % in a previous study [12]. In the present study, a

higher complication rate was expected due to inclusion of a population with a higher morbidity. To detect a decrease in number of complication from 40 % in the control group to 20 % in the GDFT group, $n = 164$ patients were needed (power 80 %, alpha 0.05, two-sided test). It was estimated that with an approximate inclusion rate of 80 patients/year in each study centre, the study could be conducted within 2 years.

Interim analysis
Due to an unexpectedly low inclusion rate, an analysis of the exclusion factors was performed after 1 year. This resulted in termination of the study. A retrospective analysis of all patients undergoing abdominal surgery within the last year and their comorbidities and surgical techniques was undertaken after approval of the institutional board.

Outcomes
The primary endpoint was the proportion of patients suffering of one or more complication within 5 days postoperatively.

After termination of the study, we decided to reject the primary outcome due to heavy underpowered sample size. To analyse reasons for exclusion, we determined the amount of excluded patients. No statistical analysis was performed of the numbers collected.

Results
Participant flow
During 1 year, $n = 732$ high-risk patients were scheduled for abdominal surgery.

Of these, $n = 341$ were not screened for inclusion. Reasons were either no investigator present or equipment missing ($n = 224$), scheduled liver or oesophagus surgery ($n = 64$) or the patient were unable to give informed consent ($n = 53$).

Of all scheduled patients, $n = 391$ patients were screened for randomisation. Of these, 64 % ($n = 249$) were excluded because a laparoscopic technique was preferred, and 24 % ($n = 95$) were excluded due to atrial fibrillation. The patient flow through the study can be seen in Fig. 1. Of all screened patients, only 7.7 % ($n = 30$) could be included in the study. The outcome data is presented by study group allocation in Table 1. A de-identified database containing all collected data of included patients is available online as an additional file (see Additional file 2).

Reason for stopped trial
After 1 year, the number of randomized patients we could include in the study was only 18 % of the estimated number we have been expected at that time. We

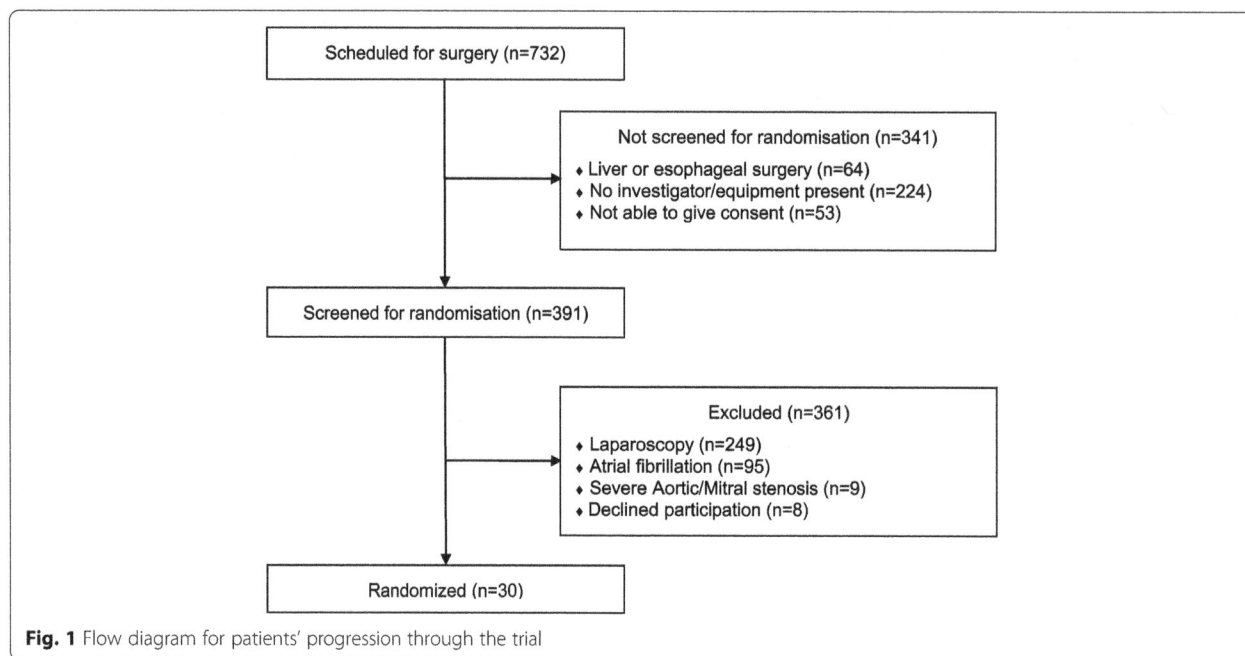

Fig. 1 Flow diagram for patients' progression through the trial

calculated that at this inclusion speed, the study would last more than 5 years and therefore decided to terminate the study early.

Discussion
Principal findings
In our study, a majority of high-risk surgical patients defined as ASA 3 and ASA 4 were not eligible for an arterial-line-based GDFT approach. The main reasons are methodological limitations of the arterial-line waveform analysis. The majority of patients had to be excluded because a laparoscopic surgical technique was preferred or due to atrial fibrillation.

This study was meant to be a prospective randomized controlled trial with a pragmatic approach to include patients. This would reflect daily routines, strengthening the study. Because the study was conducted in two tertiary hospitals, we had a high amount of high-risk surgical patients. Therefore, we expected to include enough patients in short time to run a well-powered study. Of 732 patients, 224 were not screened for randomisation due to investigator or equipment not being available. If this patient group also could have been screened, we may have had a higher number of patients randomized. However, it is to assume that the same fraction of patients would have to be excluded due to laparoscopic surgery and atrial fibrillation. Therefore, we do not believe that the total amount of patients that could be randomized would be much higher.

We terminated the study early, resulting in a heavily underpowered study. The primary outcome, postoperative morbidity, cannot be assessed since we just included 30 patients, and a statistical analysis would be meaningless. Consequently, we present just the patient flow numbers and not a complete statistical analysis of complications.

The low number of patients that could possibly benefit from GDFT is valid for our hospitals where the surgeons prefer to operate on high-risk patients with minimal invasive surgery. In hospitals that perform a higher amount of open surgery, the use of a minimal invasive GDFT approach may be more feasible.

We define the high-risk surgical patient by the ASA score to make the study pragmatic. However, other authors define "high-risk surgery" or the "high-risk patient" in different ways [13–15]. This makes comparison of trials dealing with this patient group difficult.

Maguire found in a retrospective electronic chart study of his hospital that $n = 12.308$ patients underwent surgery in 1 year, but only $n = 4.792$ (39 %) fulfilled the criteria for an arterial-line-based cardiac output monitor, and of these, only 23.2 % had an arterial-line. There was no report on how many of the patients were ASA III/IV patients [16].

Arterial-line-based waveform analysis measures hemodynamics by calculation of stroke volume variation or pulse pressure variation. However, arterial-line-based output methods are not applicable to large patient groups due to their limitations [16]. One limitation is laparoscopic procedures [17]. The increased intraabdominal pressure from the pneumoperitoneum affects dynamic parameters independently in changes of volume status [17–19]. Consequently would SVV during pneumoperitoneum increase while the blood volume do not decrease, it

Table 1 Complications (definition) within 5 days after surgery

	Intervention group	Control group
	n = 14	*n* = 16
Pulmonary		
Pneumonia (x-ray + antibiotics)	4	0
Pleural fluid (supplemental oxygen + x-ray)	0	2
Atelectasis (supplemental oxygen + x-ray)	3	1
Pneumothorax	0	0
Respiratory failure (intensive care treatment)	2	1
Pulmonary emboli (computed tomography + treatment)	0	0
Cardial		
Arrytmia (electrocardiogram + treatment or cardiologist consultation)	2	1
Coronary ischemia (electrocardiogram + troponin)	0	0
Pulmonary stasis/oedema (x-ray or treatment)	1	1
Neurological		
Postoperative delirium (treatment)	1	2
Focal neurological deficit	0	0
Infectious		
Wound infection (phlegmone + antibiotics or drainage)	0	0
Intraabdominal infection (computed tomography + antibiotics)	0	0
Central venous catheter infection	0	0
Wound rupture (operation)	0	0
Gastrointestinal (GI)		
Mechanical ileus (operation)	0	1
GI bleeding (transfusion or gastroscopy)	0	0
Paralytic ileus (unable to tolerate enteral diet > 5 days)	1	2
Others		
Renal impairment (creatinine increase > 33 %)	0	1
Impaired spontaneous voiding (catheterization > 2 times)	1	0
Venous thrombosis (treatment)	0	0
Sum of complications	15	12
Patients with at least one complication	7	7

would lead to false positive readings [20]. It is therefore not well validated in humans [21, 22]. Other limitations of waveform analysis measurements are cardiac arrhythmias and patients with severe cardiac valvulopatias [23].

Despite criticism about the evidence of the effect of goal-directed therapy, one single method of minimal invasive cardiac output monitoring (Oesophagus Doppler)

has even been officially recommended in the National Institute for Health and Clinical Excellence guidelines of the UK (http://www.nice.org.uk/guidance/MTG3). This decision has been criticized due to the lack of proof [24, 25], and the method may not be superior to a strategy of a neutral balance [26]. Other studies have not found benefices in a goal-directed fluid approach [10, 12, 26–30], have not found benefit using a restrictive fluid approach [31] or even have worse outcome in physically fit patients [5].

It is biologically plausible that the right amount of fluid given at the right time increase oxygen delivery to the organs and thereby benefit patient outcome. There has been a meta-analysis confirming that a GDFT approach may decrease postoperative complications. However, many included studies are small single centre studies with a high risk of bias or methodological limitations [1, 32, 6]. The effect on outcome in these studies is mostly small. An even statistical distribution of different studies with a small effect size would consequently result in a number of studies that would show no effect or even harm. The marked overweight of studies with a small positive effect on outcome may indicate a publication bias favouring trials with positive results. This may mask limitations of the arterial-line-based GDFT method that we report. Other studies investigating high-risk surgical patients do not report the exclusion rate due to atrial fibrillation when this condition restricted the GDFT method used [5, 9].

The OPTIMIZE trial with a study population of 734 patients is the largest trial on GDFT to date. It could not show a reduction of complications after perioperative arterial-line-based GDFT. However, when including the OPTIMIZE trial in an updated Cochrane meta-analysis, it indicates a reduced complication rate [10].

Goal-directed fluid therapy may be more important in a high-risk surgery population than in a relatively healthy population. Limitations of the method with an arterial-line-based monitor may cause exclusion of a patient group who may benefit most of the treatment. In the UK, it is recommended to use an Oesophagus Doppler to guide fluid therapy preoperatively. The same limitations that apply to the arterial-line-based method (exclusion of patient with atrial fibrillation and laparoscopic procedures) would apply to this method too.

Conclusions

Our primary goal was to investigate if high-risk surgical patients benefit from SVV-guided fluid therapy. This question still remains open. A majority of our patients had to be excluded from the trial due to methodological limitations. This leaves the question whether or not an arterial-line-based cardiac output monitor is the best method to guide fluid therapy in high-risk surgical patients.

Additional files

> **Additional file 1: Study protocol.** Study protocol, Word 2010 document.
>
> **Additional file 2: De-identified SPSS database containing collected data of all randomized patients.** SPSS Statistics Data Document.

Abbreviations

ASA: American society of anesthesia score; GDFT: Goal-directed fluid therapy; SVV: Stroke volume variation.

Competing interests

The authors declare that they have no competing interests.

Authors' contribution

IJ wrote the protocol and the first draft of the manuscript. IJ, MT and AU participated in the study design and data collection. All authors wrote, read and approved the final manuscript.

Acknowledgements

This study was supported by an unrestricted grant by The Eckbo Foundations, Norway and departmental funding. We thank Dr. Gro Østgaard for supporting the study and for critical appraisal of the manuscript.

Author details

[1]Department of Clinical Medicine, University of Bergen, 5020 Bergen, Norway. [2]Department of Anaesthesia and Intensive Care, Haukeland University Hospital, 5021 Bergen, Norway. [3]Department of Anesthesiology and Intensive Care, Oulu University Hospital, PL 21, 90029 Oulu, Finland.

References

1. Grocott MP, Dushianthan A, Hamilton MA, Mythen MG, Harrison D, Rowan K, et al. Perioperative increase in global blood flow to explicit defined goals and outcomes after surgery: a Cochrane Systematic Review. Br J Anaesth. 2013;111(4):535–48. doi:10.1093/bja/aet155.
2. Ramsingh D, Alexander B, Cannesson M. Clinical review: does it matter which hemodynamic monitoring system is used? Crit Care. 2012;17(2):208.
3. Campbell B. Innovation, NICE, and CardioQ. Br J Anaesth. 2012;108(5):726–9. doi:10.1093/bja/aes122.
4. Bartha E, Davidson T, Hommel A, Thorngren KG, Carlsson P, Kalman S. Cost-effectiveness analysis of goal-directed hemodynamic treatment of elderly hip fracture patients: before clinical research starts. Anesthesiology. 2012;117(3):519–30. doi:10.1097/ALN.0b013e3182655eb2.
5. Challand C, Struthers R, Sneyd JR, Erasmus PD, Mellor N, Hosie KB, et al. Randomized controlled trial of intraoperative goal-directed fluid therapy in aerobically fit and unfit patients having major colorectal surgery. Br J Anaesth. 2011;108(1):53–62. doi:10.1093/bja/aer273.
6. Cecconi M, Corredor C, Arulkumaran N, Abuella G, Ball J, Grounds RM, et al. Clinical review: goal-directed therapy-what is the evidence in surgical patients? The effect on different risk groups. Crit Care. 2013;17(2):209. doi:10.1186/cc11823.
7. Banz VM, Jakob SM, Inderbitzin D. Review article: improving outcome after major surgery: pathophysiological considerations. Anesth Analg. 2011;112(5):1147–55. doi:10.1213/ANE.0b013e3181ed114e.
8. Lees N, Hamilton M, Rhodes A. Clinical review: goal-directed therapy in high risk surgical patients. Crit Care. 2009;13:231.
9. Benes J, Chytra I, Altmann P, Hluchy M, Kasal E, Svitak R, et al. Intraoperative fluid optimization using stroke volume variation in high risk surgical patients: results of prospective randomized study. Crit Care. 2010;14(3):R118. doi:10.1186/cc9070.
10. Pearse RM, Harrison DA, MacDonald N, Gillies MA, Blunt M, Ackland G, et al. Effect of a perioperative, cardiac output-guided hemodynamic therapy algorithm on outcomes following major gastrointestinal surgery: a randomized clinical trial and systematic review. JAMA. 2014;311(21):2181–90. doi:10.1001/jama.2014.5305.
11. Cannesson M, Aboy M, Hofer CK, Rehman M. Pulse pressure variation: where are we today? J Clin Monit Comput. 2011;25(1):45–56. doi:10.1007/s10877-010-9229-1.
12. Jammer I, Ulvik A, Erichsen C, Lodemel O, Ostgaard G. Does central venous oxygen saturation-directed fluid therapy affect postoperative morbidity after colorectal surgery? A randomized assessor-blinded controlled trial. Anesthesiology. 2010;113(5):1072–80. doi:10.1097/ALN.0b013e3181f79337.
13. Pearse R, Harrison D, James P, Watson D, Hinds C, Rhodes A, et al. Identification and characterisation of the high-risk surgical population in the United Kingdom. Crit Care. 2006;10:R81.
14. Montenij L, de Waal E, Frank M, van Beest P, de Wit A, Kruitwagen C, et al. Influence of early goal-directed therapy using arterial waveform analysis on major complications after high-risk abdominal surgery: study protocol for a multicenter randomized controlled superiority trial. Trials. 2014;15:360. doi:10.1186/1745-6215-15-360.
15. Boyd O, Grounds RM, Bennett ED. A randomized clinical trial of the effect of deliberate perioperative increase of oxygen delivery on mortality in high-risk surgical patients. JAMA. 1993;270(22):2699–707.
16. Maguire S, Rinehart J, Vakharia S, Cannesson M. Technical communication: respiratory variation in pulse pressure and plethysmographic waveforms: intraoperative applicability in a North American academic center. Anesth Analg. 2011;112(1):94–6. doi:10.1213/ANE.0b013e318200366b.
17. Duperret S, Lhuillier F, Piriou V, Vivier E, Metton O, Branche P, et al. Increased intra-abdominal pressure affects respiratory variations in arterial pressure in normovolaemic and hypovolaemic mechanically ventilated healthy pigs. Intensive Care Med. 2007;33(1):163–71. doi:10.1007/s00134-006-0412-2.
18. Tournadre JP, Allaouchiche B, Cayrel V, Mathon L, Chassard D. Estimation of cardiac preload changes by systolic pressure variation in pigs undergoing pneumoperitoneum. Acta Anaesthesiol Scand. 2000;44(3):231–5.
19. Guenoun T, Aka EJ, Journois D, Philippe H, Chevallier JM, Safran D. Effects of laparoscopic pneumoperitoneum and changes in position on arterial pulse pressure wave-form: comparison between morbidly obese and normal-weight patients. Obes Surg. 2006;16(8):1075–81. doi:10.1381/096089206778026253.
20. Michard F, Chemla D, Teboul JL. Applicability of pulse pressure variation: how many shades of grey? Crit Care. 2015;19(1):144. doi:10.1186/s13054-015-0869-x.
21. Hoiseth LO, Hoff IE, Myre K, Landsverk SA, Kirkeboen KA. Dynamic variables of fluid responsiveness during pneumoperitoneum and laparoscopic surgery. Acta Anaesthesiol Scand. 2012;56(6):777–86. doi:10.1111/j.1399-6576.2011.02641.x.
22. Jacques D, Bendjelid K, Duperret S, Colling J, Piriou V, Viale JP. Pulse pressure variation and stroke volume variation during increased intra-abdominal pressure: an experimental study. Crit Care. 2011;15(1):R33. doi:10.1186/cc9980.
23. Chew MS, Aneman A. Haemodynamic monitoring using arterial waveform analysis. Curr Opin Crit Care. 2013;19(3):234–41. doi:10.1097/MCC.0b013e32836091ae.
24. Morris C. Oesophageal Doppler monitoring, doubt and equipoise: evidence based medicine means change. Anaesthesia. 2013;68(7):684–8. doi:10.1111/anae.12306.
25. Ghosh S, Arthur B, Klein AA. NICE guidance on CardioQ(TM) oesophageal Doppler monitoring. Anaesthesia. 2011;66(12):1081–3. doi:10.1111/j.1365-2044.2011.06967.x.
26. Brandstrup B, Svendsen PE, Rasmussen M, Belhage B, Rodt SA, Hansen B, et al. Which goal for fluid therapy during colorectal surgery is followed by the best outcome: near-maximal stroke volume or zero fluid balance? Br J Anaesth. 2012;109(2):191–9. doi:10.1093/bja/aes163.
27. Srinivasa S, Taylor MH, Singh PP, Yu TC, Soop M, Hill AG. Randomized clinical trial of goal-directed fluid therapy within an enhanced recovery protocol for elective colectomy. Br J Surg. 2013;100(1):66–74. doi:10.1002/bjs.8940.
28. Srinivasa S, Taylor MH, Singh PP, Lemanu DP, MacCormick AD, Hill AG. Goal-directed fluid therapy in major elective rectal surgery. Int J Surg. 2014;12(12):1467–72. doi:10.1016/j.ijsu.2014.11.010.
29. Pestana D, Espinosa E, Eden A, Najera D, Collar L, Aldecoa C, et al. Perioperative goal-directed hemodynamic optimization using noninvasive cardiac output monitoring in major abdominal surgery: a prospective, randomized, multicenter, pragmatic trial: POEMAS Study (PeriOperative goal-directed thErapy in Major Abdominal Surgery). Anesth Analg. 2014;119(3):579–87. doi:10.1213/ANE.0000000000000295.
30. Moppett IK, Rowlands M, Mannings A, Moran CG, Wiles MD, Investigators N. LiDCO-based fluid management in patients undergoing hip fracture surgery under spinal anaesthesia: a randomized trial and systematic review. Br J Anaesth. 2015;114(3):444–59. doi:10.1093/bja/aeu386.

31. Phan TD, D'Souza B, Rattray MJ, Johnston MJ, Cowie BS. A randomised controlled trial of fluid restriction compared to oesophageal Doppler-guided goal-directed fluid therapy in elective major colorectal surgery within an Enhanced Recovery After Surgery program. Anaesth Intensive Care. 2014;42(6):752–60.

32. Hamilton MA, Cecconi M, Rhodes A. A systematic review and meta-analysis on the use of preemptive hemodynamic intervention to improve postoperative outcomes in moderate and high-risk surgical patients. Anesth Analg. 2011;112(6):1392–402. doi:10.1213/ANE.0b013e3181eeaae5.

21

Serum arterial lactate concentration predicts mortality and organ dysfunction following liver resection

Matthew G Wiggans[1,2†], Tim Starkie[3†], Golnaz Shahtahmassebi[4], Tom Woolley[3], David Birt[3], Paul Erasmus[3], Ian Anderson[3], Matthew J Bowles[1], Somaiah Aroori[1] and David A Stell[1,2*]

Abstract

Background: The aim of this study was to determine if the post-operative serum arterial lactate concentration is associated with mortality, length of hospital stay or complications following hepatic resection.

Methods: Serum lactate concentration was recorded at the end of liver resection in a consecutive series of 488 patients over a seven-year period. Liver function, coagulation and electrolyte tests were performed post-operatively. Renal dysfunction was defined as a creatinine rise of >1.5x the pre-operative value.

Results: The median lactate was 2.8 mmol/L (0.6 to 16 mmol/L) and was elevated (≥2 mmol/L) in 72% of patients. The lactate concentration was associated with peak post-operative bilirubin, prothrombin time, renal dysfunction, length of hospital stay and 90-day mortality ($P < 0.001$). The 90-day mortality in patients with a post-operative lactate ≥6 mmol/L was 28% compared to 0.7% in those with lactate ≤2 mmol/L. Pre-operative diabetes, number of segments resected, the surgeon's assessment of liver parenchyma, blood loss and transfusion were independently associated with lactate concentration.

Conclusions: Initial post-operative lactate concentration is a useful predictor of outcome following hepatic resection. Patients with normal post-operative lactate are unlikely to suffer significant hepatic or renal dysfunction and may not require intensive monitoring or critical care.

Keywords: Liver, Hepatectomy, Post-operative care

Background

Despite advances in both operative technique and peri-operative care, liver resection is associated with post-operative mortality rates of 0% to 22% (median 3.7%) [1] and morbidity rates of 12.5% to 66% including liver dysfunction [2,3], renal dysfunction [4] and bile leak [5,6]. Factors associated with peri-operative complications and death include patient age [7,8] and gender [9,10], hospital annual number of liver resections undertaken [9,11], pathologic origin of liver tumour [9,11], pre-operative liver and renal dysfunction [8,10], diabetes [12,13], chronic liver disease [7,9], and the peripheral neutrophil to lymphocyte ratio (NLR) [14]. Operative factors associated with outcome include blood loss [8,10] and transfusion [15,16], extent of liver resection [15,17], duration of surgery [18], simultaneous extrahepatic procedures [15,19], and the use of the Pringle manoeuvre [16,20].

Therefore, many factors affect outcome after liver surgery which have not been incorporated into a single scoring system. The American Society of Anesthesiologists (ASA) grade and Portsmouth Physiologic and Operative Severity Score for the enUmeration of Mortality and morbidity (P-POSSUM) scores are used in the risk prediction of many types of surgery [21,22] including liver surgery [23]. However, these scores may not be applicable to the unique stresses of liver resection. One of the main reported causes of mortality following liver resection is post-hepatectomy liver failure (PHLF) [24]. Although

* Correspondence: david.stell@nhs.net
†Equal contributors
[1]Hepatobiliary Surgery, Plymouth Hospitals NHS Trust, Derriford Hospital, Derriford Road, Plymouth, Devon PL6 8DH, UK
[2]Peninsula College of Medicine and Dentistry, University of Exeter and Plymouth University, Research Way, Plymouth, Devon PL6 8BU, UK
Full list of author information is available at the end of the article

the '50-50 criteria' of serum bilirubin of >50 μmol/L and prothrombin index (laboratory's calculated mean normal prothrombin time (PT) divided by the patient's observed PT) of <50% measured on the fifth post-operative day have been shown to be associated with death due to PHLF [2], an earlier prediction system may be clinically more useful in guiding therapy. Furthermore, failure of multiple organ systems may contribute to death following liver resection and there is a need for a global peri-operative measure to predict the risk of developing significant post-operative morbidity and death.

Lactic acid is a by-product of anaerobic metabolism that is subsequently metabolised in the liver during gluconeogenesis [25]. Hyperlactataemia has been shown to be associated with increased mortality and morbidity in a critical care setting [26,27], in patients with liver failure [28], sepsis [29] and following trauma [30]. Similar relationships have been shown in the post-operative setting following pancreatic resection [31] and other major abdominal surgery [32], cardiac surgery [33] and after hepatic transplantation [34].

The primary aim of this study was to determine if the first post-operative arterial lactate concentration ('initial lactate') is associated with adverse outcomes following liver resection including 90-day mortality, length of hospital stay (LOS), and renal and hepatic dysfunction. The secondary aim was to determine which pre- and intra-operative risk factors are associated with initial lactate concentration following liver resection.

Methods

This study was a retrospective analysis of a prospectively maintained database of all patients undergoing liver resection since July 2005. Routine patient characteristics, laboratory data and intra-operative details were retrieved. Pre-operative liver-directed chemotherapy was administered to selected patients following discussion at a regional multidisciplinary team meeting. A period of recovery of at least six weeks was allowed following cessation of chemotherapy before undertaking surgery. The P-POSSUM scoring system was used to calculate the physiological score [21]. Prior to resection, the operating surgeon makes a visual assessment of the condition of the liver parenchyma and records this as normal or abnormal. Liver resections were performed using standard techniques with a Cavitron Ultrasonic Surgical Aspirator™ (CUSA; Tyco Healthcare, Mansfield, MA, USA) dissector. Hepatic inflow occlusion was used in a minority of cases where there was excessive blood loss. Anaesthetic techniques include the routine use of invasive arterial blood pressure monitoring, central venous pressure monitoring (CVP) (using a target CVP of <5 cm H20) and epidural anaesthesia. Liver resections were defined according to the Brisbane classification [35] and the number of removed segments recorded.

Intravenous fluid replacement was minimised during the resection phase to decrease venous pressure. After removal of the surgical specimen, a pause in surgical activity is routinely planned to allow haemostasis and intravenous volume replacement with 0.9% saline or Hartmann's solution at the anaesthetist's discretion. Patients are usually returned to the High Dependency Unit (HDU) after surgery with full invasive monitoring, except for minor resections in fit patients who are returned to the general ward.

The serum lactate was recorded from an arterial blood sample taken immediately prior to abdominal closure or immediately on arrival in the HDU. The arterial lactate in the normal population is below 1.6 mmol/L whereas in a critical care setting <2 mmol/L is more commonly accepted in acutely stressed patients [36].

Serum biochemistry tests and coagulation assays were performed on all patients in the first 24 hours post-operatively and the tests repeated according to clinical course. The peak measurement of bilirubin and PT were recorded and used for analysis. A PT index of <50% corresponds to a PT >24 s. Similarly peak post-operative creatinine levels were obtained and renal dysfunction was defined according to the Risk, Injury, Failure, Loss, and End-stage kidney disease (RIFLE) criteria [37]. Renal dysfunction in categorical analyses was defined as any increase in serum creatinine of ≥1.5-fold from the pre-operative baseline. The length of hospital stay was measured from day of surgery to day of discharge and was expressed as a natural logarithm. Ninety-day mortality was recorded.

The association between initial serum lactate concentration and continuous outcomes was investigated using a multiple linear regression model as well as Spearman's rank correlation. To overcome increasing variance with the mean a natural log transformation was used. Binary variables were investigated using univariate regression. Potential associations between initial lactate concentration and pre- and intra-operative factors were tested using univariate regression or chi-square test at the level of $P < 0.25$ [38], as appropriate. Significant variables in the univariate analysis were included in the multivariate regression model and were considered to be significant if $P < 0.05$. All analyses were carried out using the statistical package R 2.1.14 [39].

Confirmation was obtained from the South West Health Research Authority that under the harmonised Guidance Approval for Research Ethics Committees (REC), REC review was not required because patient data was collected in the course of their normal hospital care and was anonymised for research purposes. No patient consent was required for this study.

Results

In the study period 501 patients underwent liver resection for whom an initial lactate measurement was available in

Table 1 Pre-operative and intra-operative characteristics of 488 patients undergoing liver resection

n = 488			Median (range)	Count (%)
Age (years)			65 (21–90)	
Gender	Female			216 (44.3)
	Male			272 (55.7)
Pathology of resected specimen	Benign			40 (8.2)
	Primary	Hepatocellular carcinoma		30 (6.1)
		Cholangiocarcinoma		36 (7.4)
		Other		35 (7.2)
	Secondary	Colorectal metastases		291 (59.6)
		Other		56 (11.5)
Pre-operative liver-directed chemotherapy	Yes			173 (35.5)
	No			315 (64.5)
Body mass index			26 (16–54)	
P-POSSUM physiologic score			16 (12–32)	
ASA grade	1			49 (10.1)
	2			315 (64.7)
	3			121 (24.8)
	4			2 (0.4)
Pre-operative diabetes	Yes			55 (11.3)
	No			433 (88.7)
Pre-operative bilirubin (µmol/L)			9 (2–162)	
Pre-operative alkaline phosphatase (U/L)			95 (34–1190)	
Pre-operative albumin (g/L)			44 (10–53)	
Pre-operative creatinine (µmol/L)			78 (40–430)	
Pre-operative glomerular filtration rate (ml/min)	≤90			158 (33.2)
	>90			318 (66.8)
Neutrophil to lymphocyte ratio (NLR)			2.47 (0.3-17.3)	
Operation number	1st			453 (92.8)
	2nd			30 (6.1)
	3rd			5 (1.0)
Surgeons assessment of liver parenchyma	Normal			314 (65.3)
	Abnormal			167 (34.7)
Surgical approach	Open			440 (90.2)
	Laparoscopic			48 (9.8)
Radiofrequency ablation (RFA) included	Yes			22 (4.5)
	No			466 (95.5)
Operation	Right hemihepatectomy			142 (29.1)
	Extended right hemihepatectomy			65 (13.3)
	Left hemihepatectomy			55 (11.3)
	Extended left hemihepatectomy			24 (4.9)
	Left lateral sectorectomy			45 (9.2)
	Wedge resection only			127 (26.0)
	Other			30 (6.1)

Table 1 Pre-operative and intra-operative characteristics of 488 patients undergoing liver resection *(Continued)*

Wedge resection included	Yes		182 (37.3)
	No		306 (62.7)
Bile duct reconstruction included	Yes		43 (8.8)
	No		445 (91.2)
Synchronous bowel procedure	Yes		22 (4.5)
	No		466 (95.5)
Curative intent	Yes		442 (90.6)
	No		46 (9.4)
Number of segments resected		4 (1–6)	
Estimated blood loss	<100 ml		2 (0.4)
	101-500 ml		240 (49.7)
	501-1000 ml		167 (34.6)
	>1000 ml		74 (15.3)
Units of red cells transfused		0 (0–26)	

488. The indications for surgery, pre-operative and operative details are shown in Table 1. Results of blood tests are shown in Table 2 and the main post-operative outcome measures are summarised in Table 3. The median number of biochemistry tests performed per patient in the first five post-operative days was 4 (0 to 6) and coagulation assays was 3 (0 to 6). It was not necessary to administer clotting factors to any surviving patients between postoperative days 1 to 5. Peak abnormalities in PT and bilirubin usually occurred early in the post-operative course and tended to improve over five days (Table 2). Post-operatively, 118 patients (24.1%) had a serum bilirubin ≥50 μmol/L. Minor abnormalities in PT were commonly noted, though only 15 patients (3.1%) developed a PT >24 s. Although a small number of patients remained jaundiced at the time of discharge, only one patient fulfilled the '50-50 criteria' at day five. The median length of hospital stay was seven days (range 2 to 78) with 90% of patients having a LOS between two and 15 days. Twelve patients (2.5%) died within 30 days of surgery and 23 died within 90 days of surgery (4.7%). The most common cause of death was liver failure, which occurred in 11 of 23 patients. Four patients died from ongoing malignancy (of whom three had undergone non-curative resections) and two patients died from sepsis without evidence of liver failure. The remaining deaths

were attributed to pulmonary embolus, heart failure, anastomotic leak following colonic resection, bleeding peptic ulcer, strangulated hernia and peritonitis.

The median initial lactate concentration was 2.8 mmol/L (inter-quartile range = 1.9 to 3.9) and 350 patients (72%) had an elevated serum lactate concentration (≥2 mmol/L) (Figure 1). There was no difference in the lactate concentration taken prior to abdominal closure (n = 380, median 2.8 mmol/L, range 0.6 to 16.0) or immediately on arrival in the HDU (n = 108, median 2.8 mmol/L, range 0.6 to 14.0). The initial lactate concentration was noted to be associated with all recorded outcome measures (Table 4). Although major abnormalities of serum bilirubin and PT were rare in our series there was a weak correlation with initial lactate for both bilirubin (coefficient 0.41, P < 0.001) and PT (coefficient 0.37, P < 0.001), which was stronger for bilirubin. Similarly, there was a weak correlation with length of hospital stay (coefficient 0.28, P < 0.001). Of note the values for length of hospital stay include only survivors, and therefore exclude some patients who are likely to have high post-operative lactate levels. Renal dysfunction after liver resection was rare in this series (7.0%) but there was a correlation with lactate concentration (Table 4). Three of 137 patients (2.2%) with an initial lactate concentration less than 2 mmol/L who

Table 2 Post-operative blood tests for 488 patients undergoing liver resection

n = 488		POD 0	POD 1	POD 2	POD 3	POD 4	POD 5
Bilirubin	Tested (%)	393 (81)	385 (79)	324 (66)	255 (52)	213 (44)	200 (41)
	Median (range)	21 (5–170)	27 (6–211)	21 (4–195)	19 (3–167)	18 (4–179)	19 (1–186)
Prothrombin time	Tested (%)	387 (79)	317 (65)	233 (48)	170 (35)	135 (28)	107 (22)
	Median (range)	16.3 (12.2-32.4)	18.0 (12–200)	18.0 (12.6-39.4)	16.1 (11.2-37.2)	15.3 (11.6-30.6)	15.4 (12.0-26.4)
Creatinine	Tested (%)	425 (87)	458 (94)	374 (77)	288 (59)	241 (49)	226 (46)
	Median (range)	70 (30–319)	70.5 (29–377)	64.5 (26–686)	60.5 (28–518)	59 (25–611)	60 (26–292)

Table 3 Post-operative outcomes for 488 patients undergoing liver resection

n = 488		Median (range)	Count (%)
Peak bilirubin (µmol/L)		29 (4–445)	
Peak prothrombin time (s)		17.6 (12.4-200)	
Length of stay (days)		7 (2–78)	
Renal dysfunction	None		450 (92.2)
	Risk (>1.5x pre-operative creatinine)		17 (3.5)
	Injury (>2x pre-operative creatinine)		12 (2.5)
	Failure (>3x pre-operative creatinine)		5 (1.0)
90-day mortality			23 (4.7)

had creatinine measured developed renal dysfunction (negative predictive value (NPV) = 0.98) compared to 8 of 29 (27.5%) patients with an initial lactate greater than 6 mmol/L (positive predictive value (PPV) = 0.28) (P = < 0.001) (Figure 2). In 322 patients with a lactate concentration ≥2 and <6 mmol/L 23 developed renal dysfunction (7.1%).

Similarly, there was a correlation between mortality in the 90-day period following liver resection and initial lactate concentration (Table 4). One of 138 patients (0.7%) with an initial lactate concentration <2 mmol/L died within this period, due to an anastomotic leak following colonic resection (NPV = 0.99), compared to eight of 29 patients with initial lactate ≥6 mmol/L (PPV = 0.28) (P = < 0.001) (Figure 3). The deaths in patients with lactate ≥6 mmol/L

were due to liver failure in four patients, sepsis without liver failure in two patients, cardiac failure in one patient and ongoing malignancy in the other. Of the remaining 322 patients with lactate concentration ≥2 and <6 mmol/L there were 14 deaths within 90 days of surgery (4.3%).

Comparison of patients with initial lactate concentrations <2 mmol/L and ≥6 mmol/L revealed there were significantly more major resections performed (P < 0.001) and more patients with pre-operative diabetes (P < 0.001) in patients with a lactate concentration ≥6 mmol/L (Table 5). There was no significant difference in the use of pre-operative chemotherapy between these two groups (P = 0.351). The proportion of patients with both renal dysfunction and who died within 90 days was significantly higher in those with lactate concentrations ≥6 mmol/L (P < 0.001).

Regression analysis revealed that a pre-operative diagnosis of diabetes mellitus, the number of liver segments resected, the operating surgeon's assessment of the health of the liver parenchyma, the operative blood loss and number of units of red cells transfused were all independently associated with initial lactate concentration at closure (Table 6). The only pre-operative factor associated with the post-operative lactate concentration was the presence of diabetes. On average, this increased the post-operative lactate concentration at any level by 20% compared to non-diabetics.

Discussion

The principal findings of this study are that higher initial serum lactate concentration after liver resection is

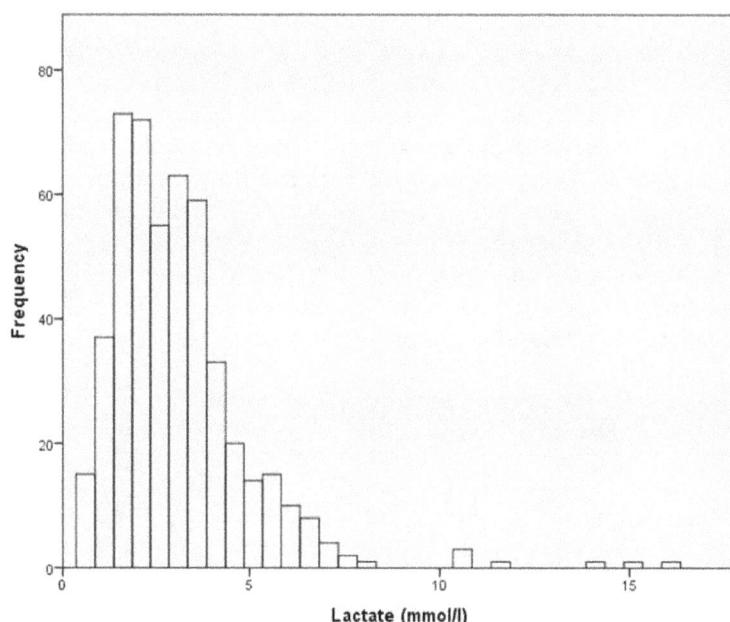

Figure 1 Distribution of arterial lactate concentration in 488 patients at the end of liver resection.

Table 4 Univariate analysis of the association between lactate and postoperative outcomes for 488 patients undergoing liver resection

n = 488	Co-efficient ± SD	P value
Peak bilirubin	0.146 ± 0.017	<0.001*
Peak prothrombin time	0.055 ± 0.002	<0.001*
Length of stay	0.046 ± 0.006	<0.001*
Renal dysfunction	0.324 ± 0.072	<0.001*
90-day mortality	0.373 ± 0.079	<0.001*

*Significant at level of P <0.05.

associated with an increased risk of mortality and renal and liver dysfunction. Both the 90-day mortality rate and the rate of renal dysfunction in patients with initial lactate concentrations greater than 6 mmol/L were 28% compared to those patients with initial lactate concentrations less than 2 mmol/L where they were 0.7% and 2.2% respectively. Similarly, higher lactate concentration was associated with higher post-operative peaks in serum bilirubin concentration and PT, as well longer lengths of hospital stay.

These findings support and extend those of an earlier study [40] by demonstrating the association of post-operative lactate with renal and hepatic dysfunction and length of hospital stay in addition to mortality. Pre-operative diabetes mellitus, the surgeon's assessment of the liver at laparotomy, the extent of liver resection, blood loss and the number of units of blood transfused are also shown to be associated with post-operative serum lactate concentration.

During cellular hypoxia pyruvate is diverted from the citric acid cycle and converted to lactate, reducing the amount of adenosine triphosphate (ATP) generated. This occurs in all metabolically active tissues including muscle, gut, liver, brain, erythrocytes and skin [41-43] and is exacerbated by intra-operative stresses including blood loss [42], endogenous release of stress hormones [44] and administration of pressor agents [45]. Liver ischaemia induced by handling of the liver during surgery and temporary inflow occlusion has been shown to lead to a rise in lactate [46]. Serum lactate can also be increased by transfusion of stored blood, which contains a higher concentration of lactate than fresh blood depending on length of storage [47]. Administration of Hartmann's solution has been shown to have a small effect on serum lactate concentration [48]. A potential weakness of this study is that details of pressor agents were not recorded, which could affect the lactate concentration. Similarly precise details regarding intravenous fluid type and volume of fluid (colloid and crystalloid) were not recorded.

In addition to being a potential source of lactate the liver is the principle location of lactate metabolism, where it is converted back to glycogen, accounting for 70% of

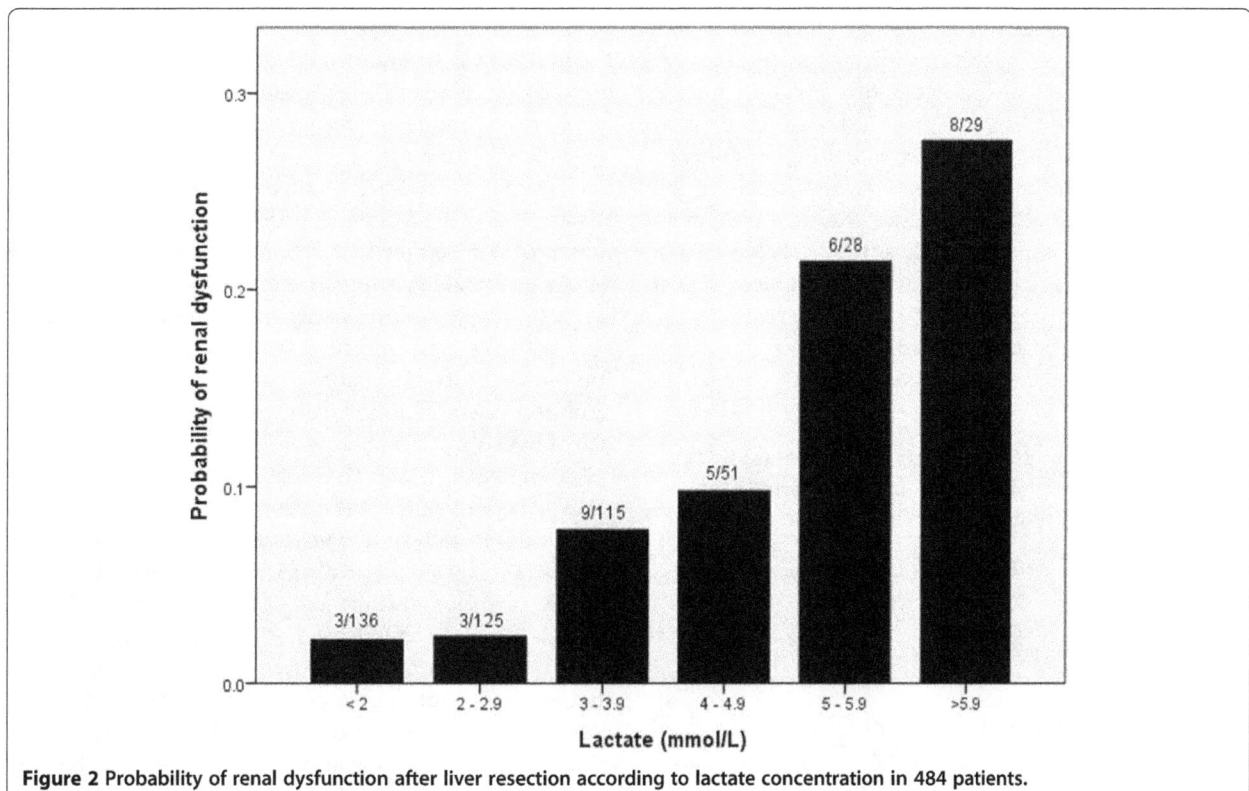

Figure 2 Probability of renal dysfunction after liver resection according to lactate concentration in 484 patients.

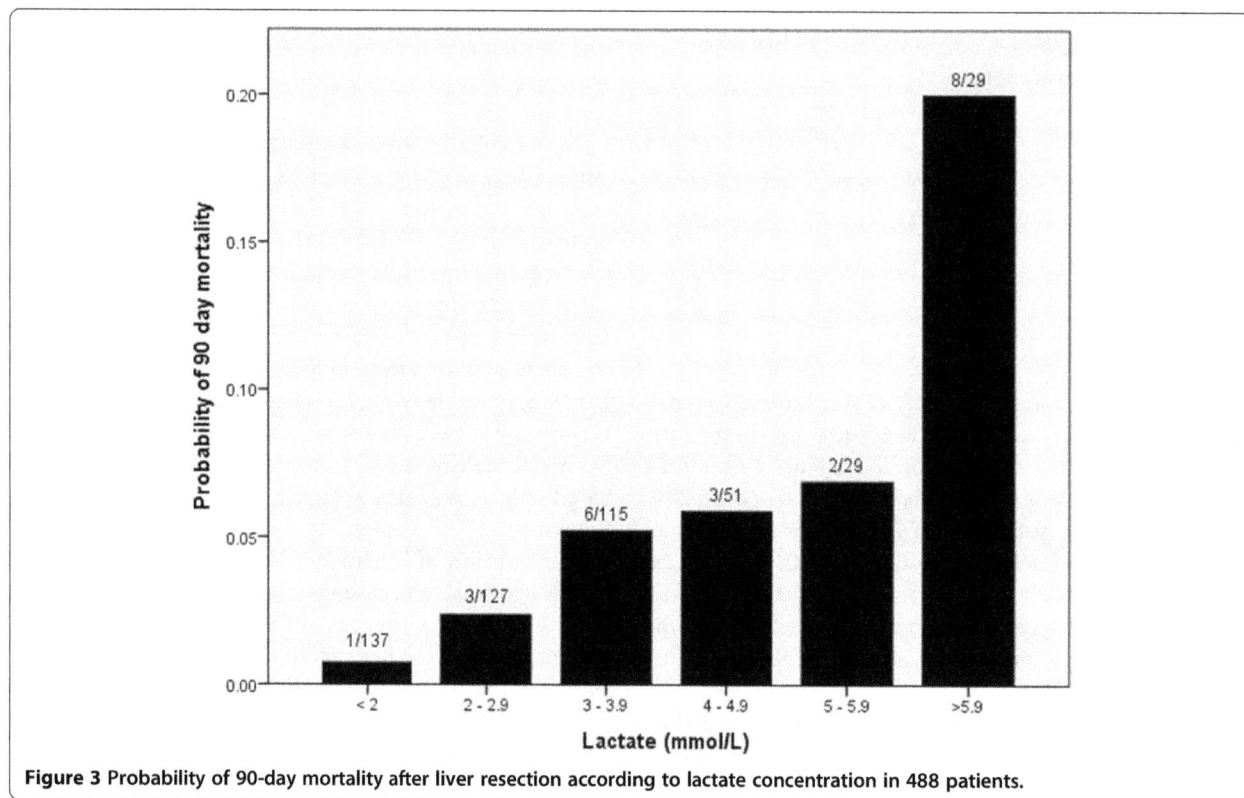

Figure 3 Probability of 90-day mortality after liver resection according to lactate concentration in 488 patients.

whole body lactate clearance [42]. No change in lactate metabolism has been demonstrated following recovery from partial hepatectomy in either rats [49] or humans [25], implying that the liver has a large functional reserve under physiological conditions of lactate production. However, the effects of intra-operative stress on hepatic glucose homeostasis have not been assessed, particularly when in combination with an extended hepatectomy. It is possible that inflow occlusion during resection and intra-operative handling of the liver lead to a temporary impairment of the ability of the liver to metabolise lactate. The finding of an association between the number of liver segments resected and the initial post-operative lactate supports this hypothesis. Diabetes is also known to be associated with impaired lactate metabolism via gluconeogenesis

Table 5 Distribution of risk factors and outcomes in 138 patients with lactate <2 mmol/L and 29 patients with lactate ≥6 mmol/L undergoing liver resection

Lactate	<2 mmol/L (n = 138)	≥6 mmol/L (n = 29)	P value
Major resection (%)	26 (18.8)	26 (89.7)	<0.001*
Pre-operative chemotherapy (%)	38 (27.5)	5 (17.2)	0.351
Pre-operative diabetes (%)	6 (4.3)	8 (27.6)	<0.001*
Post-operative renal dysfunction (%)	3 (2.2)	8 (27.6)	<0.001*
90-day mortality (%)	1 (0.7)	8 (27.6)	<0.001*

*Significant at level of P <0.05.

[42] and may account for the strong association with post-operative lactate in this series. Furthermore, the use of metformin in non-insulin-dependent diabetes has also been shown to increase lactate concentration [50]. The rise in serum lactate at the end of liver resection therefore may be due to a failure of lactate metabolism in addition to increased production during surgery.

Significantly, the use of pre-operative chemotherapy was not shown to be associated with elevation of post-operative lactate. This may be due to a policy of allowing a period of recovery after completion of pre-operative chemotherapy before undertaking surgery. Interestingly, the operating surgeon's assessment of the liver parenchyma was associated with the post-operative lactate concentration. This finding suggests that patient co-morbidity was a more common cause of abnormal liver parenchyma than the use of liver-directed chemotherapy.

An important observation of this study is the relative rarity of major hepatic dysfunction following liver resection in this series with only one patient fulfilling the '50-50' criteria [2], who subsequently recovered. Despite the infrequency of major disturbances of post-operative bilirubin and PT, there was an independent association with increasing concentration of post-operative lactate, demonstrating that even a minor degree of liver injury can lead to impaired lactate clearance or increase its production.

Renal dysfunction was also rare in this series, affecting 34 patients (7%) compared to 15% in a similar series

Table 6 Univariate and multivariate analysis of pre- and intra-operative factors associated with serum lactate concentration following liver resection in 488 patients

N = 488		Univariate analysis	Multivariate analysis	
Factor		**P value**	**Co-ef +/− SD**	**P value**
Age		0.246*		0.925
Gender		0.012*		0.129
Pathology	Benign vs. Primary	0.442		0.144
	Primary vs. Secondary	0.226*		0.878
Liver-directed chemotherapy		0.129*		0.219
Open or laparoscopic resection		0.009*		0.611
Radiofrequency ablation		0.191*		0.402
Wedge resection included		<0.001*		0.086
Bile duct reconstruction		0.004*		0.651
Number of segments resected		<0.001*	0.143 ± 0.012	<0.001†
Synchronous bowel procedure		0.516		
Surgeon's assessment of liver		<0.001*	0.185 ± 0.042	<0.001†
Redo operation	1st vs. 2nd resection	0.268		
	2nd vs. 3rd resection	0.654		
Pre-operative diabetes		<0.001*	0.204 ± 0.064	0.002†
Body mass index		0.06*		0.905
ASA grade	1 vs. 2	0.014*		0.824
	2 vs. 3	0.709		0.872
P-POSSUM physiologic score		0.054*		0.221
Hepatic fibrosis/cirrhosis		0.667		
Pre-operative bilirubin		0.320		
Pre-operative haemoglobin		0.633		
Neutrophil:lymphocyte ratio		0.400		
Pre-operative albumin		0.399		
Pre-operative alkaline phosphatase		0.014*		0.775
Pre-operative creatinine		0.392		
Pre-operative glomerular filtration rate (GFR) >90 ml/min		0.042*		0.054
Blood loss (ml)	<500 vs. 500-999	<0.001*	0.131 ± 0.038	0.013†
	500-999 vs. >1000	0.435		0.884
Units of red cells transfused		<0.001*	0.043 ± 0.011	<0.001†

*Significant at the level of 0.25 for univariate analysis and included in multivariate analysis; †significant at the level of 0.05 for multivariate analysis.

[51]. The risk factors for post-operative renal dysfunction are likely to be similar to those in other forms of abdominal surgery, including blood loss and sepsis, which are also initiating factors for anaerobic metabolism and lactate production. This supports the value of initial lactate as an early predictor of renal dysfunction. Of note, the risk of renal dysfunction appeared to rise more rapidly when the post-operative lactate rose above 5 mmol/L (Figure 2). This suggests that the kidneys are able to tolerate a degree of oxidative stress to a threshold level beyond which the risk of damage rises rapidly.

There was a weak association between initial lactate concentration and length of hospital stay in the study (Table 4). However, this may also be affected by other factors such as post-operative complications, particularly bile leaks, and degree of social support.

The strongest association demonstrated was between lactate concentration and the risk of mortality. In a similar manner to renal dysfunction, there seems to be a threshold level of post-operative lactate of approximately 6 mmol/l above which the risk of 90-day mortality rises rapidly (Figure 3). Organ dysfunction was a major contributor to mortality in the series and initial lactate concentration is a valuable global marker of poor organ function in the early post-operative period, including cardiovascular, renal and hepatic dysfunction.

Conclusions

These findings are of value in clinical practice as it may be possible to use the initial post-operative lactate concentration to determine the patient pathway in the early post-operative period. Patients with an initial post-operative lactate of less than 2 mmol/L have low rates of mortality and organ dysfunction and we are currently evaluating this criterion as a determinant of the need for post-operative critical care. In addition the correlation of post-operative lactate with subsequent organ dysfunction and mortality may allow its use as a single measure of the impact of innovations in operative technique or peri-operative care.

Abbreviations
ASA: American society of anesthesiologists; ATP: Adenosine triphosphate; CUSA: Cavitron ultrasonic surgical aspirator; CVP: Central venous pressure; HDU: High dependency unit; LOS: Length of stay; NLR: Neutrophil to lymphocyte ratio; NPV: Negative predictive value; PHLF: Post-hepatectomy liver failure; P-POSSUM: Portsmouth physiologic and operative severity score for the enUmeration of mortality and morbidity; PPV: Predictive value; PT: Prothrombin time; REC: Research ethics committee; RIFLE: Risk, injury, failure, loss, and end-stage kidney disease.

Competing interests
The authors declare that they have no competing interests.

Authors' contributions
MW and TS designed the study, collected data, analysed the data and drafted the manuscript. GS participated in the design of the study and performed the statistical analysis. TW, DB, PE, IA, SA and MB participated in the design of the study, collected data and drafted the manuscript. DS conceived the study, supervised its design and coordination and helped to draft the manuscript. All authors read and approved the final manuscript.

Authors' information
M.G. Wiggans and T. Starkie: joint first authors.

Acknowledgements
Thanks to Dr. C. Seavell, Dr. P. Davis and Dr. D. Lunn (Consultant Anaesthetists) for their work in study design and collecting lactate data.

Author details
[1]Hepatobiliary Surgery, Plymouth Hospitals NHS Trust, Derriford Hospital, Derriford Road, Plymouth, Devon PL6 8DH, UK. [2]Peninsula College of Medicine and Dentistry, University of Exeter and Plymouth University, Research Way, Plymouth, Devon PL6 8BU, UK. [3]Department of Anaesthetics, Plymouth Hospitals NHS Trust, Derriford Hospital, Derriford Road, Plymouth, Devon PL6 8DH, UK. [4]Centre for Health Statistics, Tamar Science Park, Davy Road, Plymouth, Devon PL6 8BX, UK.

References
1. Mann CD, Palser T, Briggs CD, Cameron I, Rees M, Buckles J, Berry DP: A review of factors predicting perioperative death and early outcome in hepatopancreaticobiliary cancer surgery. *HPB* 2010, **12**:380–388.
2. Balzan S, Belghiti J, Farges O, Ogata S, Sauvanet A, Delefosse D, Durand F: The "50-50 criteria" on postoperative day 5: an accurate predictor of liver failure and death after hepatectomy. *Ann Surg* 2005, **242**:824–829.
3. Schreckenbach T, Liese J, Bechstein WO, Moench C: Posthepatectomy liver failure. *Dig Surg* 2012, **29**:79–85.
4. Saner F: Kidney failure following liver resection. *Transplant Proc* 2008, **40**:1221–1224.
5. Savage AP, Malt MD: Elective and emergency hepatic resection determinants of operative mortality and morbidity. *Ann Surg* 1991, **214**:689–695.
6. Koch M, Garden OJ, Padbury R, Rahbari NN, Adam R, Capussotti L, Fan ST, Yokoyama Y, Crawford M, Makuuchi M, Christophi C, Banting S, Brooke-Smith M, Usatoff V, Nagino M, Maddern G, Hugh TJ, Vauthey J-N, Greig P, Rees M, Nimura Y, Figueras J, DeMatteo RP, Büchler MW, Weitz J: Bile leakage after hepatobiliary and pancreatic surgery: a definition and grading of severity by the International Study Group of Liver Surgery. *Surgery* 2011, **149**:680–688.
7. Alfieri S, Carrierio C, Caprino P, Di Giorgio A, Sgadari A, Crucitti F, Doglietto G: Avoiding early postoperative complications in liver surgery. A multivariate analysis of 254 patients consecutively observed. *Dig Liv Dis* 2001, **33**:341–346.
8. Jarnagin WR, Gonen M, Fong Y, DeMatteo RP, Ben-Porat L, Little S, Corvera C, Weber S, Blumgart LH: Improvement in perioperative outcome after hepatic resection: analysis of 1,803 consecutive cases over the past decade. *Ann Surg* 2002, **236**:397–406.
9. Dixon E, Schneeweiss S, Pasieka JL: Mortality following liver resection in US medicare patients: does the presence of a liver transplant program affect outcome? *J Surg Oncol* 2007, **95**:194–200.
10. Melendez J, Ferri E, Zwillman M, Fischer M, DeMatteo R, Leung D, Jarnagin W, Fong Y, Blumgart LH: Extended hepatic resection: a 6-year retrospective study of risk factors for perioperative mortality. *J Am Coll Surg* 2001, **192**:47–53.
11. Dimick J, Cowan J, Knol J, Upchurch G: Hepatic resection in the United States: indications, outcomes, and hospital procedural volumes From a nationally representative database. *Arch Surg* 2003, **138**:185–191.
12. Shimada M, Matsumata T, Akazawa K, Kamakura T, Itasaka H, Sugimachi K, Nose Y: Estimation of risk of major complications after hepatic resection. *Am J Surg* 1994, **167**:399–403.
13. Shimada M, Takenaka K, Fujiwara Y, Gion T, Shirabe K, Yanaga K, Sugimachi K: Risk factors linked to postoperative morbidity in patients with hepatocellular carcinoma. *Br J Surg* 1998, **85**:195–198.
14. Halazun KJ, Aldoori A, Malik HZ, Al-Mukhtar A, Prasad KR, Toogood GJ, Lodge JPA: Elevated preoperative neutrophil to lymphocyte ratio predicts survival following hepatic resection for colorectal liver metastases. *Eur J Surg Oncol* 2008, **34**:55–60.
15. Poon RT, Fan ST, Lo CM, Liu CL, Lam CM, Yuen WK, Yeung C, Wong J: Improving perioperative outcome expands the role of hepatectomy in management of benign and malignant hepatobiliary diseases: analysis of 1222 consecutive patients from a prospective database. *Ann Surg* 2004, **240**:698–708. discussion 708–710.
16. Benzoni E, Cojutti A, Lorenzin D, Adani GL, Baccarani U, Favero A, Zompicchiati A, Bresadola F, Uzzau A: Liver resective surgery: a multivariate analysis of postoperative outcome and complication. *Langenbecks Arch Surg* 2007, **392**:45–54.
17. Bolder U, Brune A, Schmidt S, Tacke J, Jauch KW, Löhlein D: Preoperative assessment of mortality risk in hepatic resection by clinical variables: a multivariate analysis. *Liver Transpl Surg* 1999, **5**:227–237.
18. Redaelli CA, Dufour J-F, Wagner M, Schilling M, Hüsler J, Krähenbühl L, Büchler MW, Reichen J: Preoperative galactose elimination capacity predicts complications and survival after hepatic resection. *Ann Surg* 2002, **235**:77–85.
19. Karoui M, Penna C, Amin-Hashem M, Mitry E, Benoist S, Franc B, Rougier P, Nordlinger B: Influence of preoperative chemotherapy on the risk of major hepatectomy for colorectal liver metastases. *Ann Surg* 2006, **243**:1–7.
20. Benzoni E, Lorenzin D, Baccarani U, Adani GL, Favero A, Cojutti A, Bresadola F, Uzzau A: Resective surgery for liver tumor: a multivariate analysis of causes and risk factors linked to postoperative complications. *Hepatobiliary Pancreat Dis Int* 2006, **5**:526–533.
21. Copeland GP, Jones D, Walters M: POSSUM: a scoring system for surgical audit. *Br J Surg* 1991, **78**:355–360.
22. Whiteley M, Prytherch D, Higgins B, Weaver P, Prout W: An evaluation of the POSSUM surgical scoring system. *Br J Surg* 1996, **83**:812–815.
23. Lam CM, Fan ST, Yuan AW, Law WL, Poon K: Validation of POSSUM scoring systems for audit of major hepatectomy. *Br J Surg* 2004, **91**:450–454.
24. Van den Broek MAJ, OldeDamink SWM, Dejong CHC, Lang H, Malagó M, Jalan R, Saner FH: Liver failure after partial hepatic resection: definition, pathophysiology, risk factors and treatment. *Liver Int* 2008, **28**:767–780.

25. Chioléro R, Tappy L, Gillet M, Revelly JP, Roth H, Cayeux C, Schneiter P, Leverve X: Effect of major hepatectomy on glucose and lactate metabolism. Ann Surg 1999, 229:505–513.

26. Husain FA, Martin MJ, Mullenix PS, Steele SR, Elliott DC: Serum lactate and base deficit as predictors of mortality and morbidity. Am J Surg 2003, 185:485–491.

27. Khosravani H, Shahpori R, Stelfox HT, Kirkpatrick AW, Laupland KB: Occurrence and adverse effect on outcome of hyperlactatemia in the critically ill. Crit Care 2009, 13:R90.

28. Macquillan GC, Seyam MS, Nightingale P, Neuberger JM, Murphy N: Blood lactate but not serum phosphate levels can predict patient outcome in fulminant hepatic failure. Liver Transpl 2005, 11:1073–1079.

29. Bernardin G, Pradier C, Tiger F, Deloffre P, Mattei M: Blood pressure and arterial lactate level are early indicators of short-term survival in human septic shock. Intensive Care Med 1996, 22:17–25.

30. Manikis P, Jankowski S, Zhang H, Kahn RJ, Vincent JL: Correlation of serial blood lactate levels to organ failure and mortality after trauma. Am J Emerg Med 1995, 13:619–622.

31. Gruttadauria S, Marino IR, Vitale CH, Mandala L, Scott VL, Doria C: Correlation between peri-operative serum lactate levels and outcome in pancreatic resection for pancreatic cancer, preliminary report. J Exp Clin Cancer Res 2002, 21:539–545.

32. Li SH, Liu F, Zhang YT: [Initial serum lactate level as predictor of morbidity after major abdominal surgery]. Zhonghua Yi Xue Za Zhi 2008, 88:2470–2473.

33. Murtuza B, Wall D, Reinhardt Z, Stickley J, Stumper O, Jones TJ, Barron DJ, Brawn WJ: The importance of blood lactate clearance as a predictor of early mortality following the modified Norwood procedure. Eur J Cardiothorac Surg 2011, 40:1207–1214.

34. Nishimura A, Hakamada K, Narumi S, Totsuka E, Toyoki Y, Ishizawa Y, Umehara M, Yoshida A, Umehara Y, Sasaki M: Intraoperative blood lactate level as an early predictor of initial graft function in human living donor liver transplantation. Transplant Proc 2004, 36:2246–2248.

35. IHPBA: The Brisbane 2000 terminology of hepatic anatomy and resections. HPB 2000, 2:333–339.

36. Mizock BA: Lactic acidosis. Dis Mon 1989, 35:233–300.

37. Bellomo R, Ronco C, Kellum JA, Mehta RL, Palevsky P: Acute renal failure - definition, outcome measures, animal models, fluid therapy and information technology needs: the second international consensus conference of the Acute Dialysis Quality Initiative (ADQI) group. Crit Care 2004, 8:R204–R212.

38. Agresti A: An Introduction to Categorical Data Analysis Second Edition. Hoboken, New Jersey: John Wiley & Sons; 2002.

39. R Foundation for Statistical Computing. http://www.r-project.org/.

40. Watanabe I, Mayumi T, Arishima T, Takahashi H, Shikano T, Nakao A, Nagino M, Nimura Y, Takezawa J: Hyperlactemia can predict the prognosis of liver resection. Shock 2007, 28:35–38.

41. Handy J: Lactate - the bad boy of metabolism, or simply misunderstood? Curr Anaesth Crit Care 2006, 17:71–76.

42. Phypers B, Pierce JM: Lactate physiology in health and disease. Contin Educ Anaesth Crit Care Pain 2006, 6:128–132.

43. Theodoraki K, Arkadopoulos N, Fragulidis G, Voros D, Karapanos K, Markatou M, Kostopanagiotou G, Smyrniotis V: Transhepatic lactate gradient in relation to liver ischemia/reperfusion injury during major hepatectomies. Liver Transpl 2006, 12:1825–1831.

44. James JH, Luchette FA, McCarter FD, Fischer JE: Lactate is an unreliable indicator of tissue hypoxia in injury or sepsis. Lancet 1999, 354:505–508.

45. Luchette FA, Jenkins WA, Friend LA, Su C, Fischer JE, James JH: Hypoxia is not the sole cause of lactate production during shock. J Trauma 2002, 52:415–419.

46. Pietsch UC, Herrmann ML, Uhlmann D, Busch T, Hokema F, Kaisers UX, Schaffranietz L: Blood lactate and pyruvate levels in the perioperative period of liver resection with Pringle manoeuver. Clin Hemorheol Microcirc 2010, 44:269–281.

47. Uvizl R, Klementa B, Adamus M, Neiser J: Biochemical changes in the patient's plasma after red blood cell transfusion. Signa Vitae 2011, 6:64–71.

48. Shin WJ, Kim YK, Bang JY, Cho SK, Han SM, Hwang GS: Lactate and liver function tests after living donor right hepatectomy: a comparison of solutions with and without lactate. Acta Anaesthesiol Scand 2011, 55:558–564.

49. Petenusci SO, Freitas TC, Roselino ES, Migliorini RH: Glucose homeostasis during the early stages of liver regeneration in fasted rats. Can J Physiol Pharmacol 1983, 61:222–228.

50. Davis TM, Jackson D, Davis WA, Bruce DG, Chubb P: The relationship between metformin therapy and the fasting plasma lactate in type 2 diabetes: The Fremantle Diabetes Study. Br J Clin Pharmacol 2001, 52:137–144.

51. Slankamenac K, Breitenstein S, Held U, Beck-Schimmer B, Puhan MA, Clavien P-A: Development and validation of a prediction score for postoperative acute renal failure following liver resection. Ann Surg 2009, 250:720–728.

Preoperative cardiopulmonary exercise testing in England – a national survey

Sam Huddart[1*], Emily L Young[1], Rebecca-Lea Smith[2], Peter JE Holt[3,4] and Pradeep K Prabhu[1]

Abstract

Background: Cardiopulmonary exercise testing (CPET) has become well established in the preoperative assessment of patients presenting for major surgery in the United Kingdom. There is evidence supporting its use in risk-stratifying patients prior to major high-risk surgical procedures.
We set out to establish how CPET services in England have developed since the only survey on this subject was undertaken in 2008 (*J Intensive Care Soc* 2009, 10:275–278).

Methods: Availability of preoperative CPET and contact details were collected via a telephone survey and email invites to complete the online survey were sent to all contacts. The survey was live during March and April 2011.

Results: We received 123 (74%) responses from the 166 emails that were sent out. In total, 32% (53/166) of all adult anesthetic departments in England have access to preoperative CPET services and a further 4% (6) were in the process of setting up services. The number of departments offering preoperative CPET, including those in the process of setting up services, has risen from 42 in 2008 to 59 in 2011, a rise of over 40%. Only 61% of the clinics are run by anesthetists and 39% of clinics have trained cardiorespiratory technicians assisting in the performance of the test. Most of the clinics (55%) rely solely on a bicycle ergometer. Vascular surgical patients are the largest group of patients tested, and the majority of tests are run to a symptom-limited maximum. We estimate that 15,000 tests are performed annually for preoperative assessment in England. Only 37% of respondents were confident that the tests performed were being billed for.

Conclusions: CPET is increasing in popularity as a preoperative risk assessment tool. There remains a lack of consistency in the way tests are reported and utilized. The results highlight the extent and diversity of the use of preoperative CPET and the potential for further research into its use in unstudied patient groups.

Keywords: Cardiopulmonary exercise testing, Exercise testing, Preoperative assessment, Preoperative risk assessment, National survey

Background

Cardiopulmonary exercise testing (CPET) has become well established in the preoperative assessment of patients presenting for major surgery in the United Kingdom. There is some evidence to support the use of CPET-derived variables for risk stratification and allocation to an appropriate level of post-operative care in many major surgical specialties [1-18], although there are no published randomized control trials. To date there has been one published survey into the use of preoperative cardiopulmonary exercise testing (PCPET) in England (performed in 2008, published in 2009) [19]. This survey identified 30 units in England that provided PCPET services for preoperative assessment, and a further 12 units in the process of setting up a service. We set out to determine how PCPET services have progressed since the 2008 survey and to ascertain the wider interest in PCPET in England.

Methods

The survey was conducted in two main stages. The first stage involved telephoning anesthetic secretaries in every NHS trust in England. This way, we hoped to find out how many departments performed PCPET, and to obtain contact details for a named consultant responsible for the service. The second stage involved sending a link to

* Correspondence: samhuddart@nhs.net
[1]Department of Anaesthesia, Royal Surrey County Hospital, Guildford GU2 7XX, UK
Full list of author information is available at the end of the article

an online survey to each of these contacts. The National Research Ethics Service (NRES) has confirmed that, in accordance with their guidelines, the survey does not require formal ethical approval.

Telephone survey

We accessed the NHS England website in December 2010 [20]. This website lists details of all 168 NHS trusts in England, 159 of which provide surgical services for adult patients. We contacted these trusts by telephone and identified 166 functionally separate anesthesia departments providing services for surgical procedures in adults. We contacted the anesthetic secretaries for all of these departments by telephone asking if preoperative CPET is available in their department and for contact details of the clinician responsible for either CPET or preoperative assessment.

Online survey

We composed the survey using an online survey tool (http://www.surveymonkey.com). For the majority of questions, we used a multiple-choice format with an additional free-text option for comments. Not all questions were compulsory for submission of the completed survey. The survey questions and structure are shown in Additional files 1 and 2.

The survey was sent to each identified email contact as a link within the email. A maximum of three reminder emails were sent over the following four weeks. The survey was live in March and April 2011.

Repeat telephone survey

Some of the secretaries contacted in the original telephone survey did not know if their department had access to PCPET. If we did not receive a response to the online survey and were originally unsure if they had PCPET services, we re-contacted them by telephone, so that we could confirm the total number of departments in England with PCPET services.

Results

We contacted all 166 (100%) anesthesia departments by telephone. In total (after the repeat telephone survey described above) we identified 53 departments who offer PCPET (32%).

Online survey

We received a total of 128 responses to the survey. Five of these were duplicate responses from individuals in the same department. Only the first response received from each of these departments was included in the analysis. As such our overall response rate was 74% (123/166).

We received 49 (40% of total) responses from departments that offer PCPET and 74 (60% of total)

responses from departments without access to PCPET services.

Departments without PCPET services (*n* = 74)

Thirty-five (47%) of those who responded have made an attempt to set up PCPET services that was unsuccessful. The reasons given for failed attempts included: financial (43%), perceived lack of clinical need (11%) and insufficient evidence of benefit (6%).

Thirty-three departments (45%) have not attempted to set up a service. Reasons stated for this included: financial constraints or lack of resources (39%), inappropriate case mix (9%), training issues (3%), lack of support from other departments (3%) and conflicting evidence for clinical benefit (3%).

Six departments (8%) are in the process of setting up a peri-operative CPET service.

The survey responses rates are summarized in Figure 1.

Departments with PCPET services (*n* = 49)

The majority of respondents to the survey were anesthetists (90%), the remainder being clinical scientists (6%) and physicians (4%).

Logistical aspects of PCPET services

Forty-five respondents (92%) indicated that testing is performed in-house. One department refers patients to a private CPET clinic as well as testing patients in-house themselves.

The majority of tests are conducted by anesthetists. Some are conducted by a variety of other clinicians and non-clinicians (Figure 2). Three respondents do not have any assistance during testing (6%) and 19 (39%) are assisted by a trained cardio-respiratory technician. Other assistance during testing includes: operating department practitioners (14%), pre-assessment nurse (14%), nursing auxiliary (6%), anesthetic practitioner (2%), physicians' assistants in anesthesia (2%) and research nursing staff (2%).

Clinics are operated in a variety of locations: in the pre-assessment clinic (39%), in the respiratory laboratory/clinic (27%), in the cardiology department (12%), in a ward area (4%), in the outpatients department (4%), in a research laboratory (2%) and on the intensive care unit (2%). The responsibility for maintenance, cleaning and sterilization of reusables and stocking of disposables lies with the clinician (20%), technician (49%) or a nurse (10%).

Clinical aspects of PCPET services

Referrals for CPET are received from multiple sources. Departments receive referrals from surgical colleagues (76%), anesthetic colleagues (69%), the pre-assessment clinic (67%) and from multi-disciplinary team meetings (35%). Interestingly only 22% of departments include

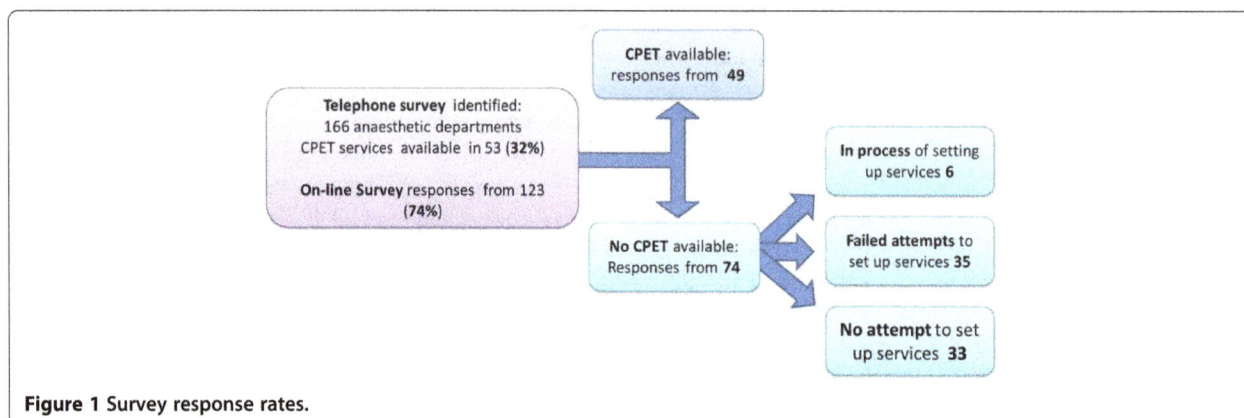

Figure 1 Survey response rates.

strict predetermined criteria as a part of their referral pathway. Of the total, 8% reported receiving referrals from cardiologists and respiratory physicians.

Twenty-four (49%) departments consent their patients verbally for PCPET, 11 (22%) require formal written consent and seven (14%) do not consent their patients prior to testing. This is a significant deviation from the practice in most cardiology exercise labs, where formal consent is not obtained prior to a treadmill test.

All respondents have access to a cycle ergometer for testing. However, the majority (55%) of departments only have access to a cycle ergometer, thereby limiting the range of patients who are physically able to perform the test. In addition to a cycle ergometer, eight (16%) departments have access to a hand crank ergometer and seven (14%) have access to a treadmill ergometer. One department (2%) has access to bicycle, hand crank and treadmill ergometers.

A variety of sub-specialty patient groups are tested, as depicted in Figure 3. Other patient groups tested are pediatric cardiology, ICU follow-up and adult congenital heart disease follow-up (Figure 3).

The majority of respondents use the anaerobic threshold (AT) (90%), Ve/VCO2 (71%), peak VO2 (59%), and Ve/VO2 (31%) to risk-stratify patients. A variety of other CPET-derived parameters were also reported as being used for risk stratification. For example: onset of ischemia, oxygen pulse, heart rate response, blood pressure response, desaturation, ventilator limitation, VO2/work rate slope and Ve/VCO2 slope.

The majority of respondents run their tests to the patients' symptom limited maximum (71%). This provides evidence for the need for a clinician to be present during the test on the grounds of safety. Some terminate tests after the patient has exercised to their anaerobic threshold (14%) or to their target peak VO2 (6%). Other responses

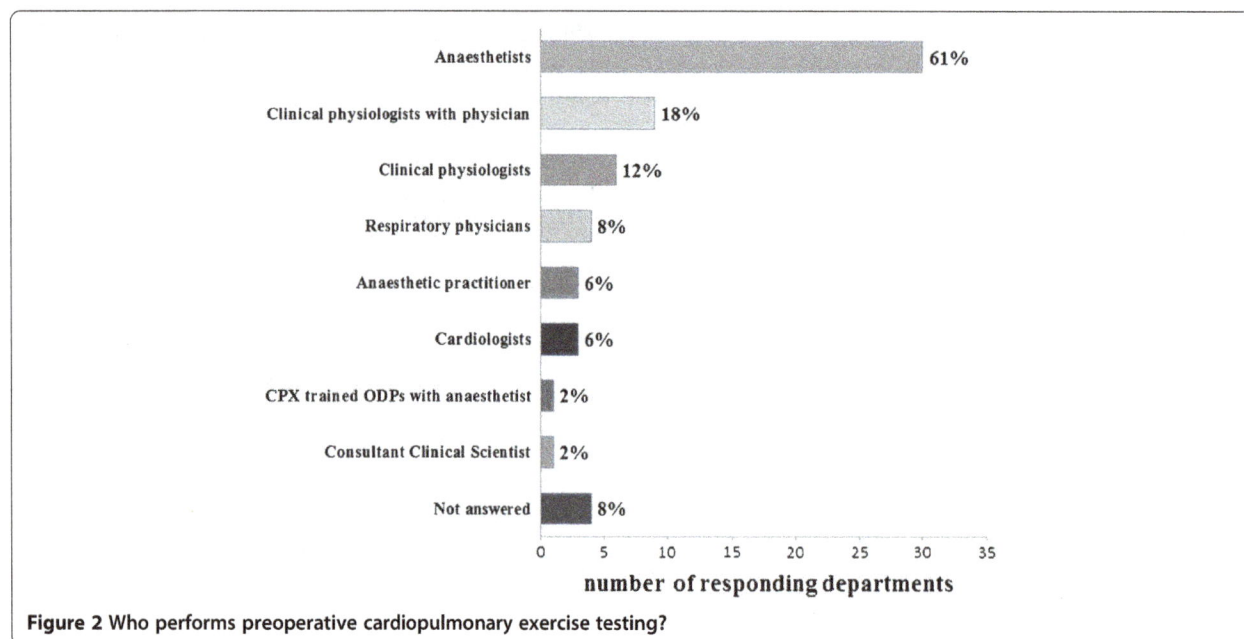

Figure 2 Who performs preoperative cardiopulmonary exercise testing?

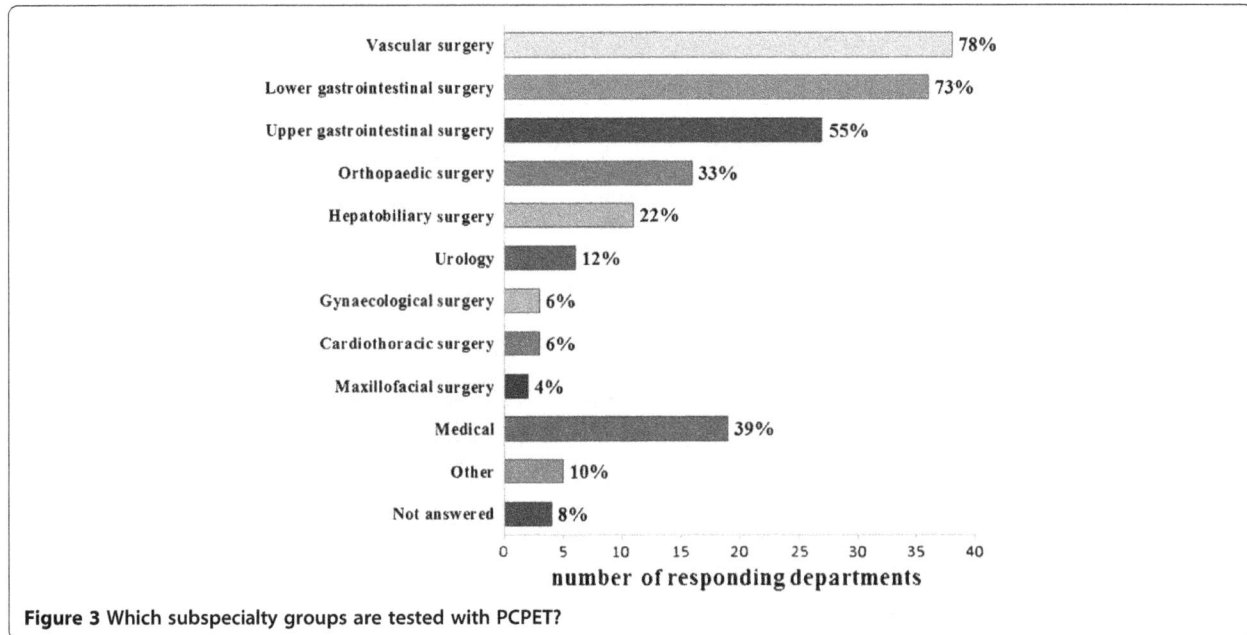

Figure 3 Which subspecialty groups are tested with PCPET?

include achieving predicted maximal heart rate and ischemic ECG changes.

The majority of respondents use the results for individual patient risk stratification and counseling (86%) and to allocate patients to an appropriate level of post-operative care (84%). Some departments use the results to determine the level of intraoperative monitoring (47%). Other uses reported by respondents include: for clinical diagnostics, to modify surgical procedure (in support of funding applications for less invasive procedures in high risk cases) and to assess the need for pre-optimization.

The majority do not recommend cancellation of an individual case based on the CPET result (55%). However, 33% of respondents do recommend cancellation of cases based on individual CPET results. There were many comments left for this question implying that the decision to cancel cases is more complex than this. The comments highlighted that CPET results advise risk and that the final decision lies with the patient, surgeon and, in some cases, the anesthetist. Some respondents felt strongly that the decision to cancel a case is not for the CPET clinic.

The median number of tests performed per clinic session was 3 (range 0.5-7.5, mean 3.2, mode 3, SD 7.3). The median number of PCPET clinic sessions per month was 6 (range 0.5-40, mean 8.4, mode 4, SD 1.5). Of the 53 departments identified by the telephone survey we received 49 responses. Of these 42 gave estimates regarding the output of testing services. If we substitute mode values (most conservative estimate) for missing data we estimate that over 15,000 PCETs are performed each year in England (Figure 4).

Administrative and managerial aspects of PCPET services

We were keen to find out how the administrative aspects of these clinics were managed. The questions ranged from organizing appointments to calibrating and validating the equipment and getting the reports to the referring clinician.

Appointments are arranged using written, formal appointment letters with an information leaflet in the majority of cases (76%). Other methods include: by telephone (8%) or written, formal appointment letters without information leaflet (8%).

The PCPET equipment is owned either by anesthetic departments (51%), respiratory departments (20%), cardiology departments (10%), clinical measurement/physiology departments (4%), surgical departments (2%) or clinical research facilities (2%).

Respondents reported a variety of administrative support as part of their service infrastructure. These include: departmental secretary (39%), pre-assessment clinic staff (27%) and own secretary (10%). Several respondents commented that administrative tasks are undertaken by clinicians. Nine services (18%) have no administrative support.

Where anesthetists perform PCPET, the majority of sessions are considered as a clinical professional activity (51%) in job plans. Some sessions are in supporting professional activity time (12%), and others in the clinicians' own time (8%).

The majority of tests performed are logged onto the hospitals' patient administration systems (67%); 12% are not logged and 10% of respondents did not know if tests were logged.

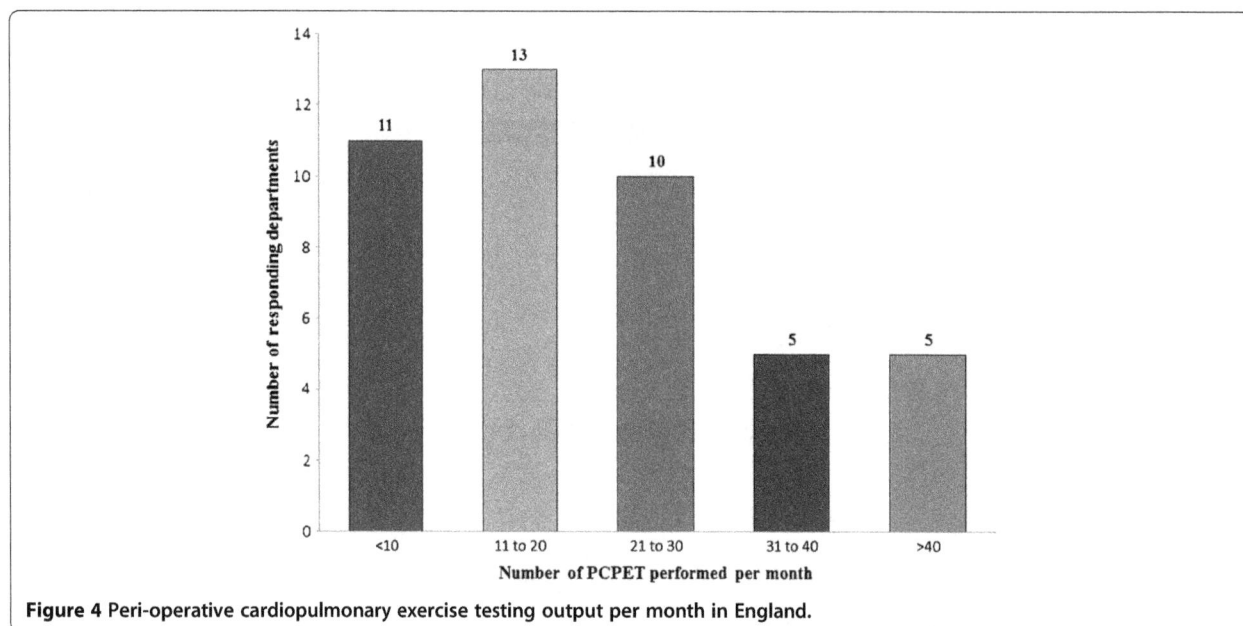

Figure 4 Peri-operative cardiopulmonary exercise testing output per month in England.

The primary care trust (PCT) is billed for the patients tested in only 37% of departments. No payment is received for testing in 31% of responding departments and 24% of respondents did not know if the PCT was billed.

Discussion and conclusion

We contacted 100% of individual anesthetic departments and identified 32% with CPET services and 4% in the process of setting up. In the 2008 survey Simpson *et al.* contacted 89% of trusts in England by telephone and received a 66% response rate when asking about the availability of CPET [1]. The higher response rate in our survey could be attributed to persistence with the telephone survey, the inclusion of a repeat telephone survey and accessibility of the online survey. The number of departments offering CPET has increased from 17% in 2008 to 32% in 2011 (while those in the process of setting up increased from 23% in 2008 to 36% in 2011). However, the 2008 survey may well have underestimated the availability of CPET due to their lower response rate. It is also unknown if any departments in the process of setting up a service were indeed successful. The 2008 survey was structured as nine open questions and sent as an email attachment. The authors commented that some responses were brief and lacked detail. In contrast our survey was online and included mostly multiple-choice questions with the opportunity for comment where appropriate. We believe this method increases the consistency of responses. However, we acknowledge that this style of questioning can be leading and may not collect some details of uncommon practice. The 2008 survey identified specific thresholds for parameters used for risk stratification, our survey did not. We have shown

that the majority of patients tested have vascular, lower gastrointestinal or upper gastrointestinal symptoms. It appears that there is an extrapolation of the evidence to other unstudied surgical groups. The published evidence shows that different CPET parameters have variable predictive power in different sub-specialties [2-18]. Therefore, we believe extrapolating specific evidence to unstudied patient groups is not advisable.

We were surprised to find that the responses from departments without PCPET suggest that there is a desire to have these services in the majority of departments, but that the primary obstacles are financial. Some departments may not have the high-risk case load to justify their own service, although this was not commented on by any respondents. The results suggest that there is an interest in PCPET in the majority of anesthetic departments, but that the perceived obstacles are the financial implications of setting up such a service. However, the survey was targeted at those with an interest in preoperative assessment. This group may be more enthusiastic and not represent the views of all anesthetists.

Not all questions in the survey were compulsory. While this ensured a better response rate overall, we did receive responses with some unanswered questions. The median number of unanswered responses per question was four (8%) (range 4–9, mean 4.9, SD 1.2) and this accounts for the shortfall in percentages of responses given in the results section.

There are a number of patient groups in whom PCPET does not have published outcome correlation data. These include patients requiring hepatobiliary, maxillofacial, gynecological or urological surgery. This highlights the importance of and potential for, further research into PCPET and post-operative outcomes, particularly in unstudied groups.

Departments use a wide variety of PCPET parameters to risk-stratify individual patients. Some parameters used are well established in the literature as good predictors of outcome (for example AT and Ve/VCO2) [2-11,14-18]. However, some studies suggest that AT is not a consistently strong predictor across all surgical groups [12,13]. Other parameters are also used to predict risk without published evidence, for example oxygen pulse. The variability of parameters used by respondents seems to reveal confusion over how results should be used to guide management. This is reflected in the inconsistencies of the reported predictive power of individual parameters published in the literature [2-18]. It would be interesting to know how many respondents use combinations of parameters or individual parameters alone (e.g. AT, Ve/VCO$_2$, peak VO$_2$ or Ve/VO$_2$) to risk-stratify patients.

Results are used for individual patient risk stratification and to allocate patients to the appropriate post-operative level of care. Some departments reported using results to determine the level of intra-operative monitoring. We are not aware of any specific evidence supporting this practice. One department reported using the results to support applications for funding for less invasive surgery (e.g. endovascular aortic aneurysm repair) in cases identified as high-risk cases by PCPET; again we are not aware of any evidence supporting this.

There appears to be controversy regarding the recommendation to cancel patients based on PCPET results. The majority of departments (55%) do not recommend cancellation of individual cases solely on the basis of PCPET results. A third of departments do recommend cancellation on the basis of PCPET results. The comments suggest that those who cancel patients on the basis of test results do so in conjunction with surgical colleagues and other clinical patient information available to them.

We were surprised to see the estimated number of tests performed in England per year is in excess of 15,000. Since we used modal values for missing data it is likely to be a conservative estimate. The numbers given in the survey responses do not necessarily take into account seasonal variations in output (e.g. bank holidays, annual leave and cancellations) and therefore may be overestimates. Even if we assume a month of testing is lost to these factors, the estimate is still in excess of 14,000 tests performed per year in England.

The number of tests, and the breadth of specialty groups in which testing is used, represents an exciting opportunity for collaborative research. Recent national attempts to establish communication and data sharing between departments will be a welcome step towards this goal (National PCPET Meeting, July 2011).

We were surprised to see that not all services are appropriately remunerated for the tests performed. Of respondents, 31% reported receiving no funding for tests from the PCT. Indeed a further 24% of respondents did not know if payment for tests was received from the PCT. We perceive this as being one of the key messages from the survey. Given that a significant proportion of respondents have indicated financial constraints as being the major hurdle in setting up these services, we were surprised to find that more than half the existing services were not generating income from their tests.

The survey has demonstrated the rapid growth of PCPET as a preoperative risk assessment tool in England. It has identified financial constraints as the main obstacle in setting up new services. This is despite clear evidence that there is significant national interest in having PCPET services available for the preoperative risk assessment of high-risk patients. We hope the results of the survey will add to the evidence presented in support of future attempts to establish new services.

Additional files

Additional file 1: CPET survey flow chart. Additional file 1 - CPET survey flowchart.docx.

Additional file 2: Cardiopulmonary exercise testing survey questions and structure. Additional file 2 - CPET survey structure and content.docx. This additional content details the survey structure and content. It contains a flow chart of the survey structure and a list of the survey questions and answer options. This report is independent research supported by the National Institute for Health Research (NIHR) Clinical Scientist – (NIHR CS-011-008). The views expressed in this publication are those of the author(s) and not necessarily those of the NHS, the National Institute for Health Research or the Department of Health.

Abbreviations
AT: anaerobic threshold; CPET: cardiopulmonary exercise testing; ECG: electrocardiogram; NHS: National Health Service; PCPET: preoperative cardiopulmonary exercise testing; PCT: primary care trust; Ve/VCO2: ventilatory equivalents for carbon dioxide; Ve/VO2: ventilatory equivalents for oxygen; VO2: oxygen consumption (liters per minute).

Authors' contributions
SH co-wrote and designed the survey (with PKP), collected contact details and data, coordinated the data collection, interpreted data and drafted the manuscript. ELY collected contact details and data, independently validated data interpretation and helped in the draft of the manuscript. RS collected contact details and data, independently validated data interpretation and helped in the draft of the manuscript. PJEH independently validated data interpretation and helped in the draft of the manuscript. PKP conceived of the study, co-wrote and designed the survey with SH, coordinated data collection, independently validated data interpretation, drafted the manuscript and supervised the project. All authors read and approved the final manuscript.

Authors' information
SH, RS and ELY are anesthetic trainees at the St Georges School of Anaesthesia, London, UK. PH is an NIHR Clinical Scientist at the St George's Vascular institute and is currently working at the Queen Elizabeth Hospital, Adelaide, Australia. PKP is a consultant anesthetist and cardiopulmonary

exercise testing lead at the Royal Surrey County Hospital, Guildford, Surrey, UK.

The results of this survey were presented by the authors as a poster and an oral presentation at the 4th National CPET Forum, the Institute of Education, London on 6 July 2011.

Acknowledgments

We would like all of the clinicians and support staff who responded to the surveys. In addition we thank Professor M Grocott and Dr W Fawcett for their invaluable advice on the writing of this manuscript.

Author details

¹Department of Anaesthesia, Royal Surrey County Hospital, Guildford GU2 7XX, UK. ²Department of Anaesthesia, Mount Sinai Hospital, Toronto, Canada. ³St George's Vascular Institute, London, UK. ⁴The Queen Elizabeth Hospital, Adelaide, Australia.

References

1. Carlisle J, Swart M: **Mid-term survival after abdominal aortic aneurysm surgery predicted by cardiopulmonary exercise testing.** *Br J Surg* 2007, **94**(8):966–969.
2. Mancini DM, Eisen H, Kussmaul W, Mull R, Edmunds LH, Wilson JR: **Value of peak exercise oxygen consumption for optimal timing of cardiac transplantation in ambulatory patients with heart failure.** *Circulation* 1991, **83**(3):778–786.
3. Older P, Hall A, Hader R: **Cardiopulmonary exercise testing as a screening test for perioperative management of major surgery in the elderly.** *Chest* 1999, **116**(2):355–362.
4. Swart M, Carlisle JB: **Case-controlled study of critical care or surgical ward care after elective open colorectal surgery.** *Br J Surg* 2012, **99**(2):295–299.
5. Wilson RJ, Davies S, Yates D, Redman J, Stone M: **Impaired functional capacity is associated with all-cause mortality after major elective intra-abdominal surgery.** *Br J Anaesth* 2010, **105**(3):297–303.
6. Snowden CP, Prentis JM, Anderson HL, Roberts DR, Randles D, Renton M, Manas DM: **Submaximal cardiopulmonary exercise testing predicts complications and hospital length of stay in patients undergoing major elective surgery.** *Ann Surg* 2010, **251**(3):535–541.
7. Hightower CE, Riedel BJ, Feig BW, Morris GS, Ensor JE Jr, Woodruff VD, Daley-Norman MD, Sun XG: **A pilot study evaluating predictors of postoperative outcomes after major abdominal surgery: physiological capacity compared with the ASA physical status classification system.** *Br J Anaesth* 2010, **104**(4):465–471.
8. McCullough PA, Gallagher MJ, Dejong AT, Sandberg KR, Trivax JE, Alexander D, Kasturi G, Jafri SM, Krause KR, Chengelis DL, Moy J, Franklin BA: **Cardiorespiratory fitness and short-term complications after bariatric surgery.** *Chest* 2006, **130**(2):517–525.
9. Epstein SK, Freeman RB, Khayat A, Unterborn JN, Pratt DS, Kaplan MM: **Aerobic capacity is associated with 100-day outcome after hepatic transplantation.** *Liver Transpl* 2004, **10**(3):418–424.
10. Nugent AM, Riley M, Megarry J, O'Reilly MJ, MacMahon J, Lowry R: **Cardiopulmonary exercise testing in the pre-operative assessment of patients for repair of abdominal aortic aneurysm.** *Ir J Med Sci* 1998, **167**(4):238–241Y.
11. Nagamatsu Y, Shima I, Yamana H, Fujita H, Shirouzu K, Ishitake T: **Preoperative evaluation of cardiopulmonary reserve with the use of expired gas analysis during exercise testing in patients with squamous cell carcinoma of the thoracic esophagus.** *J Thorac Cardiovasc Surg* 2001, **121**(6):1064–1068.
12. Forshaw MJ, Strauss DC, Davies AR, Wilson D, Lams B, Pearce A, *et al*: **Is cardiopulmonary exercise testing a useful test before esophagectomy?** *Ann Thorac Surg* 2008, **85**(1):294–299.
13. Junejo MA, Mason JM, Sheen AJ, Moore J, Foster P, Atkinson D, Parker MJ, Siriwardena AK: **Cardiopulmonary exercise testing for preoperative risk assessment before hepatic resection.** *Br J Surg* 2012, **99**(8):1097–1104.
14. Ausania F, Snowden CP, Prentis JM, Holmes LR, Jaques BC, White SA, French JJ, Manas DM, Charnley RM: **Effects of low cardiopulmonary reserve on pancreatic leak following pancreaticoduodenectomy.** *Br J Surg* 2012, **99**(9):1290–1294.

15. Prentis JM, Trenell MI, Jones DJ, Lees T, Clarke M, Snowden CP: **Submaximal exercise testing predicts perioperative hospitalization after aortic aneurysm repair.** *J Vasc Surg* 2012, **56**:1564–1570.
16. Colson M, Baglin J, Bolsin S, Grocott MP: **Cardiopulmonary exercise testing predicts 5 yr survival after major surgery.** *Br J Anaesth* 2012. Epub ahead of print.
17. Hennis PJ, Meale PM, Hurst RA, O'Doherty AF, Otto J, Kuper M, Harper N, Sufi PA, Heath D, Montgomery HE, Grocott MP: **Cardiopulmonary exercise testing predicts postoperative outcome in patients undergoing gastric bypass surgery.** *Br J Anaesth* 2012, **109**:566–571.
18. Society BT, Party IW: **Guidelines on the selection of patients with lung cancer for surgery.** *Thorax* 2001, **56**(2):89–108.
19. Simpson JC, Sutton H, Grocott MPW: **Cardiopulmonary exercise testing – a survey of current use in England.** *J Intensive Care Soc* 2009, **10**:275–278.
20. *A-Z List of All NHS Acute (Hospital) Trusts in England.* http://www.nhs.uk/servicedirectories/pages/acutetrustlisting.aspx.

23

Protocol-directed insulin infusion sliding scales improve perioperative hyperglycaemia in critical care

Man Lin Hui[1], Arun Kumar[2] and Gary G Adams[3*]

Abstract

Perioperative hyperglycaemia is associated with poor outcomes in patients undergoing cardiac surgery. Frequent postoperative hyperglycaemia in cardiac surgery patients has led to the initiation of an insulin infusion sliding scale for quality improvement.

A systematic review was conducted to determine whether a protocol-directed insulin infusion sliding scale is as safe and effective as a conventional practitioner-directed insulin infusion sliding scale, within target blood glucose ranges.

A literature survey was conducted to identify reports on the effectiveness and safety of an insulin infusion protocol, using seven electronic databases from 2000 to 2012: MEDLINE, CINAHL, EMBASE, the Cochrane Library, the Joanna Briggs Institute Library and SIGLE. Data were extracted using pre-determined systematic review and meta-analysis criteria.

Seven research studies met the inclusion criteria. There was an improvement in overall glycaemic control in five of these studies. The implementation of protocols led to the achievement of blood glucose concentration targets more rapidly and the maintenance of a specified target blood glucose range for a longer time, without any increased frequency of hyperglycaemia. Of the seven studies, four used controls and three had no controls.

In terms of the meta-analysis carried out, four studies revealed a failure of patients reaching target blood glucose levels ($P < 0.0005$) in the control group compared with patients in the protocol group. The risk of hypoglycaemia was significantly reduced ($P < 0.00001$) between studies.

It can be concluded that the protocol-directed insulin infusion sliding scale is safe and improves blood glucose control when compared with the conventional practitioner-directed insulin infusion sliding scale. This study supports the adoption of a protocol-directed insulin infusion sliding scale as a standard of care for post-cardiac surgery patients.

Keywords: Hyperglycaemia, Perioperative, Protocol-directed insulin infusion, Sliding scales

Review

Introduction

Hyperglycaemia is a problem associated with blood glucose levels in excess of 10 mmol/l; it is a common occurrence in cardiac surgery patients and is associated with adverse outcomes [1]. Prolonged hyperglycaemia increases the risk of infection and contributes to higher mortality and morbidity. Mounting evidence documents the beneficial effects of tight glycaemic control on patients' recoveries [2] and highlights the importance of avoiding hyperglycaemic-related complications in coronary artery bypass graft patients, for effective postoperative glycaemic control.

Temporary hyperglycaemia during stress is often helpful and helps to provide more glucose to prepare the individual for action [3]. However, hyperglycaemia in a critically ill [4] or postoperative patient [5] may have various detrimental effects on the host's defence system: blood glucose levels >180 mg/dl (10 mmol/l) have a

* Correspondence: Gary.adams@nottingham.ac.uk
[3]Insulin and Diabetes Experimental Research (IDER) Group, Faculty of Medicine and Health Science, University of Nottingham, Clifton Boulevard, Nottingham NG7 2RD, UK
Full list of author information is available at the end of the article

compromising effect on the immune system [6]; the immune responsiveness of the mononuclear phagocytic
cells is depressed; neutrophil function is impaired; the
inflammatory response is exaggerated; and the immune
system is weakened, thus increasing susceptibility to infection [7]. Recent evidence has proved that perioperative (intraoperative plus postoperative) hyperglycaemia is
directly correlated with the development of deep sternal
wound infection, increased mortality and morbidity, and
increased hospital stay [8]. Furnary [6] reported that the
rate of wound infection was doubled when blood glucose
levels were between 180 mg/dl (10 mmol/l) and 216 mg/
dl (12 mmol/l), fourfold when they were between 216
mg/dl (12 mmol/l) and 252 mg/dl (14 mmol/l) and even
sixfold when over 252 mg/dl (14 mmol/l); when blood
glucose levels were maintained at below 180 mg/dl (10
mmol/l), there was no increase in the rate of wound infection [6].

Treating hyperglycaemia in hospitalized patients has
proven to be beneficial [9]. However, normoglycaemia
after cardiac surgery is usually difficult to maintain and
requirements for insulin after cardiac surgery with cardiopulmonary bypass are much higher than after other
operations.

Because the use of the cardiopulmonary bypass ma-
chine necessitates the administration of catecholamines
and corticosteroids during and after cardiac surgery, the
patient's insulin resistance status changes continuously,
thus altering the patient's insulin response and causing
fluctuations in glycaemia.

Recognizing the detrimental impact of hyperglycaemia
on postoperative surgical wound infection and the importance of glycaemic control in cardiac surgery patients
is important and appropriate in managing hyperglycaemic control. To address this issue, a systematic review was carried out to examine the effectiveness and
safety of the protocol-directed insulin infusion sliding
scale variable rate intravenous insulin infusion on this
population group.

Design of the study

The electronic databases MEDLINE and CINAHL were
searched to identify keywords and index terms used in
describing relevant studies. Keywords used in the preliminary searching process included: 'insulin infusion
sliding scale', 'open-heart surgery', 'practitioner-directed'
and 'protocol-directed'.

A more detailed and extensive search was then conducted across a number of electronic databases to ensure that the majority of studies within the inclusion
criteria were recruited (Figure 1). Databases that cover
the healthcare literature and clinical trials were searched.
To increase the coverage of all relevant evidence, different databases were used in the searching process:

MEDLINE, CINAHL, the Cochrane Library, the Joanna
Briggs Institute (JBI) Library, and EMBASE. To identify
published studies that are not available electronically,
hand searching was also done. In addition, as it can take
more than a year for some studies to be published, and
these studies may not be searchable in electronic databases, a manual journal search was also performed.

Unpublished studies were sought, to overcome or reduce publication bias, using the System of Information
on Grey Literature in Europe (SIGLE) database.

The bibliographies and reference lists from the
recruited articles were consulted to identify additional
studies for possible inclusion in this review.

The outcomes of interest are the effectiveness and
safety of the insulin infusion sliding scale in controlling
blood glucose level. The efficiency of an insulin infusion
sliding scale in controlling blood glucose levels and reducing them to within the normal range plays a large
role in dictating the scale's use in clinical practice. So efficiency was set as one of the outcome of interest. In
addition, any insulin infusion sliding scale used to lower
the blood glucose level may induce hypoglycaemia,
which can lead to devastating effects, such as irreversible
neurologic deficit [10]. Therefore, safety of an insulin infusion scale is another important factor that needs to be
taken into consideration.

To prevent publication bias, all published and unpublished studies that were written in English and met the
inclusion criteria were included. In addition, to identify
only the most up-to-date studies, only those published
after 2000 were included.

Type of participant

All adult patients, over 18 years old who had undergone
open-heart surgery with blood glucose level >180 mg/dl
(10 mmol/l) and needed insulin therapy, with or without
comorbidities will be eligible for inclusion, except those
patients who developed diabetes ketoacidosis.

Of the 239 potentially relevant articles identified during
the primary search, and after screening all titles and
abstracts, 229 clearly did not meet the inclusion criteria
and were therefore excluded. Hard copies of all potentially
relevant articles were retrieved, including those obtained
directly from the search ($n = 10$) and those obtained
through reference lists ($n = 7$). Irrelevant articles were
excluded after detailed evaluation of the full text (Figure 1).

There was usually more than one reason for excluding
each study from the analysis; these included:

1) Not all participating patients received protocol-
   directed blood glucose management (67 articles).
2) There was an irrelevant comparison group, (for
   example, a computer-based algorithm was used
   instead of a control group) (21 articles).

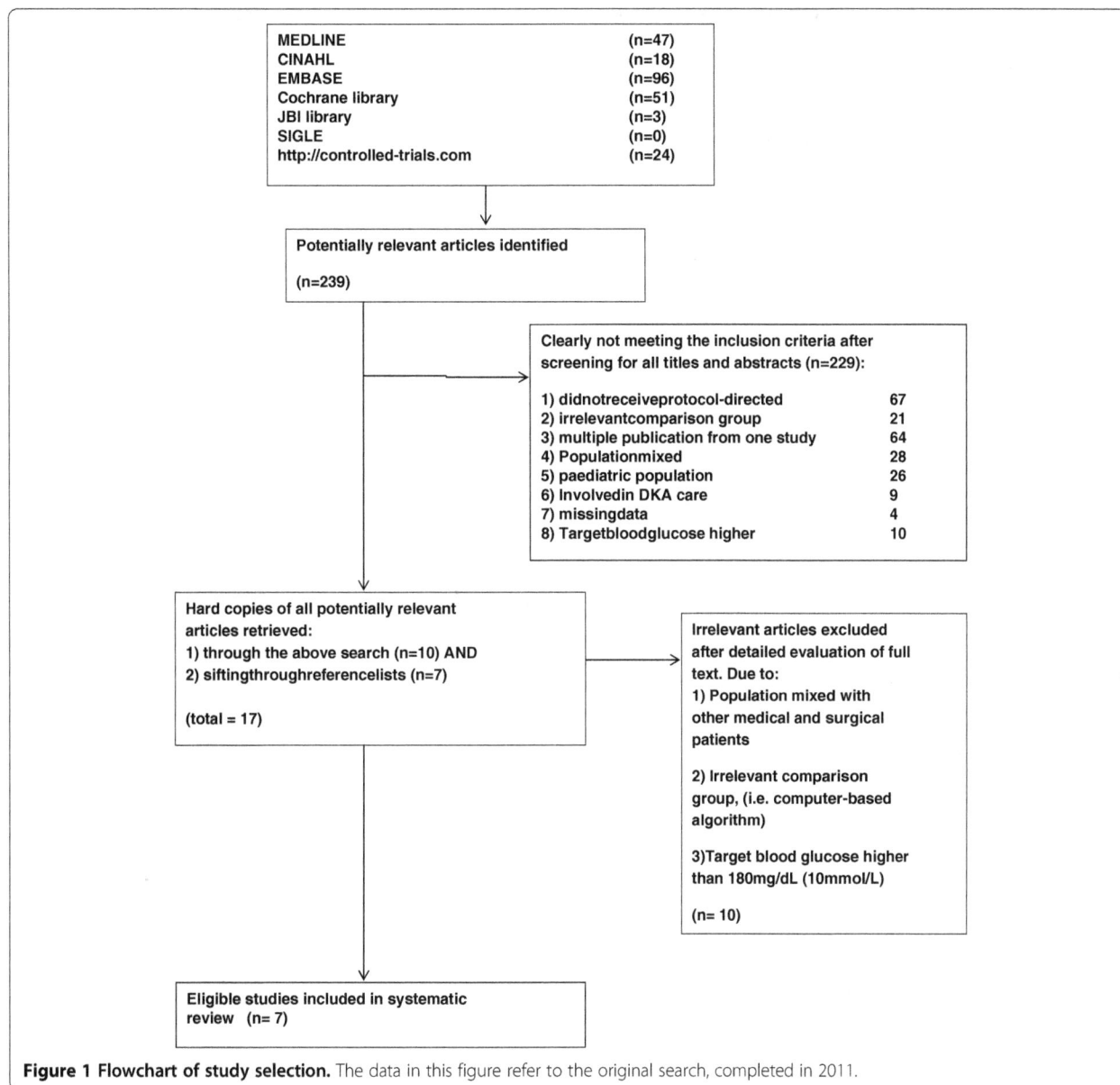

MEDLINE	(n=47)
CINAHL	(n=18)
EMBASE	(n=96)
Cochrane library	(n=51)
JBI library	(n=3)
SIGLE	(n=0)
http://controlled-trials.com	(n=24)

Potentially relevant articles identified

(n=239)

Clearly not meeting the inclusion criteria after screening for all titles and abstracts (n=229):

1) didnotreceiveprotocol-directed	67
2) irrelevantcomparison group	21
3) multiple publication from one study	64
4) Populationmixed	28
5) paediatric population	26
6) Involvedin DKA care	9
7) missingdata	4
8) Targetbloodglucose higher	10

Hard copies of all potentially relevant articles retrieved:
1) through the above search (n=10) AND
2) siftingthroughreferencelists (n=7)

(total = 17)

Irrelevant articles excluded after detailed evaluation of full text. Due to:
1) Population mixed with other medical and surgical patients

2) Irrelevant comparison group, (i.e. computer-based algorithm)

3)Target blood glucose higher than 180mg/dL (10mmol/L)

(n= 10)

Eligible studies included in systematic review (n= 7)

Figure 1 Flowchart of study selection. The data in this figure refer to the original search, completed in 2011.

3) Data from one study were used in more than one publication (in the form of quality of life data) (64 articles).
4) The population studied included other medical and surgical patients (28 articles).
5) The report studied a paediatric population (26 articles).
6) The patients studied were receiving diabetes ketoacidosis care (9 articles).
7) There were missing data for patients receiving study medication (4 articles).
8) The target blood glucose was higher than 180 mg/dl (10 mmol/l) (10 articles).

This left seven studies eligible for systematic review (Table 1).

Description of interventions
Interventions of interest will be limited to the use of the protocol-directed insulin infusion sliding scale; (2) a newly developed insulin infusion protocol; or a protocol modified from an existing protocol. For comparison, a practitioner-directed insulin infusion sliding scale and a conventional simple insulin infusion sliding scale will be included. Studies examining other types of insulin infusion sliding scale (such as computer-directed scales) will be excluded.

Table 1 Protocol-directed insulin infusion improve perioperative hyperglycaemia in critical care

Reference	Number of patients	Method	Target blood glucose concentration	Frequency of measurement	Frequency of hyperglycaemia	Main results
Zimmerman et al. (2004) [16]	168 postoperative cardiothoracic surgical intensive care patients	A nurse-driven insulin infusion protocol was developed and implemented in postoperative cardiothoracic surgical intensive care patients with or without diabetes.	80 to 150 mg/dl (4.4 to 8.3 mmol/l)	Every 1 to 4 hours	12 patients (7.1%) <40 mg/dl (2.2 mmol/l)	Findings showed percentage and time of blood glucose measurements within the tight glycaemic control range (control 47% vs. protocol 61%; $P = 0.001$),
		This before-and-after cohort study used two periods of measurement: a 6-month baseline period prior to the initiation of the insulin			28 patients (16.7%) <65 mg/dl (3.6 mmol/l)	Area under curve (AUC) of glucose exposure >150 mg/dl (8.3mmol/l) vs. time for the first 24 hours of the insulin infusion (control 28.4 vs. protocol 14.8; $P < 0.001$), median time to blood glucose <150 mg/dl (8.3mmol/l) (control 9.4 h vs. protocol 2.1h; $P < 0.001$), and percentage blood glucose <65 mg/dl (3.6 mmol/l) as a marker for hypoglycaemia (control 9.8% vs. protocol 16.7%; NS).
		infusion protocol (control group, $n = 174$) followed by a 6-month intervention period, in which the protocol was used (protocol group, $n = 168$).				
Tamaki et al. (2008) [17]	40 cardiac surgery patients	The Yale insulin infusion protocol was modified by taking into consideration the characteristics of Japanese diabetics and the hospital environment.	80 to 140 mg/dl (4.4 to 7.8 mmol/l)	Every 30 min to every 2 hours	Blood glucose values <60 mg/dl (3.3mmol/l) 0.5% ± 5.9%	Analyses of 1,656 blood glucose measurements during insulin infusion revealed that the percentage of samples that showed achievement of target blood glucose level (80 to 140 mg/dl (4.4 to 7.8 mmol/l)) was higher under protocol (78 ± 15%, $n = 870$) than control (57 ± 23%, $n = 786$, $P < 0.0001$).
		The modified protocol was tested in 40 type-2 diabetic patients after elective open-heart surgery, compared with 35 type-2 diabetic patients under empirical blood glucose control.				On the other hand, the fraction of samples with blood glucose <60 mg/dl (3.3 mmol/l) was comparable in the two groups (protocol: 0.5 ± 5.9‰, control: 5.1 ± 18.5‰).
						None of the patients with hypoglycaemia showed significant clinical adverse effects.
Caddell et al. (2010) [18]	100 cardiovascular surgery patients	Prospective data were gathered on 100 consecutive cardiovascular surgery patients managed with standard insulin infusion protocol and 100 patients managed with an insulin-resistance-guided protocol. Clinical characteristics and glycaemic indices were analyzed for the two groups. Primary outcomes included: percentage of time spent in the target range; number of hypoglycaemic and hyperglycaemic episodes; time to achievement of target blood	80 to 110 mg/dl (4.4 to 6.1 mmol/l)	Hourly	<70 mg/dl (3.9 mmol/l): 0.12 event per patient	The insulin-resistance guided protocol resulted in significant improvements, including increased percentage of time spent in the normoglycaemic range (82.5% vs. 65.8%, $P < 0.001$), reduced rate of hypoglycaemic episodes (0.12 vs. 0.99, $P < 0.01$), reduced rate of hyperglycaemic episodes (capillary blood glucose >126 mg/dl (7 mmol/l): 4.8 vs. 8.2, $P < 0.01$), and reduced time to the first measurement in the target range. Total daily dose of insulin was mildly increased,

Table 1 Protocol-directed insulin infusion improve perioperative hyperglycaemia in critical care *(Continued)*

		glucose concentration; and total daily dose of insulin required.				but failed to reach statistical significance (92.48 vs. 82.64 units, $P = 0.32$).
					<40 mg/dl (2.2 mmol/l): 0.04 event per patient	
Leibowitz et al. (2010) [31]	203 cardiac surgery patients	Patients with diabetes mellitus or random blood glucose >150 mg/dl were treated in the intensive care unit with intravenous insulin, followed by a multi-injection protocol consisting of four glargine-aspart insulin injections in the ward, with a glycaemic target of 110 to 150 mg/dl (6.1 to 8.3 mml/l).	110 to 150 mg/dl (6.1 to 8.3 mmol/l)	Every 20 min to every 4 hours	3% patients with blood glucose <60mg/dl (3.3 mmol/l)	During the intervention, mean blood glucose ± SD was 151 ± 19 mg/dl (8.4 ± 1.1 mmol/l) and 157 ± 32 mg/dl (8.7 ± 1.8 mmol/l) in the intensive care unit and ward, respectively, vs. 166 ± 27 mg/dl (9.2 ± 1.5 mmol/l) and 184 ± 46 mg/dl (10.2 ± 2.6 mmol/l) during the control period ($P < 0.0001$). The incidence of hypoglycaemia (blood glucose less than 60 mg/dl) was low and similar in the two groups (2.5% control vs. 3% intervention). Intensive insulin treatment decreased the risk for infection from 11% to 5% (56% risk reduction, $P = 0.018$), mainly by reducing the incidence of graft harvest site infection (6.9% vs. 2.5%, $P = 0.034$). The incidence of atrial fibrillation after coronary artery bypass graft surgery decreased from 30% to 18% (39% risk reduction; $P = 0.042$).
		The study cohort ($n = 410$) consisted of consecutive patients undergoing cardiothoracic surgery. Control patients ($n = 207$) were admitted during the first 8 months *(CONTROL GROUP)* The intervention group of patients ($n = 203$) were operated on during the following 8 months. The main outcome measures were glycaemic control and the rate of postsurgery infection.				
Goldberg et al. (2004) [24]	118 cardiothoracic intensive care unit patients	A standardized, intensive insulin infusion protocol was used for all patients admitted to two cardiothoracic intensive care unit s. Hourly blood glucose levels, relevant baseline variables, and clinical interventions were collected prospectively from the active hospital chart and cardiothoracic intensive care unit nursing records.	100 to 139 mg/dl (5.6 to 7.7 mmol/l)	Hourly	Five blood glucose values (0.2%) <60 mg/dl (3.3 mmol/l)	The insulin infusion protocol was used 137 times in 118 patients. The median time required to reach target blood glucose levels (100 to 139 mg/dl (5.6 to 7.7 mmol/l)) was 5 hours. Once blood glucose levels decreased below 140 mg/dl, 58% of 2242 subsequent hourly blood glucose values fell within the target range, 73% within a 'clinically desirable' range of 80 to 199 mg/dl (4.4 to 11 mmol/l). Only five (0.2%) blood glucose values were less than 60 mg/dl (3.3 mmol/l),

Table 1 Protocol-directed insulin infusion improve perioperative hyperglycaemia in critical care *(Continued)*

						with no associated adverse clinical events.
					Lowest recorded blood glucose value: 48 mg/dl (2.7 mmol/l)	
Lecomte *et al.* (2008) [25]	651 cardiac surgery patients	483 nondiabetics and 168 diabetics scheduled for cardiac surgery with cardiopulmonary bypass were recruited.	80 to 110 mg/dl (4.4 to 6.1 mmol/l)	Every 30 min to every 2 hours	Blood glucose values <60mg/dl (3..3 mmol/l)	18,893 blood glucose measurements were made during and after surgery. During surgery, the mean glucose level in nondiabetic patients was within targeted levels except during (112 ± 17 mg/dl (6.2 ± 0.9mmol/l)) and after rewarming (113 ± 19 mg/dl (6.3 ± 1.1mmol/l)) on cardiopulmonary bypass.
		To anticipate rapid perioperative changes in insulin requirement or sensitivity during surgery, a dynamic algorithm presented in tabular form, with rows representing blood glucose ranges and columns representing insulin dosages based on the patients' insulin sensitivity was developed. The algorithm adjusts insulin dosage based on blood glucose level and the projected insulin sensitivity (for example, reduced sensitivity during cardiopulmonary bypass and normalizing sensitivity after surgery).			In nondiabetic patients: 0.16%	In diabetics, blood glucose was decreased from 121 ± 40 mg/dl (6.7 ± 2.2 mmol/l) at anaesthesia induction to 112 ± 26 mg/dl (6.2 ± 1.4 mmol/l) at the end of surgery (*P* < 0.05), with 52.9% of patients achieving the target.
					In diabetic patients: 0.22%	In the intensive care unit, the mean glucose level was within the targeted range at all times, except for diabetics on arrival at the intensive care unit (113 ± 24 mg/dl (6.3 ± 1.3mmol/l)).
					Lowest recorded blood glucose value: 40 mg/dl	Of all blood glucose measurements (operating room and intensive care unit), 68.0% were within the target, with 0.12% of measurements in nondiabetics and 0.18% in diabetics below 60 mg/dl (3.3 mmol/l). Hypoglycaemia <50 mg/dl (2.8mmol/l) was avoided in all but four (0.6%) patients (40 mg/dl (2.2mmol/l) was the lowest observed value).
					(2.2mmol/l)	
Studer *et al.* (2010) [26]	230 cardiac surgery patients	230 consecutive patients (mean ± SD age: 67 ± 11 years; diabetic patients: *n* = 62) undergoing cardiac surgery (coronary artery bypass grafting: *n* = 137; 20% off-pump) or intrathoracic aortic (*n* = 10) surgery were included.	100 to 139 mg/dl (5.6 to 7.7 mmol/l)	Every 1 to 3 hours	Blood glucose <75 mg/dl (4.2 mmol/l): Postoperative day 1: 12 patients (5.3%)	All patients received postoperative insulin therapy. Patients spent 57.3% and 69.7% of time within the blood glucose target range on postoperative days 1 and 2, respectively. The percentage of time was significantly higher in nondiabetics than in diabetics. Mean blood glucose

Table 1 Protocol-directed insulin infusion improve perioperative hyperglycaemia in critical care *(Continued)*

		measurements per patient intraoperatively, on postoperative days 1 and 2 were 4 ± 1, 10 ± 2 and 7 ± 2, respectively. No patient experienced any severe hypoglycaemic events (blood glucose <50 mg/dl (2.8mmol/l)).
Blood glucose control was managed according to an insulin therapy protocol, described by Goldberg *et al.* [24], in use for 6 months. Insulin infusion rate and frequency of blood glucose monitoring were adjusted according to: (1) the current blood glucose	Postoperative day 2: 7 patients (3.1%).	
value; (2) the previous blood glucose value; and (3) the current insulin infusion rate. Efficacy was assessed by the percentage of time spent at the target blood glucose level (100 to 139 mg/dl (5.6 to 7.7mmol/l)) intraoperatively and during the first two postoperative days.	Blood glucose <50 mg/dl (2.78%): 0 patients (0%)	

Type of analysis

The objective of this study was to conduct a systematic review to determine whether a protocol-directed insulin infusion sliding scale is as safe and effective as the practitioner-directed insulin infusion sliding scale in bringing blood glucose values within the target range in a practical and real-life setting.

To minimize any errors and subjective judgement in the decision process, a critical appraisal instrument developed from the Joanna Briggs Institute (JBI-MAStARI) was used to appraise the methodological validity and quality of the studies independently [11]. This checklist required the authors to rate each individual study into one of three levels of credibility [12].

Data extraction was carried out by two reviewers independently to minimize errors. Data were extracted and stored using the standardized data extraction tool developed by JBI-MAStARI. Inconsistency in extracted data was settled by discussion between two reviewers. Where an agreement could not be reached, the problem was referred to a third reviewer for a decision.

Meta-analysis was carried out where appropriate and pooled using meta-analytical methods within Review Manager (RevMan) Version 5.1 software. No ethical approval was needed for this study.

Permission was obtained to use the databases and data within this study.

No ethical approval was required.

Results and discussion

Perioperative hyperglycaemia has been shown to be associated with adverse surgical outcomes in cardiac surgery patients [13,14]. Effective hyperglycaemic treatment is, therefore, of significant benefit in all patients after cardiac surgery [15]. Here, we present the results of a number of studies where protocol-directed insulin infusions improve perioperative hyperglycaemia in critical care. These are divided into those with and without the use of controls in their studies.

The studies carried out by Zimmerman *et al.* [16], Tamaki *et al.* [17], Caddell *et al.* [18] and Leibowitz *et al.* [19] all showed positive correlations between the ability to attain target blood glucose levels and the infusion regimen used when compared with the controls.

This is exemplified in the study of Zimmerman *et al.* [16], who examined 168 (protocol group) and 174 (control group) patients in the cardiothoracic intensive care unit. The results clearly showed that the target blood glucose range was achieved within 2.1 hours of treatment compared with those patients on the standard sliding scale, where it took 9.4 hours to achieve the target blood glucose range, a significance level of $P < 0.001$. Moreover, 61% of all blood glucose measurements were within the target range (protocol group) compared with 47% (control group). Furthermore, the protocol group remained within the target range for longer (65.4%) compared with the control group (54.6%).

The glycaemic level in the protocol group may be lower than observed, owing to the administration of corticosteroids and their ability to aggravate hyperglycaemic status [20]. Nevertheless, the results demonstrated that implementation of the protocol led to a significant improvement in glycaemic control. The speed with which this control was achieved, however, is controversial because this study was associated with the highest level of hypoglycaemia among all seven studies. This indicates that too-rapid lowering of blood glucose levels could be dangerous in cardiac diabetic surgery patients, which is supported by a randomized controlled trial of 10,251 patients that demonstrated that rapidly lowering blood glucose concentrations in patients with type 2 diabetes might harm patients by precipitating hypoglycaemia [21]. The safety of this particular protocol is, however, called into question when 16.7% of patients in the protocol group were subjected to levels of <65 mg/dl (3.6 mmol/l) or less compared with 9.8% of patients in the control group.

In another protocol versus control study, Tamaki and co-workers evaluated the effectiveness and safety of a modified Yale insulin infusion protocol [17], to maintain blood glucose levels at 80 to 140 mg/dl (4.4 to 7.8 mmol/l) in 40 Japanese diabetic patients who had undergone cardiac surgery. The rate of change of insulin infusion was modified to ensure effective and safe use for Asian patients [22].

Once again, there was a positive correlation between the treatments used in the protocol group compared with those used in the control group. The patients in the protocol group reached their target blood glucose levels more quickly (3.1 ± 2.1 hours) compared with the control group (5.0 ± 3.3 hours). In addition, of the total 870 blood glucose measurements, 78 ± 15% were within the target range (protocol group) compared with 57 ± 23% of the total 786 measurements in the control group (P <0.0001).

Although this supports the work carried out by Zimmerman et al. [16], Tamaki's work is still the only study carried out on Asian cardiac surgery patients, and it is difficult to correlate these results directly with those carried out in countries that utilize alternative protocols. Moreover, the small sample size of this study limited the generalizability of this particular study and the ability to capture the true clinical impact on this population.

Caddell et al. [18] introduced an insulin-resistance guided protocol, which demonstrated similar findings to those obtained in the Zimmerman and Tamaki studies. Caddell's group showed that the insulin-resistance guided protocol led to more rapid and effective blood glucose control in cardiac surgery patients with target blood glucose levels of 80 to 110 mg/dl (4.4–6.1 mmol/l) in the first 24 hour postoperative period.

In the protocol group, 65% of patients reached target blood glucose ranges within 3 hours compared with 65% of the patients (control group), who reached the target range within 9 hours, (P < 0.01). Additionally, patients in the protocol group maintained their blood glucose concentration within the target range longer (82.5% (19.8 hours)) than the control group (65.8% (15.7 hours)), a significance level of P < 0.001.

The principal strength of Leibowitz's study [19] over the Zimmerman, Tamaki and Caddell studies is the comparatively large number of patients. The study cohort consisted of 410 patients undergoing cardiothoracic surgery. The control patients (n = 207) were admitted during the first 8 months, whereas the intervention group of patients (n = 203) were operated on during the following 8 months.

The percentage of patients maintaining a target blood glucose level of 110 to 150 mg/dl (6.1 to 8.3 mmol/l) was 55% (protocol group) and 39% (control group) (P < 0.0001), although the effective achievement of target blood glucose control resulted in a small increase in the frequency of hypoglycaemia (3% vs. 2.5%), which was not considered significant. Nevertheless, the frequency of hypoglycaemia was still lower than that observed in other studies, which used the same target blood glucose range (110 to 150 mg/dl (6.1 to 8.3 mmol/l)) and was associated with 5% of hypoglycaemic events in cardiac care unit patients [23].

Three studies that were carried out without the use of controls were those of Goldberg et al. [24], Lecomte et al. [25] and Studer et al. [26]. Although no controls were used, insulin infusion protocols were used to obtain target blood glucose levels of 100 to 139 mg/dl (5.6 to 7.7 mmol/l), 80 to 110 mg/dl (4.4 to 6.1 mmol/l) and 100 to 139 mg/dl (5.6 to 7.7 mmol/l), respectively.

Goldberg's group [24] investigated the use of an insulin infusion protocol in 118 patients (protocol group). The median time required to achieve the target glycaemic level was 5 hours. When blood glucose levels fell below 140 mg/dl (7.8 mmol/l), 58% of 2242 subsequent hourly blood glucose values fell within the target range. The strength and effectiveness of Lecomte's study [25] stemmed from the large number of patients (651 patients) included, in addition to the homogeneity of the sample population. Results showed that the protocol achieved the target blood glucose level faster than Goldberg's, in 3 hours (72.4% = nondiabetic) and (66.2% = diabetic patients). Studer's study [26] demonstrated that under treatment conditions, nondiabetic patients achieved a better glycaemic control with a lower incidence of hypoglycaemic events than diabetic patients and is consistent with a previous study [27]. There were only four observed cases of hypoglycaemia in Lecomte's study [25] and there were no associated adverse clinical episodes in the work carried out by Goldberg's group [24].

The effectiveness and safety of these protocols rests with the fact that clinicians have pre-existing knowledge of previous blood glucose values, current blood glucose values and current insulin infusion rates, and this is confirmed by the meta-analysis of the four studies with controls [16-19], which showed that the percentage failure of patients reaching target blood glucose levels demonstrated a significant difference ($P < 0.0005$) from patients failing to achieve target blood glucose levels in the control group compared with patients treated by protocol (Additional file 1: Table S2).

Owing to the stress of surgery and the use of catecholamine and steroids during the perioperative period, patient's blood glucose values can fluctuate immediately postoperatively [28]. Therefore, a dynamic protocol that regulates insulin dosage according to the relative change of blood glucose concentration, rather than one absolute blood glucose value is of great important in achieving tight glycaemic control effectively without increasing the risk of hypoglycaemia.

Intensive insulin management [29] is often required to optimize glycaemic control but this can be associated with insulin mismanagement, and severe hypoglycaemia is possible [30]. Hypoglycaemia, which requires emergency medical assistance, is commonplace in patients with longstanding insulin-treated type 1 and type 2 diabetes. Left untreated, severe hypoglycaemia can result in morbidity and death. Severe hypoglycaemia [31] can be prevented by utilizing appropriate medications and medication regimens [32], and effective glucose monitoring strategies [33] and technologies [34]. This is fully supported by our meta-analysis on the risk of hypoglycaemia on the studies and the subgroup (Additional file 2: Table S3) examined, in which the risk of hypoglycaemia was significantly reduced compared with control ($P < 0.00001$) between studies that used an insulin infusion protocol.

Conclusion

Perioperative hyperglycaemia is associated with poor outcomes in patients undergoing cardiac surgery. Frequent postoperative hyperglycaemia in cardiac surgery patients has led to the instigation of a quality improvement insulin infusion sliding scale. A systematic review was conducted, to determine whether a protocol-directed insulin infusion sliding scale was as safe and effective as conventional practitioner-directed insulin infusion sliding scales. Seven research studies met the inclusion criteria. Five studies compared their insulin infusion protocols to the previous blood glucose management practice. Overall glycaemic control showed an improvement in all five studies. Of the seven

studies, four used controls and three had no controls. Implementation of protocols led to blood glucose concentrations being achieved more readily. Moreover, blood glucose ranges were maintained for a longer time, without any increased frequency of hyperglycaemia.

Key messages

- The protocol-directed insulin infusion sliding scale is a safe and effective method.
- Blood glucose control is improved when compared with the conventional practitioner-directed insulin infusion sliding scale.
- This study supports the adoption of a protocol-directed insulin infusion sliding scale as a standard of care for post-cardiac surgery patients.
- An effective protocol should be based on the velocity of glycaemic changes and patient's insulin sensitivity.
- The current blood glucose level, previous blood glucose levels and relative change of blood glucose levels between two consecutive measurements, as well as the patient's insulin resistance status, are clinically important and should be used as parameters of care, instead of relying solely on the latest blood glucose level itself to adjust insulin infusion rates.

Abbreviations
JBI: Joanna Briggs Institute; SIGLE: Open System for Information on Grey literature in Europe.

Competing interests
The authors have no competing interests.

Authors' contributions
Conception and design: MLH/GGA; Analysis and interpretation: MLH/GGA; Drafting the manuscript for important intellectual content:MLH/AK/GGA. All authors read and approved the final manuscript.

Author details
[1]The Queen Elizabeth Hospital, 30 Gascoigne Road, Kowloon, Hong Kong. [2]Faculty of Medicine and Health Science, University of Nottingham, Clifton Boulevard, Nottingham NG7 2RD, UK. [3]Insulin and Diabetes Experimental Research (IDER) Group, Faculty of Medicine and Health Science, University of Nottingham, Clifton Boulevard, Nottingham NG7 2RD, UK.

References
1. Knapik P, Nadziakiewicz P, Urbanska E, Saucha W, Herdynska M, Zembala M: Cardiopulmonary bypass increase postoperative glycaemia and insulin consumption after coronary surgery. *Ann Thorac Surg* 2009, **87**:1859–1865.

2. Haga K, McClymont KL, Clarke S, Grounds RS, Ng KYB, Glyde DW, Loveless RJ, Carter GH, Alston RP: The effects of tight glycaemic control, during and after cardiac surgery, on patient mortality and morbidity: a systematic review and meta-analysis. *J Cardiothorac Surg* 2011, **6**(3):1–10.

3. Shine T, Uchikado M, Crawford CC, Murray MJ: Importance of perioperative blood glucose management in cardiac surgical patients. *Asian Cardiovasc Thorac Ann* 2007, **15**(6):534–538.

4. Van den Berghe G, Wouters P, Weekers F, Verwaest C, Bruyninckx F, Schetz M, Vlasselaers D, Ferdinande P, Lauwers P, Bouillon R: Intensive insulin therapy in critically ill patients. *N Eng J Med* 2001, **345**:1359–1367.

5. Stojković A, Koracević G, Perisić Z, Krstić N, Pavlović M, Todorović L, Glasnović J, Burazor I, Apostolović S, Nikolić G, Kostić T, Branković N: The influence of stress hyperglycemia on the prognosis of patients with acute myocardial infarction and temporary electrical cardiac pacing. *Srp Arh Celok Lek* 2010, **138**(7–8):430–435.

6. Furnary AP: Clinical benefits of tight glycaemic control: focus on the perioperative setting. *Best Pract Res Clin Anaesthesiol* 2009, **23**:411–420.

7. Hanazaki K, Maeda H, Okabayashi T: Relationship between perioperative glycaemic control and post-operative infections. *World J Gastroenterol* 2009, **15**(33):4122–4125.

8. Ljungqvist O, Nygren J, Soop M, Thorell A: Metabolic perioperative management: novel concepts. *Curr Opin Crit Care* 2005, **11**(4):295–299.

9. Clement S, Braithwaite SS, Magee MF, Ahmann A, Smith EP, Schafer RG, Hirsh IB: Management of diabetes and hyperglycaemia in hospitals. *Diabetes Care* 2004, **27**(2):553–591.

10. Brown G, Dodeck P: Intravenous insulin nomogram improves blood glucose control in the critically ill. *Crit Care Med* 2001, **29**:1714–1719.

11. Pope C, Mays N, Popay J: *Synthesizing Qualitative and Quantitative Health Evidence. A Guide to Methods.* Maidenhead: Open University Press; 2007.

12. Bruce N, Pope D, Stanistreet D: *Quantitative Methods for Health Research: A Practical Interactive Guide to Epidemiology and Statistics.* Chichester: Wiley; 2009.

13. Estrada C, Young JA, Nifong LW, Chitwood WR: Outcomes and perioperative hyperglycaemia in patients with or without diabetes mellitus undergoing coronary artery bypass grafting. *Ann Thorac Surg* 2003, **75**:1392–1399.

14. May AK, Kauffmann RM, Collier BR: The place for glycemic control in the surgical patient. *Surg Infect (Larchmt)* 2011, **12**(5):405–418.

15. Desai SP, Henry LL, Holmes SD, Hunt SL, Martin CT, Hebsur S, Ad N: Strict versus liberal target range for perioperative glucose in patients undergoing coronary artery bypass grafting: a prospective randomized controlled trial. *J Thorac Cardiovasc Surg* 2012, **143**(2):318–325.

16. Zimmerman CR, Mlynarek ME, Jordan JA, Rajda CA, Horst HM: An insulin infusion protocol in critically ill cardiothoracic surgery patients. *Ann Pharmacother* 2004, **38**(7–8):1123–1129.

17. Tamaki M, Shimizu T, Kanazawa A, Tamura Y, Hanzawa A, Ebato C, Itou C, Yasunari E, Sanke H, Abe H, Kawai J, Okayama K, Matsumoto K, Komiya K, Kawaguchi M, Inagaki N, Watanabe T, Kanazawa Y, Hirose T, Kawamori R, Watada H: Efficacy and safety of modified Yale insulin infusion protocol in Japanese diabetic patients after open-heart surgery. *Diabetes Res Clin Pract* 2008, **81**:296–302.

18. Caddell KA, Komanapalli CB, Slater MS, Hagg D, Tibayan FA, Smith S, Ahmann A, Guyton SW, Song HK: Patient-specific insulin-resistance-guided infusion improves glycemic control in cardiac surgery. *Ann Thorac Surg* 2010, **90**(6):1818–1823.

19. Leibowitz G, Raizman E, Brezis M, Glaser B, Raz I, Shapira O: Effects of moderate intensity glycemic control after cardiac surgery. *Ann Thorac Surg* 2010, **90**(6):1825–1832.

20. Agarwal D, Jeloka T, Sharma AP, Sharma RK: Steroid induced diabetes mellitus presenting as diabetic ketoacidosis. *Indian J Nephrol* 2002, **12**:122–123.

21. ACCORD SG: Action to Control Cardiovascular Risk in Diabetes (ACCORD) trial: design and methods. *Am J Cardiol* 2007, **99**(suppl):21i–33i.

22. Torrens J, Skurnick J, Davidow AL, Korenman SG, Santoro N, Soto-Greene M, Lasser N, Weiss G: Ethnic differences in insulin sensitivity and beta-cell function in premenopausal or early perimenopausal women without diabetes: the Study of Women's Health Across the Nation (SWAN). *Diabetes Care* 2004, **27**:354–361.

23. Barth MM, Oyen LJ, Warfield KT, Elmer JL, Evenson LK, Tescher AN, Kuper PJ, Bannon MP, Gajic O, Farmer JC: Comparison of a nurse initiated insulin infusion protocol for intensive insulin therapy between adult surgical trauma, medical and coronary care intensive care patients. *BMC Emerg Med* 2007, **7**(14):1–9.

24. Goldberg PA, Sakharova OV, Barrett PW, Falko LN, Roussel MG, Bak L, Blake-Holmes D, Marieb NJ, Inzucchi SE: Improving glycemic control in the cardiothoracic intensive care unit: clinical experience in two hospital settings. *J Cardiothorac Vasc Anesth* 2004, **18**(6):690–697.

25. Lecomte P, Foubert L, Nobels F, Coddens J, Nollet G, Casselman F, Crombrugge PV, Vandenbroucke G, Cammu G: Dynamic tight glycemic control during and after cardiac surgery is effective, feasible, and safe. *Anesth Analg* 2008, **107**(1):51–58.

26. Studer C, Sankou W, Penfornis A, Pili-Floury S, Puyraveau M, Cordier A, Etievent JP, Samain E: Efficacy and safety of an insulin infusion protocol during and after cardiac surgery. *Diabetes Metab* 2010, **36**(1):71–78.

27. Scheurn L, Baetz B, Cawley MJ, Fitzpatrick R, Cachecho R: Pharmacist designed and nursing-driven insulin infusion protocol to achieve and maintain glycaemic control in critical care patients. *J Trauma Nurs* 2006, **13**(3):140–145.

28. Prieto-Sanchez L: Hyperglycaemia in-hospital management. *Therapeutic Advances in Endocrinology and Metabolism* 2011, **2**(1):3–7.

29. Chima RS, Schoettker P, Varadarajan KR, Kloppenborg E, Hutson TK, Brilli RJ, Repaske DR, Seid M: Reduction in hypoglycemic events in critically ill patients on continuous insulin following implementation of a treatment guideline. *Qual Manag Health Care* 2012, **21**(1):20–28.

30. Unger J: Comparing the efficacy, safety, and utility of intensive insulin algorithms for a primary care practice. *Diabetes Ther* 2011, **2**(1):40–50.

31. Buehler AM, Cavalcanti A, Berwanger O, Figueiro M, Laranjeira LN, Zazula AD, Kioshi B, Bugano DG, Santucci E, Sbruzzi G, Guimaraes HP, Carvalho VO, Bordin SA: Effect of tight blood glucose control versus conventional control in patients with type 2 diabetes mellitus: a systematic review with meta-analysis of randomized controlled trials. *Cardiovasc Ther* 2011. doi:10.1111/j.1755-5922.2011.00308.x.

32. Mauras N, Beck R, Xing D, Ruedy K, Buckingham B, Tansey M, White NH, Weinzimer SA, Tamborlane W, Kollman C, The Diabetes Research in Children Network (DirecNet) Study Group: A randomized clinical trial to assess the efficacy and safety of real-time continuous glucose monitoring in the management of type 1 diabetes in young children aged 4 to <10 years. *Diabetes Care* 2012, **34**:204–210.

33. Joubert M, Reznik Y: Personal continuous glucose monitoring (CGM) in diabetes management: Review of the literature and implementation for practical use. *Diabetes Res Clin Pract* 2012, **96**:294–305.

34. Moghissi E, Korytkowski MT, Dinardo M, Einhorn D, Hellman R, Hirsch IB, Inzucchi SE, Ismail-Beigi F, Kirkman MS, Umpierrez GE: American Association of Clinical Endocrinologists and American Diabetes Association consensus statement on impatient glycaemic control. *Diabetes Care* 2009, **32**(6):1119–1131.

24

Less invasive methods of advanced hemodynamic monitoring: principles, devices, and their role in the perioperative hemodynamic optimization

Christos Chamos[1*], Liana Vele[2], Mark Hamilton[3] and Maurizio Cecconi[3]

Abstract

The monitoring of the cardiac output (CO) and other hemodynamic parameters, traditionally performed with the thermodilution method via a pulmonary artery catheter (PAC), is now increasingly done with the aid of less invasive and much easier to use devices. When used within the context of a hemodynamic optimization protocol, they can positively influence the outcome in both surgical and non-surgical patient populations. While these monitoring tools have simplified the hemodynamic calculations, they are subject to limitations and can lead to erroneous results if not used properly. In this article we will review the commercially available minimally invasive CO monitoring devices, explore their technical characteristics and describe the limitations that should be taken into consideration when clinical decisions are made.

Keywords: Minimally invasive monitoring, Pulse pressure analysis, Lithium dilution, Transpulmonary thermodilution, Oesophageal doppler, Gas rebreathing, Transthoracic bioimpendance, Goal-directed therapy

Introduction

The need for the precise quantification of cardiac output (CO) in high-risk surgical patients, both in the operative room and the intensive care unit, is vital in modern medical practice. While up to 20 years ago CO had to be estimated from the PAC, nowadays new, less invasive techniques are available. When used together with perioperative protocols aiming at improving CO and oxygen delivery (DO2), their use is referred to as hemodynamic optimization or goal-directed therapy (GDT) [1].

Much has changed since the introduction of the pulmonary artery catheter (PAC) by Swan and Ganz in 1970 for the measurement of CO using the thermodilution method. Although in the context of moderate and high-risk surgery the beneficial effect of the PAC combined with goal directed therapy (GDT) has been established in a recent meta-analysis [2], the invasive nature of the insertion of the catheter and a considerable number of complications that

follow its use (infection, arrhythmias, thrombosis, and pulmonary artery rupture) have led to a decline in its popularity, and prompted the scientific community to search for alternative methods that could substitute the PAC.

The term 'minimally invasive cardiac monitoring' encompasses all the methods and devices that calculate the cardiac output without the need of inserting a PAC, ranging from methods almost non-invasive to marginally less invasive than the PAC. These include the pulse pressure analysis, the transpulmonary thermodilution, the indicator dilution, the esophageal Doppler, the thoracic electrical bioimpedance, the carbon dioxide rebreathing, and the echocardiography. Since each one of these devices utilizes a different method of estimating the cardiac output, the clinician should be aware of their distinct features, their limitations but also the sources of potential error that stem for their use.

Review

Pulse pressure analysis

The pulse pressure analysis uses the arterial waveform, obtained either from an arterial catheter or a finger

* Correspondence: hamos1977@yahoo.gr
[1]Senior clinical fellow in cardiac anaesthesia, St George's Healthcare NHS Trust, London, UK
Full list of author information is available at the end of the article

probe, in order to calculate the stroke volume (SV) and the systemic vascular resistance (SVR).

Its principles first described by Erlanger and Hooker in 1904 [3], pulse pressure analysis is based on the hypothesis that the SV is proportional to the arterial pulse pressure. However, a major drawback was the fact that the compliance of the aortic wall is non-linear rather than linear, being high at low distending pressures but decreasing more rapidly at higher pressures, preventing this way the overstretching of the vessel wall.

This and the fact that the compliance is also age-related, prevented any straightforward correlation of the pressure to the volume [4]. Only in 1983 and after the development of an algorithm by Wesseling et al. [5] to compensate for this non-linearity, did it become possible to calculate the SV by integrating the area under the curve of the systolic phase of the arterial waveform, and calculating the CO by simply multiplying the SV with the heart rate (HR) Figure 1.

One should always keep in mind that the pulse pressure method relies heavily on an optimal arterial pressure tracing, making an under- or over-damped arterial waveform a potential source of errors in calculation. Moreover, the pulse pressure systems necessitate an arterial wave that is purely reflective of the forward SV. As a consequence, situations in which the arterial wave is distorted either by artifact or a physiologic phenomenon (intra-aortic balloon counterpulsation, aortic regurgitation) will lead to inaccuracies [6]. Finally, the discrepancy in the compliance of the aorta compared to more peripheral parts of the arterial tree distorts the pattern of the arterial waveform and requires a careful interpretation of the measured values.

A variety of commercial systems that make use of the pulse pressure analysis method are available and they are divided in two groups, depending on the way that they are

calibrated. Monitors that are 'autocalibrated' consist of the FloTrac/Vigileo, the Pulsioflex, the LidCO rapid, and the recently introduced Nexfin and esCCO monitors. On the other hand, there are devices that are externally calibrated: the PiCCOplus and the recently developed EV1000 use the transpulmonary thermodilution method, while the LidCO plus utilizes the lithium dilution technique for the same purpose. Moreover, apart from being useful tools in CO calculations, these monitors can also help predict the fluid responsiveness, as will be discussed later in this review article.

Uncalibrated devices
Connected to a standard indwelling arterial catheter, the FloTrac sensor (Edwards Lifesciences, Irvine, CA, USA) uses an upgraded algorithm that derives the SV from the pulse pressure (PP) of the arterial waveform, after correcting for the compliance and the resistance of the arterial system.

A similar pulse pressure analysis method is used by the ProAQT sensor which is incorporated in the Pulsioflex monitor (Pulsion Medical Systems, Munich, Germany). Utilizing an existing peripheral arterial catheter and analyzing the arterial waveform 250 times per second, a start value for CO trend monitoring is determined after the patient's characteristics are inserted to the system. To increase accuracy, a CO value measured by another method (for example by echocardiography) can be entered and thus the system can be externally calibrated.

As for the LidCO rapid system (LidCO Ltd, Cambridge, UK), it is based on the same algorithm as the LidCO plus monitor (which will be described later), but instead of thermodilution it relies on nomograms for the calculation of the CO.

One of the latest additions to the field of minimally invasive CO monitoring is the Nexfin monitor (BMEYE, Amsterdam, The Netherlands). Rather than a minimally invasive monitor, it is a completely non-invasive method of determining the patient's hemodynamic parameters, as the need for an invasive arterial catheter is obviated. The monitor is connected to the patient by wrapping an inflatable cuff around the middle phalanx of the finger. The pulsating finger artery is 'clamped' to a constant volume by applying a varying counter pressure equivalent to the arterial pressure resulting in a pressure waveform. The finger arterial pressure is then reconstructed into brachial arterial pressure waveform using a transfer function and a level correction based on a vast clinical database. The resulting brachial pressure waveform serves as the basis for determining continuous CO. Real-time continuous CO and other hemodynamic parameters are derived by a novel pulse contour method (Nexfin CO-Trek®), which is based on the systolic

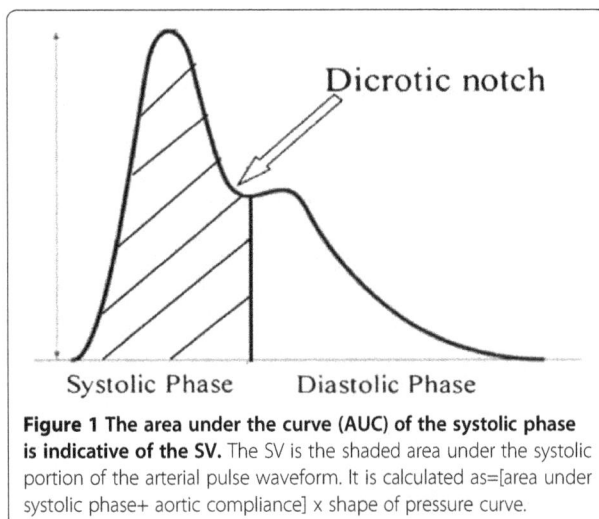

Figure 1 The area under the curve (AUC) of the systolic phase is indicative of the SV. The SV is the shaded area under the systolic portion of the arterial pulse waveform. It is calculated as=[area under systolic phase+ aortic compliance] x shape of pressure curve.

pressure area and a physiological three-element Windkessel model individualized for each patient. Moreover, the presence of a co-oximeter enables the non-invasive calculation of hemoglobin, from which the oxygen delivery index (DO_2I) is derived.

For completion purposes, we should also mention the latest entry in the pulse pressure analysis field, under the name of esCCO (Nihon Kohden, Tokyo, Japan). Also being a non-invasive monitor, it uses a new technology that derives the CO using the Pulse Wave Transit Time (PWTT), which is obtained by the pulse oximetry and the ECG signals of each cardiac cycle. The rationale behind this is that animal studies have shown a strong correlation between the SV and the PWTT. The only up-to-date validation study has demonstrated a clinically unacceptable performance of the device when compared to the CO values obtained with transthoracic echocardiography [7].

The accuracy of the pulse pressure analysis method in estimating CO has been extensively investigated against CO calculations by the thermodilution method using the PAC. This holds true particularly for the FloTrac/Vigileo monitoring. In one of the most recent meta-analyses, Mayer et al. [8] showed improved correlation between the Flotrac/Vigileo and the thermodilution method when the new generation software was used, as opposed to the initially poor correlation with previous generation softwares. Also, the SVV calculated with this method showed good performance in predicting fluid responsiveness in septic shock patients [9]. On the other hand, it appears that the CO calculated by the FloTrac/Vigileo has a less accurate correlation with the one derived by the PAC when changes are induced by norepinephrine administration [10], and also tends to be overestimated compared to a continuous cardiac output calculation with a PAC when used in off-pump coronary artery bypass surgery (CABG) [11]. A discrepancy in measurements also appears when the FloTrac/Vigileo is used to calculate hemodynamic parameters in open aortic abdominal aneurysm (AAA) repair [12] compared with echocardiography derived measurements.

Given its straightforward setup and use, it seems that the FloTrac/Vigileo is a useful tool correlating well with the gold standard of the thermodilution method with the PAC, in patients with a regular rhythm and stable respiratory pattern and mechanics, hospitalized in an environment with less abrupt hemodynamic changes as is the intensive therapy unit (ITU). While awaiting for further studies to assess this relationship, a more cautious approach should be adopted when it is used to assess the CO in patients that rely on substantial inotropic or vasopressor support or in environments and settings with rapid dynamic changes, as in the operating room (OR).

Despite its relatively short presence in the market, the non-invasive Nexfin monitor has also been validated against the traditional methods of CO calculation, yielding positive results so far. Two different research groups demonstrated a reasonable correlation of CO values obtained by the Nexfin when they were compared with those calculated by transpulmonary thermodilution, both in the setting of cardiac surgery [13,14]. The same good agreement appears when the Nexfin derived CO values are compared to those measured by Doppler echocardiography, either from the transthoracic [15] or the esophageal route [16]. Adding to these studies the lack of invasiveness and the ease of use, the Nexfin monitor appears to be an alternative method of calculating hemodynamics where the traditional invasive approach is difficult or undesirable.

Calibrated devices

The PiCCOplus monitor (Pulsion Medical Systems, Munich, Germany), which is based on the pulse pressure analysis to provide continuous real-time assessment of the CO, uses the transpulmonary thermodilution for intermittent calibration, being until recently the only device to incorporate this method in a commercial application. This method is based on the same principle as the traditional thermodilution but spares the need for a PAC insertion. The technique starts with the injection of a cold injectate in the superior vena cava (SVC) via a central venous catheter (CVC) which mixes with the ambient blood and travels through the right heart, the pulmonary vasculature and the left heart before reaching the aorta. A thermistor in the aorta or a major arterial branch measures the blood temperature and a thermodilution curve of temperature over time, similar to that from the PAC-based method but having a delayed peak temperature change, is plotted. The CO is measured by the thermodilution equation:

$$CO = \frac{(T_B - T_I) \times K}{\int_0^\infty \Delta T_B(t) dt}$$

here T_B=blood temperature, T_I=injectate temperature, and K=−computation constant (Figure 2).

The PiCCOplus monitor also provides information on variables as the global end-diastolic volume (GEDV) [17], which is an estimate of the preload much more reliable than the CVP, the intrathoracic blood volume (ITBV), the extravascular lung water (EVLW), and the pulmonary vascular permeability index (PVPI). The combination of the last two variables could potentially help in diagnosing pulmonary edema and distinguishing between the hydrostatic and inflammatory forms of the condition [18]. This comes at the cost of needing a CVC for injection of the cold indicator and a thermistor-

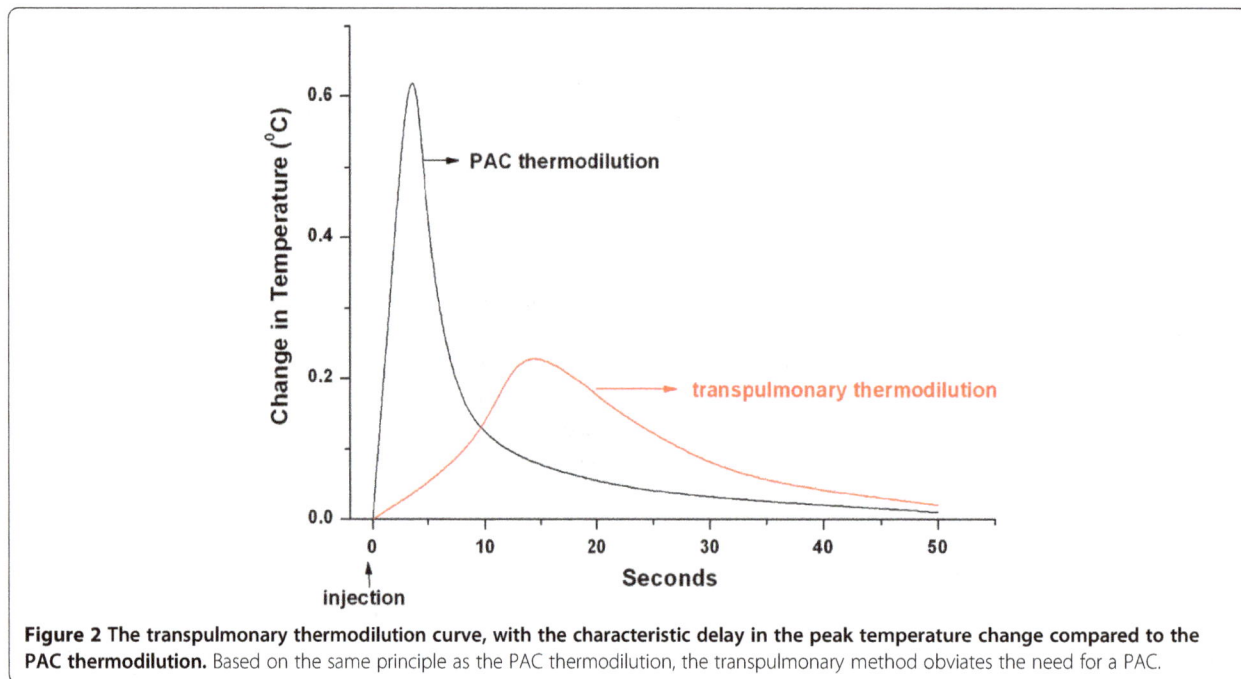

Figure 2 The transpulmonary thermodilution curve, with the characteristic delay in the peak temperature change compared to the PAC thermodilution. Based on the same principle as the PAC thermodilution, the transpulmonary method obviates the need for a PAC.

tipped catheter in a central artery (femoral, axillary, or brachial), this way being a more invasive method than the FloTrac/Vigileo and the LidCO monitors.

Since a pulse contour method is used for continous CO display, the same limitations as in the FloTrac/Vigileo monitor apply for the PiCCOplus (IABP counterpulsation, significant aortic regurgitation, arrhythmias). Sources of potential errors that are specific for the transpulmonary thermodilution come from the fact that the PiCCOplus estimates the CO of the left heart whereas the PAC thermodilution that of the right side. These should be identical in ideal conditions, however a discrepancy is encountered in the presence of intracardiac and intrapulmonary shunts. Moreover, conditions related to indicator loss in the tissues (that is, in the presence of pulmonary edema) or recirculation will lead to a discrepancy of the calculated CO compared to the one derived by the PAC thermodilution, although these two phenomena may actually cancel each other [19].

Regarding the reliability of the method, it appears that there is good correlation of the CO measurements obtained with the PiCCOplus compared to other methods. Two studies performed on pediatric animal models by the same scientific team showed a significant correlation when the transpulmonary thermodilution derived values were juxtaposed to those obtained with an ultrasound probe around the main pulmonary artery, both in normal cardiac anatomy and in the presence of a left-to-right shunt [20,21].

An older study confirms the good performance of the transpulmonary thermodilution even during substantial

variations in vascular tone and hemodynamics [22]. Taking these under consideration and calibrating the device according to the manufacturer's advice, it is reasonable to consider the PiCCOplus as a reliable, less invasive substitute method to the PAC.

The latest entry in the area of minimally invasive CO monitoring using the transpulmonary thermodilution comes from Edwards Lifesciences, which developed the EV1000/VolumeView monitor (Edwards Lifesciences, Irvine, CA, USA). Needing, as the PiCCOplus does, a specific to the set central arterial catheter and using a patented for the company algorithm, it also displays volumetric parameters as the EVLW and GEDV but also a new variable named the global ejection fraction (GEF). A recent clinical validation study proved the interchangeability of this new method to the PiCCOplus monitor, with VolumeView scoring better in the calculation of GEDV [23].

The last of the calibrated CO monitors is the LidCOplus (LidCO Ltd, Cambridge, UK) that utilizes the lithium dilution technique. Based on the pulse power rather than the pulse pressure analysis via the PulseCO algorithm, which does not rely on the arterial waveform morphology, and needing only a peripheral arterial catheter, the LidCOplus technology uses the lithium dilution to intermittently calibrate the system. Specifically, boluses of 0.5-2 mL of lithium chloride are each time injected through a peripheral or central line and the lithium concentration is measured through aspiration of blood from the arterial catheter, using a Li^+-sensitive electrode attached to the catheter that generates a voltage [24]. Since the electrode has a low sensitivity for distinguishing lithium from sodium, a correction factor is applied for sodium plasma levels and a baseline voltage is determined that helps differentiate the concentration of the two cations. Once the lithium dilution curve is obtained, the CO is calculated using the Stewart-Hamilton equation, again with a correction for packed cell volume. The main advantage of lithium as an indicator is that it does not naturally occur in plasma and therefore can generate a high signal-to-noise ratio when used with a sensitive electrode, followed by a rapid redistribution time and an insignificant first-pass loss from the circulation [25].

Apart from the expected lack of accuracy of the LidCOplus technology in a patient already on lithium treatment, the other interference that should be taken into account is the use of bolus doses of muscle relaxant drugs in the operative and intensive care setting. High peak doses of these drugs can cross-react with the lithium sensor as they incorporate a positively charged quaternary ammonia ion that can be detected by the sensor and thus lead to an overestimation of the CO. Muscle relaxant agents which are not compatible with the LidCOplus monitor are atracurium and rocuronium, whereas suxamethonium, vecuronium, and pancuronium can be used provided that a time interval of 15–30 minutes elapses between their bolus administration and the LidCOplus calibration.

The consistency of the CO measurement with the LidCOplus technology compared to the traditionally established thermodilution method with the PAC, has been investigated in a number of validation studies. In one of the most recent studies by Mora et al. [26], the lithium dilution method showed good correlation and marginal bias (0.28 L/min) with the thermodilution method in patients with impaired left ventricular function after cardiac surgery. This good correlation was corroborated by Costa et al. [27] when they validated the LidCOplus against intermittent thermodilution measurements in patients with hyperdynamic conditions. On the other hand, the uncalibrated pulse power analysis using the Pulse CO algorithm performed less well when used in comparison to the PAC based thermodilution in patients undergoing CABG [28] or when used in very dynamic conditions such as the clamping and unclamping of the aorta in AAA surgery [29]. Concluding, the LidCOplus technology appears to be a reliable substitute to the more invasive thermodilution method via the PAC, provided that the system is calibrated in regular intervals when an absolute value rather than a simple trend of the CO is required.

Esophageal Doppler monitor

The Esophageal Doppler (ED) monitor, which is based on the Doppler effect in order to measure the velocity of blood flow, was first introduced in the 1970s as a non-invasive means to measure CO. The velocity is calculated from the following equation:

$$V(cf_d)/(2f_0\cos\theta)$$

where v is the blood flow velocity, c is the speed of sound in tissue, f_d is the frequency shift, f_0 is the frequency of the emitted ultrasound, and θ is the angle between the ultrasound beam and the direction of the blood flow. If the flow of blood in the descending aorta is known, this figure can be used to estimate the stroke volume and hence the cardiac output. The esophageal Doppler measures the velocity of blood in the descending aorta in centimeters per second (cm/s). In order to convert this figure into blood flow in milliliters per second (mL/s), the diameter of the aorta needs to be known. This is derived from published nomograms based on age, sex, weight, and height (Deltex, West Sussex, England) or through direct ultrasound measurement (Arrow's HemoSonic® Reading, PA, USA). The ED also has the ability to measure the corrected flow time (FT_c) as a measure of cardiac preload. The FT_c is the duration of flow during systole corrected for a heart rate of 60 beats per minute. It is unclear as to whether the FTc or SV should be used to guide fluid therapy, but it appears that the ability to respond to a fluid challenge is best determined by FTc. Several studies have compared FT_c with other indices such as pulmonary artery occlusion pressure and have found good agreement between the two [30-32].

There are some limitations to the usage of ED. First, the ED only measures descending aortic blood flow, which may not always be constant due aortic pathology or compression or due to abnormal upper to lower body blood flow distribution. Also, the aortic cross-sectional area is not constant, due to changes in pulse pressure, vascular tone, aortic compliance, volume status, or catecholamine use. Due to the fact that the radius of the aorta is squared in the final CO equation, even small changes in aortic area can significantly affect CO determinations [33]. Moreover, the probe position is critical to obtain accurate measurement for both blood flow measurement and aortic cross-sectional measurement. The Doppler beam must be within 20° of axial flow to obtain a good measure of aortic blood flow. Even small misalignments of the ultrasound beam with blood flow will lead to underestimation of flow when using the Doppler equation [34,35]. Finally, the equation assumes that the flow is laminar and any turbulent flow in the aorta will reduce measurement accuracy.

There have been studies that have compared ED measurements of CO with PAC-derived thermodilution CO.

Dark and Singer performed a literature review regarding the validity of ED monitoring as a measure of CO in critically ill adults, concluding that the ED monitor has high validity in tracking changes in CO [36]. In addition, other studies have shown that using ED to guide fluid administration improved patients' management. Sinclair et al. conducted a randomized controlled trial of patients undergoing femoral fracture repair. Patients were randomized to either routine care or ED-guided fluid loading. The patients in the ED group had a shorter hospital stay [37]. A similar trial conducted by Venn et al. showed that the ED-monitored patients had less intraoperative hypotension and were considered fit for discharge earlier [38]. Noblett et al. [39] performed a double-blind randomized control trial of Doppler-guided fluid therapy *versus* anesthetist-directed fluid therapy in 108 patients undergoing elective colorectal resection. They found that despite both groups of patients receiving the same volume of intraoperative fluids, the group managed with the ED had a shorter hospital stay and lower morbidity rates than the control group. Interestingly, patients in the intervention group also had lower levels of interleukin-6, which suggested an attenuated inflammatory response to surgery, perhaps due to the improved organ perfusion. In a study by Wakeling et al. patients recovered gut function significantly faster and suffered significantly less gastrointestinal and overall morbidity [40]. These overwhelming data in support of the ED led the National Institute for Health and Clinical Excellence (NICE) to release guidelines in 2011 advocating the use of this technology [41].

A completely non-invasive Doppler technology, the USCOM (Ultrasound CO monitor, USCOM, Sydney, Australia), is also available which uses Doppler technology to measure CO from a suprasternal Doppler probe. This technology has been studied in a few patient population groups (mostly stable ICU patients) and has shown reasonable correlation with PAC [42,43].

Thoracic electrical bioimpedance
Variations in the electrical impedance of the thorax to an alternating current which occur synchronously with the cardiac cycle were observed nearly 40 years ago. The first use of this phenomenon to measure SV and CO was described by Nyboer [44], and Kubicek and colleagues [45] introduced the technique into clinical practice in 1966.

Electrical bioimpedance involves the analysis of intrabeat variations in transthoracic voltage in response to the applied high frequency transthoracic current. Two commercial devices based on electrical bioimpedance use electrodes attached to an endotracheal tube (ECOM, Conmed Corp, Utica, NY, USA) or the skin (BioZ, Cardio-Dynamics, San Diego, CA, USA). Pulsatile changes in

thoracic blood volume result in changes in electrical impedance. The rate of change of impedance during systole is measured and an estimate of the SV and the CO is derived from a mathematical equation.

Sources of potential inaccuracies include motion artifacts, electrical interference, cardiac arrhythmias, heart and lung pathologies (as chest deformities, pulmonary edema, pleural and pericardial effusions, intracardiac shunts), and foreign bodies (as chest tubes). Clinical trials of TEB have been shown to be reliable in young healthy volunteers, but in septic or surgical patients, the results have been inconsistent [46-48].

Bioreactance
Recently, bioreactance (NICOM, Cheetah Medical Ltd, Maidenhead, Berkshire, UK), a modification of thoracic bioimpedance, has been introduced. Bioreactance refers to the electrical resistance, capacitive and inductive properties of blood and biological tissue that induce phase shifts between an applied electrical current and the resulting voltage signal. In contrast to bioimpedance, the bioreactance technique analyzes the frequency spectra variations of the delivered oscillating current. When blood flows out of the heart, phase shifts occur if alternating currents are applied across the patient's chest. Such phase shifts are conceptually similar to a frequency modulation as used in radio transmission. The phase shifts are measured continuously and have been shown to relate almost linearly to blood flow in the aorta. This results in less interfering from the electrical noise, patient movement, respiratory effort, lead placement, and body mass index.

In addition to cardiac output, mean bioreactance measurements are indicative of the total thoracic fluid content (TFC). TFC is affected by both intravascular and extravascular fluid in the chest cavity and although it does not correlate with pulmonary artery wedge pressure (PAWP), its changes are very reliable indicators of the changes in intravascular or extravascular fluid volume [49]. In a study of patients undergoing cardiac surgery, the bioreactance did well initially in determining CO when compared with PAC, however, during the immediate postoperative period, the correlation was not as robust [50].

It appears that the new generation of devices might be better than the first generation TEB machines, although there are still limitations regarding their accuracy in measuring CO during dynamic conditions.

Gas rebreathing
The partial carbon dioxide (CO_2) rebreathing technique uses the Fick principle applied to the CO_2 in order to estimate CO non-invasively. The NICO monitor (Novametrix Medical Systems, Inc., Wallingford, CT, USA) imple-

ments intermittent partial rebreathing through a specific disposable rebreathing loop. The monitor consists of a CO_2 sensor, a disposable airflow sensor and a pulse oximeter. CO_2 production (VCO_2) is calculated from minute ventilation and its CO_2 content, whereas the arterial CO_2 content ($CacO_2$) is estimated from end-tidal CO_2, with adjustments for the slope of the CO_2 dissociation curve and the degree of dead space ventilation. The partial rebreathing reduces CO_2 elimination and increases end-tidal CO_2. Measurements under normal and rebreathing conditions allow one to omit the venous CO_2 content ($CvCO_2$) measurement in the Fick equation, because $CvCO_2$ does not change during this brief period of rebreathing [51].

$$CO=VCO_2/(CvCO_2\text{-}CaCO_2)$$

While the technique is easy to use, the correlation between the NICO and standard thermodilution has been shown to be adversely affected in spontaneously breathing patients, which limits the number of suitable candidates [52,53]. Partial rebreathing has been shown to be more accurate in less critically ill patients with normal alveolar gas exchange when compared with PAC thermodilution [54,55]. Severe chest trauma, significant intrapulmonary shuntdead-space ventilation, low minute ventilation, and high CO may all reduce accuracy [56]. There have been no reports on the device when used in hemodynamically unstable patients [57]. Moreover, the partial-rebreathing technique only measures the CO and does not provide information on the intravascular volume status or fluid responsiveness. For these reasons, partial gas rebreathing is limited in its clinical applicability.

Transesophageal echocardiography

Widely used in the cardiac operative and postoperative setting to demonstrate cardiac anatomy and identify pathology, the transesophageal echocardiography (TOE) has been impractical in assisting with continuous CO measurements outside the operative theater because of the size of the probe and the limitations that come with it. However, the recent development of a miniaturized 5 mm TOE probe (ClariTEE Probe, ImaCor Inc., Garden City, NY, USA) that can stay indwelled for up to 72 hours, has enabled hemodynamic management of the critically ill patients [58]. Although not a CO monitoring *per se*, the ClariTEE uses a monoplane transducer that enables the operator to acquire basic views of the heart (ascending aortic short-axis, four-chamber, and transgastric short-axis) that, combined with a software tool, offer continuous calculations of the ventricular size and systolic performance. Moreover, echocardiography

derived measurements of the stroke volume can help in the assessment of fluid responsiveness [59]. Validation studies are pending.

Predicting fluid responsiveness

The assessment of intravascular volume status of an individual has been traditionally performed with static parameters, mainly filling pressures such as CVP and PAWP, which reflect the preload of the right and the left ventricles, respectively. It is now acknowledged that these values correlate poorly with the intravascular volume and the response to a fluid bolus [60], hence there has been a shift to more dynamic indices such as the stroke volume variation (SVV) and the pulse pressure variation (PPV).

All the devices that use the pulse pressure analysis method for CO monitoring, also calculate those two parameters. Based on the effect of the cyclic variation of intrathoracic pressures with respiration on the preload of the left ventricle and using appropriate algorithms, the beat to beat variation of the SV and the pulse pressure (PP) is calculated. Specifically, positive pressure ventilation induces cyclic changes in vena cava blood flow, pulmonary artery flow, and aortic blood flow.

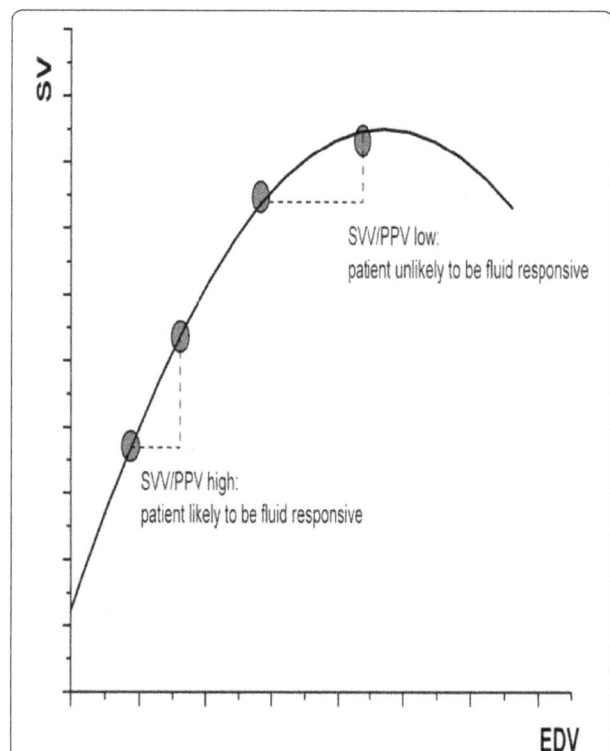

Figure 3 Correlation of fluid responsiveness with SVV/PPV variables. As a general rule, the higher the SVV/PPV values, the more fluid responsive the patient will be. The correlation can only be applied to mechanically ventilated patients.

During inspiration, vena cava blood flow decreases (venous return decreases) and, according to the Frank-Starling relationship, pulmonary artery flow decreases. Approximately three beats later this decrease in pulmonary artery flow is transmitted to the left ventricle inducing a decrease in SV and aortic PP. As a general rule, values of SVV >10% and PPV >13% are indicative of patients that will probably respond to the administration of fluids, while lower values indicate the opposite. The basic limitation is that the above calculations can only be applied to mechanically ventilated patients, as the correlation in spontaneously breathing individuals is weaker. Moreover, for optimal results the tidal volume (TV) should be >8 mL/Kg of body weight, the patient should be in sinus rhythm, and the chest must be closed [61] (Figure 3).

More recently, a new index called the Pleth Variability Index (PVI) may help with the prediction of fluid responsiveness. The PVI is continuously calculated by the new non-invasive Masimo monitor (Masimo Corporation, Irvine, CA, USA), a device that resembles the traditional pulse oximeter. The monitor measures first the change during a respiratory cycle of the Perfusion Index (PI), which is the ratio of non-pulsatile to pulsatile blood flow through the peripheral capillary bed, and then calculates the PVI from the following formula:

$$PVI=[(PImax-PImin)/PImax]x100$$

The greater the PVI value is, the more likely the patient will respond to fluid administration [62]. As is the case with SVV and PVV, one should always bear in mind the same limitations before taking clinical decisions regarding the hemodynamic optimization of patients (Table 1).

Goal-directed therapy

All the above methods of quantifying the CO have the potential to reduce the morbidity and mortality of the patients if they are integrated into appropriate protocols that guide the therapeutic interventions. The use of CO measurements to guide fluid administration and inotropic therapy, optimizing this way the tissue perfusion and cellular oxygenation has been given the broad term goal-directed therapy (GDT). Its beneficial effects demonstrated as early as the late 1970s by the seminal work of Shoemaker and his team [63,64], it is now accepted

Table 1 Overview and classification of minimally invasive CO monitors

Modality	Available devices	Requirements	Additional values
Pulse pressure analysis			
-Uncalibrated devices	Flo/Trac-Vigileo	Standard arterial line	GEDV, EVLW
	Pulsioflex	Standard arterial line	
	LidCO rapid	Standard arterial line	
-Calibrated devices	LidCO plus	Standard arterial line	
	PiCCOplus	Standard arterial line	
		Central venous line	
	Volumeview	Standard arterial line	
		Central venous line	GEDV, EVLW, GEF
Doppler			
-Transesophageal	CardioQ/CardioQ-OCM	Transesophageal probe	FTc
-Transthoracic	USCOM	Transthoracic probe	
Echocardiography	ClariTEE	Miniaturized transesophageal probe	
Gas rebreathing	NICO	Disposable rebreathing circuit	
Bioimpedance/ Bioreactance			
-Thoracic electrical bioimpedance			
- Bioreactance	BioZ	Specific electrodes	
	NICOM	Specific electrodes	
Non-invasive monitors			
	Nexfin	Finger probe	Hb
	Masimo	Specific pulse oximeter	PVI
	esCCO	ECG/ specific pulse oximeter	PWTT

that GDT reduces complications and improves outcome rates in both surgical [2,65,66] and non-surgical populations [67]. With increasing availability of a variety of minimally invasive CO monitors, one should expect the GDT to be widely implemented for the hemodynamic optimization of various patients' groups, especially when questions regarding the cost-effectiveness of the method are adequately addressed.

Conclusions

A whole array of minimally invasive devices and monitors that can reliably calculate trends in the CO without the need for a PAC are now available to the clinicians. Needing only peripheral or central arterial catheters or only a finger probe, as is the case in the Nexfin and Masimo monitors, they can give reliable measurements of CO and of dynamic indices such as the SVV and the PPV, provided that their limitations are taken into account.

Additional tools in the area of minimal invasiveness are the OD, with its use strongly advocated by recent NICE guidelines, and the less widely used gas rebreathing and thoracic bioimpedance methods. Last, the introduction of a miniaturized TOE probe may revolutionize the management of ITU patients, providing real-time information on cardiac anatomy and function.

The integration of these devices into therapeutic protocols enables the clinician to apply GDT and guide the inotropic support and fluid administration in a rational way, reducing this way the mortality and morbidity of the patients.

Abbreviations

AAA: Abdominal aortic aneurysm; BP: Blood pressure; CABG: Coronary artery bypass grafting; CI: Cardiac Index; CO: Cardiac output; CVC: Central venous catheter; CVP: Central venous pressure; DO2: Oxygen delivery; DO2I: Oxygen delivery index; ED: Esophageal Doppler; EPCI: Ejection phase contractility index; EVLW: Extravascular lung water; FT_C: Corrected flow time; GDT: Goal-directed therapy; GEDV: Global end-diastolic volume; GEF: Global ejection fraction; HR: Heart rate; IABP: Intra-aortic Balloon Pump; ITBV: Intrathoracic blood volume; ITU: Intensive Therapy Unit; NICE: National Institute for Health and Clinical Ecxellence; OR: Operating room; PAC: Pulmonary artery catheter; PP: Pulse pressure; PAWP: Pulmonary artery wedge pressure; PWTT: Pulse wave transition time; PI: Perfusion index; PPV: Pulse pressure variation; PVI: Pleth Variability Index; PVPI: Pulmonary vascular permeability index; SV: Stroke volume; SVC: Superior vena cava; TEB: Thoracic electrical bioimpedance; TOE: Transesophageal echocardiography; TV: Tidal volume; VEPT: Volume of electrically participating tissues; VET: Ventricular ejection time.

Competing interests

CC and LV declare no competing interests. MH has received lecture fees and expenses from Deltex Medical, Edwards Lifescienses, LidCO. MC has received honoraria, travel expenses, or unrestricted educational grants from LiDCO, Edwards Lifesciences, Deltex, Cheetah, Masimo, and Bmeye; he is part of the medical advisory board of Applied Physiology.

Authors' contributions

CC has drafted the manuscript apart from the sections for the esophageal Doppler, the thoracic electrical bioimpedance, the bioreactance, and the gas rebreathing. LV has written the sections for the esophageal Doppler, the thoracic electrical bioimpedance, the bioreactance, and the gas rebreathing. MH has critically reviewed the manuscript. MC has conceived and critically

reviewed the manuscript. All authors have read and approved the final version of the manuscript.

Author details
[1]Senior clinical fellow in cardiac anaesthesia, St George's Healthcare NHS Trust, London, UK. [2]Specialist registrar in anaesthesia, Croydon Health Services NHS Trust, London, UK. [3]Consultant and honorary senior lecturer in anaesthesia and intensive care medicine, St George's Healthcare NHS Trust, London, UK.

References

1. Cecconi M, Rhodes A: Within five years cardiac output monitoring will be included in the minimum monitoring standards for major surgery. *Bulletin of the Royal College of Anaesthetists* 2012, **76**:31–33.
2. Hamilton MA, Cecconi M, Rhodes A: A systematic review and meta-analysis on the use of preemptive hemodynamic intervention to improve postoperative outcomes in moderate and high-risk surgical patients. *Anesth Analg* 2011, **112**:1392–1402.
3. Erlanger J, Hooker DR: An experimental study of blood pressure and of pulse-pressure in man. *Johns Hopkins Hosp Rep* 1904, **12**:145–378.
4. van Lieshout JJ, Wesseling KH: Editorial II: Continuous cardiac output by pulse contour analysis? *Br J Anaesth* 2001, **86**:467–468.
5. Wesseling KH, de Wit B, Weber JAP, Ty SN: A simple device for the continuous measurement of cardiac output. *Adv Cardiovasc Phys* 1983, **5**:16–52.
6. Breukers SM, Sepehrkhouy S, Spiegelenberg SR, Groeneveld AB: Cardiac output measured by a new arterial pressure waveform analysis method without calibration compared with thermodilution after cardiac surgery. *J Cardiothorac Vasc Anesth* 2007, **21**:632–635.
7. Bataille B, Bertuit M, Mora M, Mazerolles M, Cocquet P, Masson B, Moussot PE, Ginot J, Silva S, Larché J: Comparison of esCCO and transthoracic echocardiography for non-invasive measurement of cardiac output intensive care. *Br J Anaesth* 2012, **109**:879–886.
8. Mayer J, Boldt J, Poland R, Peterson A, Manecke GR Jr: Continuous arterial pressure waveform-based cardiac output using the FloTrac/Vigileo: a review and meta-analysis. *J Cardiothorac Vasc Anesth* 2009, **23**:401–406.
9. Khwannimit B, Bhurayanontachai R: Prediction of fluid responsiveness in septic shock patients: comparing stroke volume variation by FloTrac/Vigileo and automated pulse pressure variation. *Eur J Anaesthesiol* 2012, **29**:64–69.
10. Monnet X, Anguel N, Jozwiak M, Richard C, Teboul JL: Third-generation FloTrac/Vigileo does not reliably track changes in cardiac output induced by norepinephrine in critically ill patients. *Br J Anaesth* 2012, **108**:615–622.
11. Jeong YB, Kim TH, Roh YJ, Choi IC, Suh JH: Comparison of uncalibrated arterial pressure waveform analysis with continuous thermodilution cardiac output measurements in patients undergoing elective off-pump coronary artery bypass surgery. *J Cardiothorac Vasc Anesth* 2010, **24**:767–771.
12. Kusaka Y, Yoshitani K, Irie T, Inatomi Y, Shinzawa M, Ohnishi Y: Clinical comparison of an echocardiograph-derived versus pulse counter-derived cardiac output measurement in abdominal aortic aneurysm surgery. *J Cardiothorac Vasc Anesth* 2012, **26**:223–226.
13. Fischer MO, Avram R, Cârjaliu I, Massetti M, Gérard JL, Hanouz JL, Fellahi JL: Non-invasive continuous arterial pressure and cardiac index monitoring with Nexfin after cardiac surgery. *Br J Anaesth* 2012, **109**:514–521.
14. Broch O, Renner J, Gruenewald M, Meybohm P, Schöttler J, Caliebe A, Steinfath M, Malbrain M, Bein B: A comparison of the Nexfin® and transcardiopulmonary thermodilution to estimate cardiac output during coronary artery surgery. *Anaesthesia* 2012, **67**:377–383.
15. van der Spoel A, Voogel AJ, Folkers A, Boer C, Bouwman RA: Comparison of noninvasive continuous arterial waveform analysis (Nexfin) with transthoracic Doppler echocardiography for monitoring of cardiac output. *J Clin Anesth* 2012, **24**:304–309.
16. Chen G, Meng L, Alexander B, Tran NP, Kain ZN, Cannesson M: Comparison of noninvasive cardiac output measurements using the Nexfin monitoring device and the esophageal Doppler. *J Clin Anesth* 2012, **24**:275–283.

17. Michard F, Alaya S, Zarka V, Bahloul M, Richard C, Teboul JL: Global end-diastolic volume as an indicator of cardiac preload in patients with septic shock. *Chest* 2003, 124:1900–1908.

18. Kushimoto S, Taira Y, Kitazawa Y, Okuchi K, Sakamoto T, Ishikura H, Endo T, Yamanouchi S, Tagami T, Yamaguchi J, Yoshikawa K, Sugita M, Kase Y, Kanemura T, Takahashi H, Kuroki Y, Izumino H, Rinka H, Seo R, Takatori M, Kaneko T, Nakamura T, Irahara T, Saito N, Watanabe A, The PiCCO Pulmonary Edema Study Group: The clinical usefulness of extravascular lung water and pulmonary vascular permeability index to diagnose and characterize pulmonary oedema: a prospective multicenter study on the quantitative differential diagnostic definition for acute lung injury/ acute respiratory distress syndrome. *Crit Care* 2012, 16:R232.

19. Reuter DA, Huang C, Edrich T, Shernan SK, Eltzschig HK: Cardiac output monitoring using indicator-dilution techniques: basics, limits, and perspectives. *Anesth Analg* 2010, 110:799–811.

20. Lemson J, de Boode WP, Hopman JC, Singh SK, van der Hoeven JG: Validation of transpulmonary thermodilution cardiac output measurement in a pediatric animal model. *Pediatr Crit Care Med* 2008, 9:313–319.

21. Nusmeier A, de Boode WP, Hopman JC, Schoof PH, van der Hoeven JG, Lemson J: Cardiac output can be measured with the transpulmonary thermodilution method in a paediatric animal model with a left-to-right shunt. *Br J Anaesth* 2011, 107:336–343.

22. Wouters PF, Quaghebeur B, Sergeant P, Van Hemelrijck J, Vandermeersch E: Cardiac output monitoring using a brachial arterial catheter during off-pump coronary artery bypass grafting. *J Cardiothorac Vasc Anesth* 2005, 19:160–164.

23. Kiefer N, Hofer CK, Marx G, Geisen M, Giraud R, Siegenthaler N, Hoeft A, Bendjelid K, Rex S: Clinical validation of a new thermodilution system for the assessment of cardiac output and volumetric parameters. *Crit Care* 2012, 16:R98.

24. Drummond KE, Murphy E: Minimally invasive cardiac output monitors. *Contin Educ Anaesth Crit Care Pain* 2012, 12:5–10.

25. Rhodes A, Sunderland R: Arterial pulse pressure analysis: the LiDCOplus system. In *Functional Hemodynamic Monitoring Update in Intensive Care and Emergency Medicine*. Edited by Pinsky MR, Payen D. Berlin: Springer; 2005:183–192.

26. Mora B, Ince I, Birkenberg B, Skhirtladze K, Pernicka E, Ankersmit HJ, Dworschak M: Validation of cardiac output measurement with the LiDCO™ pulse contour system in patients with impaired left ventricular function after cardiac surgery. *Anaesthesia* 2011, 66:675–681.

27. Costa MG, Della Rocca G, Chiarandini P, Mattelig S, Pompei L, Barriga MS, Reynolds T, Cecconi M, Pietropaoli P: Continuous and intermittent cardiac output measurement in hyperdynamic conditions: pulmonary artery catheter vs. lithium dilution technique. *Int Care Med* 1008, 34:257–263.

28. Broch O, Renner J, Höcker J, Gruenewald M, Meybohm P, Schöttler J, Steinfath M, Bein B: Uncalibrated pulse power analysis fails to reliably measure cardiac output in patients undergoing coronary artery bypass surgery. *Crit Care* 2011, 15:R76.

29. Beattie C, Moores C, Thomson AJ, Nimmo AF: The effect of anaesthesia and aortic clamping on cardiac output measurement using arterial pulse power analysis during aortic aneurysm repair. *Anaesthesia* 2010, 65:1194–1199.

30. DiCorte CJ, Latham P, Greilich PE, Cooley MV, Grayburn PA, Jessen ME: Esophageal Doppler monitor determinations of cardiac output and preload during cardiac operations. *Ann Thorac Surg* 2000, 69:1782–1786.

31. Madan AK, UyBarreta VV, Aliabadi-Wahle S, Jesperson R, Hartz RS, Flint LM, Steinberg SM: Esophageal Doppler ultrasound monitor versus pulmonary artery catheter in the hemodynamic management of critically ill surgical patients. *J Trauma* 1999, 46:607–611. discussion 11–12.

32. Mythen MG, Webb AR: Perioperative plasma volume expansion reduces the incidence of gut mucosal hypoperfusion during cardiac surgery. *Arch Surg* 1995, 130:423–429.

33. Cariou A, Monchi M, Joly LM, Bellenfant F, Claessens YE, Thebert D, Brunet F, Dhainaut JF: Noninvasive cardiac output monitoring by aortic blood flow determination: evaluation of the Sometec Dynemo-3000 system. *Crit Care Med* 1998, 26:2066–2072.

34. Freund PR: Transesophageal Doppler scanning versus thermodilution during general anesthesia. An initial comparison of cardiac output techniques. *Am J Surg* 1987, 153:490–494.

35. Lefrant JY, Bruelle P, Aya AG, Saissi G, Dauzat M, de La Coussaye JE, Eledjam JJ: Training is required to improve the reliability of esophageal Doppler to

36. measure cardiac output in critically ill patients. *Intensive Care Med* 1998, 24:347–352.

36. Dark PM, Singer M: The validity of trans-esophageal Doppler ultrasonography as a measure of cardiac output in critically ill adults. *Intensive Care Med* 2004, 30:2060–2066.

37. Sinclair S, James S, Singer M: Intraoperative intravascular volume optimisation and length of hospital stay after repair of proximal femoral fracture: randomised controlled trial. *BMJ* 1997, 315:909–912.

38. Venn R, Steele A, Richardson P, Poloniecki J, Grounds M, Newman P: Randomized controlled trial to investigate influence of the fluid challenge on duration of hospital stay and perioperative morbidity in patients with hip fractures. *Br J Anaesth* 2002, 88:65–71.

39. Noblett SE, Snowden CP, Shenton BK, Horgan AF: Randomized clinical trial assessing the effect of Doppler-optimized fluid management on outcome after elective colorectal resection. *Br J Surg* 2006, 93:1069–1076.

40. Wakeling HG, McFall MR, Jenkins CS, Woods WG, Miles WF, Barclay GR, Fleming SC: Intraoperative oesophageal Doppler guided fluid management shortens postoperative hospital stay after major bowel surgery. *Br J Anaesth* 2005, 95:634–642.

41. Ghosh S, Arthur B, Klein AA: NICE guidance on CardioQ(TM) oesophageal Doppler monitoring. *Anaesthesia* 2011, 66:1081–1083.

42. Tan HL, Pinder M, Parsons R, Roberts B, van Heerden PV: Clinical evaluation of USCOM ultrasonic cardiac output monitor in cardiac surgical patients in intensive care unit. *Br J Anaesth* 2005, 94:287–291.

43. Chand R, Mehta Y, Trehan N: Cardiac output estimation with a new Doppler device after off-pump coronary artery bypass surgery. *J Cardiothorac Vasc Anesth* 2006, 20:315–319.

44. Nyboer J: Plethysmography. Impedance. In *Medical Physics, Volume 2*. Edited by Glasser O. Chicago, IL: Year Book Pub; 1950:736–743.

45. Kubicek WG, Karegis JN, Patterson RP, Witsoe DA, Matteson RH: Development and evaluation of an impedance cardiac output system. *Aerosp Med* 1966, 37:1208–1212.

46. Barin E, Haryadi DG, Schookin SI, Westenskow DR, Zubenko VG, Beliaev KR, Morozov AA: Evaluation of a thoracic bioimpedance cardiac output monitor during cardiac catheterization. *Crit Care Med* 2000, 28:698–702.

47. Imhoff M, Lehner JH, Lohlein D: Noninvasive whole-body electrical bioimpedance cardiac output and invasive thermodilution cardiac output in high-risk surgical patients. *Crit Care Med* 2000, 28:2812–2818.

48. Raaijmakers E, Faes TJ, Scholten RJ, Goovaerts HG, Heethaar RM: A meta-analysis of three decades of validating thoracic impedance cardiography. *Crit Care Med* 1999, 27:1203–1213.

49. Raval NY, Squara P, Cleman M, Yalamanchili K, Winklmaier M, Burkhoff D: Multicenter evaluation of noninvasive cardiac output measurement by bioreactance technique. *J Clin Monit Comput* 2008, 22:113–119.

50. Guzzi L, Jaffe MB, Orr JA: Clinical evaluation of a new non-invasive method of cardiac output measurement – preliminary results in CABG patients. *Anesthesiology* 1998, 89:A543.

51. Berton C, Cholley B: Equipment review: New techniques for cardiac output measurement – oesophageal Doppler, Fick principle using carbon dioxide, and pulse contour analysis. *Crit Care Med* 2002, 6:216–221.

52. Odenstedt H, Stenqvist O, Lundin S: Clinical evaluation of a partial CO2 rebreathing technique for cardiac output monitoring in critically ill patients. *Acta Anaesthesiol Scand* 2002, 46:152–159.

53. Rocco M, Spadetta G, Morelli A, Dell'Utri D, Porzi P, Conti G, Pietropaoli P: A comparative evaluation of thermodilution and partial CO2 rebreathing techniques for cardiac output assessment in critically ill patients during assisted ventilation. *Intensive Care Med* 2004, 30:82–87.

54. Kotake Y, Moriyama K, Innami Y, Shimizu H, Ueda T, Morisaki H, Takeda J: Performance of noninvasive partial CO2 rebreathing cardiac output and continuous thermodilution cardiac output in patients undergoing aortic reconstruction surgery. *Anesthesiology* 2003, 99:283–288.

55. Rocco M, Spadetta G, Morelli A, Dell'Utri D, Porzi P, Conti G, Pietropaoli P: A comparative evaluation of thermodilution and partial CO_2 rebreathing techniques for cardiac output assessment in critically ill patients during assisted ventilation. *Intensive Care Med* 2004, 30:82–87.

56. Tachibana K, Imanaka H, Takeuchi M, Takauchi Y, Miyano H, Nishimura M: Noninvasive cardiac output measurement using partial carbon dioxide - rebreathing is less accurate at settings of reduced minute ventilation and when spontaneous breathing is present. *Anesthesiology* 2003, 98:830–837.

57. Nilsson LB, Eldrup N, Berthelsen PG: **Lack of agreement between thermodilution and carbon dioxide-rebreathing cardiac output.** *Acta Anaesthesiol Scand* 2001, **45**:680–685.

58. Wagner CE, Bick JS, Webster BH, Selby JH, Byrne JG: **Use of a miniaturized transesophageal echocardiographic probe in the intensive care unit for diagnosis and treatment of a hemodynamically unstable patient after aortic valve replacement.** *J Cardiothorac Vasc Anesth* 2012, **26**:95–97.

59. Charron C, Caille V, Jardin F, Vieillard-Baron A: **Echocardiography measurement of fluid responsiveness.** *Curr Opin Crit Care* 2006, **12**:249–254.

60. Kumar A, Anel R, Bunnell E, Habet K, Zanotti S, Marshall S, Neumann A, Ali A, Cheang M, Kavinsky C, Parrillo JE: **Pulmonary artery occlusion pressure and central venous pressure fail to predict ventricular filling volume, cardiac performance, or the response to volume infusion in normal subjects.** *Crit Care Med* 2004, **32**:691–699.

61. Cannesson M, Aboy M, Hofer CK, Rehman M: **Pulse pressure variation: Where are we today?** *J Clin Monit Comput* 2010, **25**:45–56.

62. Cannesson M, Desebbe O, Rosamel P, Delannoy B, Robin J, Bastien O, Lehot JJ: **Pleth variability index to monitor the respiratory variations in the pulse oximeter plethysmographic waveform amplitude and predict fluid responsiveness in the operating theatre.** *Br J Anaesth* 2008, **101**:200–206.

63. Shoemaker WC, Czer LSC: **Evaluation of the biologic importance of various hemodynamic and oxygen transport variables.** *Crit Care Med* 1979, **7**:424–429.

64. Shoemaker WC, Appel PL, Kram HB, Waxman K, Lee TS: **Prospective trial of supranormal values of survivors as therapeutic goals in high-risk surgical patients.** *Chest* 1988, **94**:1176–1186.

65. Pearse R, Dawson D, Fawcett J, Rhodes A, Grounds RM, Bennett ED: **Early goal-directed therapy after major surgery reduces complications and duration of hospital stay. A randomised, controlled trial [ISRCTN38797445].** *Crit Care* 2005, **9**:R687–R693.

66. Aya HD, Cecconi M, Hamilton M, Rhodes A: **Goal-directed therapy in cardiac surgery: a systematic review and meta-analysis.** *Br J Anaesth* 2013, **110**:510–517.

67. Rivers E, Nguyen B, Havstad S, Ressler J, Muzzin A, Knoblich B, Peterson E, Tomlanovich M, Early Goal-Directed Therapy Collaborative Group: **Early goal-directed therapy in the treatment of severe sepsis and septic shock.** *N Engl J Med* 2001, **345**:1368–1377.

Permissions

All chapters in this book were first published in PM, by BioMed Central; hereby published with permission under the Creative Commons Attribution License or equivalent. Every chapter published in this book has been scrutinized by our experts. Their significance has been extensively debated. The topics covered herein carry significant findings which will fuel the growth of the discipline. They may even be implemented as practical applications or may be referred to as a beginning point for another development.

The contributors of this book come from diverse backgrounds, making this book a truly international effort. This book will bring forth new frontiers with its revolutionizing research information and detailed analysis of the nascent developments around the world.

We would like to thank all the contributing authors for lending their expertise to make the book truly unique. They have played a crucial role in the development of this book. Without their invaluable contributions this book wouldn't have been possible. They have made vital efforts to compile up to date information on the varied aspects of this subject to make this book a valuable addition to the collection of many professionals and students.

This book was conceptualized with the vision of imparting up-to-date information and advanced data in this field. To ensure the same, a matchless editorial board was set up. Every individual on the board went through rigorous rounds of assessment to prove their worth. After which they invested a large part of their time researching and compiling the most relevant data for our readers.

The editorial board has been involved in producing this book since its inception. They have spent rigorous hours researching and exploring the diverse topics which have resulted in the successful publishing of this book. They have passed on their knowledge of decades through this book. To expedite this challenging task, the publisher supported the team at every step. A small team of assistant editors was also appointed to further simplify the editing procedure and attain best results for the readers.

Apart from the editorial board, the designing team has also invested a significant amount of their time in understanding the subject and creating the most relevant covers. They scrutinized every image to scout for the most suitable representation of the subject and create an appropriate cover for the book.

The publishing team has been an ardent support to the editorial, designing and production team. Their endless efforts to recruit the best for this project, has resulted in the accomplishment of this book. They are a veteran in the field of academics and their pool of knowledge is as vast as their experience in printing. Their expertise and guidance has proved useful at every step. Their uncompromising quality standards have made this book an exceptional effort. Their encouragement from time to time has been an inspiration for everyone.

The publisher and the editorial board hope that this book will prove to be a valuable piece of knowledge for researchers, students, practitioners and scholars across the globe.

List of Contributors

Rebecca M Speck, Mark D Neuman and Lee A Fleisher
Department of Anesthesiology and Critical Care, University of Pennsylvania, 3400 Spruce Street, Philadelphia, PA 19104, USA

Rebecca M Speck
Department of Biostatistics and Epidemiology, University of Pennsylvania, 423 Guardian Drive, Blockley Hall, Philadelphia, PA 19104-6021, USA

Andrew R Bond
Department of Anesthesia, Brigham and Women's Hospital, 75 Francis StreetBoston, MA 02115, USA

John Whittemore Stokes
Vanderbilt University School of Medicine, 2215 Garland Avenue (Light Hall), Nashville, TN 37232, USA

Jonathan Porter Wanderer and Matthew David McEvoy
Multispecialty Adult Anesthesiology, Vanderbilt University Medical Center, 1301 Medical Center Drive, 4648 The Vanderbilt Clinic, Nashville, TN 37232-5614, USA

Onyi C. Onuoha and Michael B. Hatch
Department of Anesthesiology and Critical Care, Perelman School of Medicine at the University of Pennsylvania, 3400 Spruce Street Dulles 680, Philadelphia, PA 19104, USA

Todd A. Miano
Center for Clinical Epidemiology and Biostatistics, Perelman School of Medicine, University of Pennsylvania, Philadelphia, Pennsylvania, USA

Lee A. Fleisher
Department of Anesthesiology and Critical Care, Perelman School of Medicine, Senior Scholar, Leonard Davis Institute, University of Pennsylvania, Philadelphia, Pennsylvania, USA

Benjamin Harris
Academic Department of Critical Care, Queen Alexandra Hospital, Southwick Hill Road, Cosham, Portsmouth PO6 3LY, UK

Christian Schopflin
Anaesthetic Department, Queen Alexandra Hospital, Southwick Hill Road, Cosham, Portsmouth PO6 3LY, UK

Clare Khaghani
Anaesthetic Department, Royal Hampshire County Hospital, Romsey Road, Winchester, Hampshire SO22 5DG, UK

Mark Edwards
Anaesthetic Department Mail Point 24, University Hospital Southampton NHS Foundation Trust, Tremona Road, Southampton SO16 6YD, UK

Timothy E. Miller and Charles S. Brudney
Department of Anesthesiology, Duke University Medical Center, Durham, NC 27710, USA

Martin Bunke
Department of Medical Affairs, Grifols, 79 TW Alexander Dr. Bldg. 4101, Research Triangle Park, NC 27709, USA

Paul Nisbet
One Research, LLC, 1150 Hungry Neck Blvd., Suite C-303, Charleston, SC 29464, USA

Alex Wickham
Department of Anaesthetics, Imperial College Healthcare NHS Trust, London, UK

David Highton
Neurocritical Care, the National Hospital for Neurology and Neurosurgery, University College London Hospitals, Queen Square, London, UK

Daniel Martin
Division of Surgery and Interventional Science, Royal Free Hospital, University College London, Pond Street, London NW3 2QG, UK
Royal Free Perioperative Research, Department of Anaesthesia, Royal Free Hospital, Pond Street, London NW3 2QG, UK

Kamlesh Patel, Fatemeh Hadian, Aysha Ali, Graham Broadley, Kate Evans, Claire Horder, Marianne Johnstone, Fiona Langlands, Jake Matthews, Prithish Narayan, Priya Rallon, Charlotte Roberts, Sonali Shah and Ravinder Vohra
West Midlands Research Collaborative, Academic Department of Surgery, School of Cancer Sciences, University of Birmingham, Birmingham B15 2TH, UK

Ravinder Vohra
Nottingham Oesophago-Gastric Unit, Nottingham University Hospitals, Nottingham, UK

Lisa Loughney, Malcolm A. West, Graham J. Kemp, Michael PW. Grocott and Sandy Jack
Anaesthesia and Critical Care Research Area, NIHR Respiratory Biomedical Research Unit, University Hospital Southampton NHS Foundation Trust, CE93, MP24, Tremona Road, Southampton SO16 6YD, UK

Lisa Loughney
MedEx Research Cluster, School of Health and Human Performance, Dublin City University, Dublin, Ireland

Malcolm A. West
Academic Unit of Cancer Sciences, Faculty of Medicine, University of Southampton, Southampton, UK

Borislav D. Dimitrov
Academic Unit of Primary Care and Population Sciences, Faculty of Medicine, University of Southampton, Southampton, UK

Graham J. Kemp
Department of Musculoskeletal Biology and MRC – Arthritis Research UK Centre for Integrated research into Musculoskeletal Ageing (CIMA), Faculty of Health and Life Sciences, University of Liverpool, Liverpool, UK

Charles R. Horres, Richard E. Moon, Timothy E. Miller and Stuart A. Grant
Department of Anesthesiology, Duke University, DUMC 3094, Durham, NC 27710, USA

Mohamed A. Adam, Zhifei Sun and Julie K. Thacker
Department of Surgery, Duke University, Durham, USA

Solomon Aronson
Department of Anesthesiology, Duke University, 201 Trent Drive, 101 Baker House, Durham, NC 27710, USA

Paul Nisbet
One Research, LLC, 1150 Hungryneck Blvd. Suite C-303, Mt. Pleasant, SC 29464, USA

Martin Bunke
Department of Medical Affairs, Grifols, 79 T.W. Alexander Drive, 4101 Research Commons, Research Triangle Park, Raleigh, NC 27709, USA

Alex Helkin, Sumeet V. Jain, Angelika Gruessner, Maureen Fleming, Leslie Kohman, Michael Costanza and Robert N. Cooney
Department of Surgery, SUNY Upstate Medical University, 750 East Adams Street, Syracuse, NY 13206, USA

Heath McAnally
Northern Anesthesia and Pain Medicine, LLC, 10928 Eagle River Rd #240, Eagle River, AK 99577, USA
Department of Anesthesiology and Pain Medicine, University of Washington, Box 356540, Seattle, WA 98195-6540, USA

David Andrew Gilhooly and Suneetha Ramani Moonesinghe
UCLH NIHR Surgical Outcomes Research Centre, Department of Anaesthesia and Perioperative Medicine, University College Hospital, London NW1 2BU, UK

David Andrew Gilhooly
Department of Applied Health and Research, 1-19 Torrington Place, London WE1C 7HB, UK

David Andrew Gilhooly and Michelle Cole
Bariatric Fellow, UCL Centre for Anaesthesia, University College London Hospital, London NW1 2BU, UK

Suneetha Ramani Moonesinghe
NIAA Health Services Research Centre, Churchill House, 35 Red Lion Square, London WC1R 4SG, UK

Darren R Raphael, Maxime Cannesson, Leslie M Garson, Shermeen B Vakharia and Zeev N Kain
Department of Anesthesiology and Perioperative Care, University of California, 333 The City Boulevard West, Suite 2150, Orange, Irvine, California 92868, USA

Ran Schwarzkopf and Ranjan Gupta
Department of Orthopedic Surgery, University of California, 101 The City Drive South Pavilion III, Building 29A Orange, Irvine, California 92868, USA

C. Groleau
Hematology Residency Program, McGill University, Montreal, Canada

S. N. Morin and A. Bessissow
Department of Medicine, Division of General Internal Medicine, McGill University Health Centre, Montreal, Canada

L. Vautour
Department of Medicine, Division of Endocrinology, McGill University Health Centre, Montreal, Canadas

A. Amar-Zifkin
Medical library, McGill University Health Centre, Montreal, Canada

Sunghye Kim
Department of Internal Medicine, Section of General Internal Medicine, Wake Forest School of Medicine, Medical Center Boulevard, Winston-Salem, NC 27157, USA

Sunghye Kim, Stephen B. Kritchevsky and Leanne Groban
Sticht Center for Healthy Aging and Alzheimer's Prevention, Wake Forest School of Medicine, Medical Center Boulevard, Winston-Salem, NC 27157, USA

Rebecca Neiberg
Division of Public Health Sciences, Department of Biostatistical Sciences, Wake Forest School of Medicine, 525 Vine, Winston-Salem, NC 27101, USA

W. Jack Rejeski and Anthony P. Marsh
Department of Health and Exercise Science, Wake Forest University, PO Box 7868, Winston-Salem, NC 27109, USA

Leanne Groban
Department of Anesthesiology, Wake Forest School of Medicine, Medical Center Boulevard, Winston-Salem, NC 27157-1009, USA

Stephanie Archer and Jane Montague
Psychology Department, Faculty of Education, Health and Science, University of Derby, Kedleston Road, Derby DE22 1GB, UK

Stephanie Archer
Centre for Patient Safety and Service Quality, Imperial College London, Medical School Building, St Mary's Campus, Norfolk Place, London W2 1PG, UK

Anish Bali
Gynaecology/Oncology, Maternity and Gynaecology Level 2, Women and Children's Services, Royal Derby Hospital, Uttoxeter Road, Derby DE22 3NE, UK

Suneetha Ramani Moonesinghe and Eleanor Mary Kate Walker
UCL/UCLH Surgical Outcomes Research Centre, University College Hospital NIHR Biomedical Research Centre, London NW1 2BU, UK

Suneetha Ramani Moonesinghe, Eleanor Mary Kate Walker and Madeline Bell
National Institute for Academic Anaesthesia's Health Services Research 2Centre, Royal College of Anaesthetists, Churchill House 35 Red Lion Square, London WC1R 4SG, UK

Raquel R Bartz and William D White
Department of Anesthesiology, Duke University Medical Center, Durham, NC, USA

Tong J Gan
Department of Anesthesiology, Stony Brook University, HSC Level 4, Rm 060, Stony Brook, NY 11794-8480, USA

Ib Jammer
Department of Clinical Medicine, University of Bergen, 5020 Bergen, Norway

Ib Jammer and Atle Ulvik
Department of Anaesthesia and Intensive Care, Haukeland University Hospital, 5021 Bergen, Norway

Mari Tuovila
Department of Anesthesiology and Intensive Care, Oulu University Hospital, PL 21, 90029 Oulu, Finland

Matthew G Wiggans, Matthew J Bowles, Somaiah Aroori and David A Stell
Hepatobiliary Surgery, Plymouth Hospitals NHS Trust, Derriford Hospital, Derriford Road, Plymouth, Devon PL6 8DH, UK

David A Stell
Peninsula College of Medicine and Dentistry, University of Exeter and Plymouth University, Research Way, Plymouth, Devon PL6 8BU, UK

Tim Starkie, Tom Woolley, David Birt, Paul Erasmus and Ian Anderson
Department of Anaesthetics, Plymouth Hospitals NHS Trust, Derriford Hospital, Derriford Road, Plymouth, Devon PL6 8DH, UK

Golnaz Shahtahmassebi
Centre for Health Statistics, Tamar Science Park, Davy Road, Plymouth, Devon PL6 8BX, UK

Sam Huddart, Emily L Young and Pradeep K Prabhu
Department of Anaesthesia, Royal Surrey County Hospital, Guildford GU2 7XX, UK

Rebecca-Lea Smith
Department of Anaesthesia, Mount Sinai Hospital, Toronto, Canada

Peter JE Holt
St George's Vascular Institute, London, UK
The Queen Elizabeth Hospital, Adelaide, Australia

Man Lin Hui
The Queen Elizabeth Hospital, 30 Gascoigne Road, Kowloon, Hong Kong

Arun Kumar
Faculty of Medicine and Health Science, University of Nottingham, Clifton Boulevard, Nottingham NG7 2RD, UK

Gary G Adams
Insulin and Diabetes Experimental Research (IDER) Group, Faculty of Medicine and Health Science, University of Nottingham, Clifton Boulevard, Nottingham NG7 2RD, UK

Christos Chamos
Senior clinical fellow in cardiac anaesthesia, St George's Healthcare NHS Trust, London, UK

Liana Vele
Specialist registrar in anaesthesia, Croydon Health Services NHS Trust, London, UK

Mark Hamilton and Maurizio Cecconi
Consultant and honorary senior lecturer in anaesthesia and intensive care medicine, St George's Healthcare NHS Trust, London, UK

Index

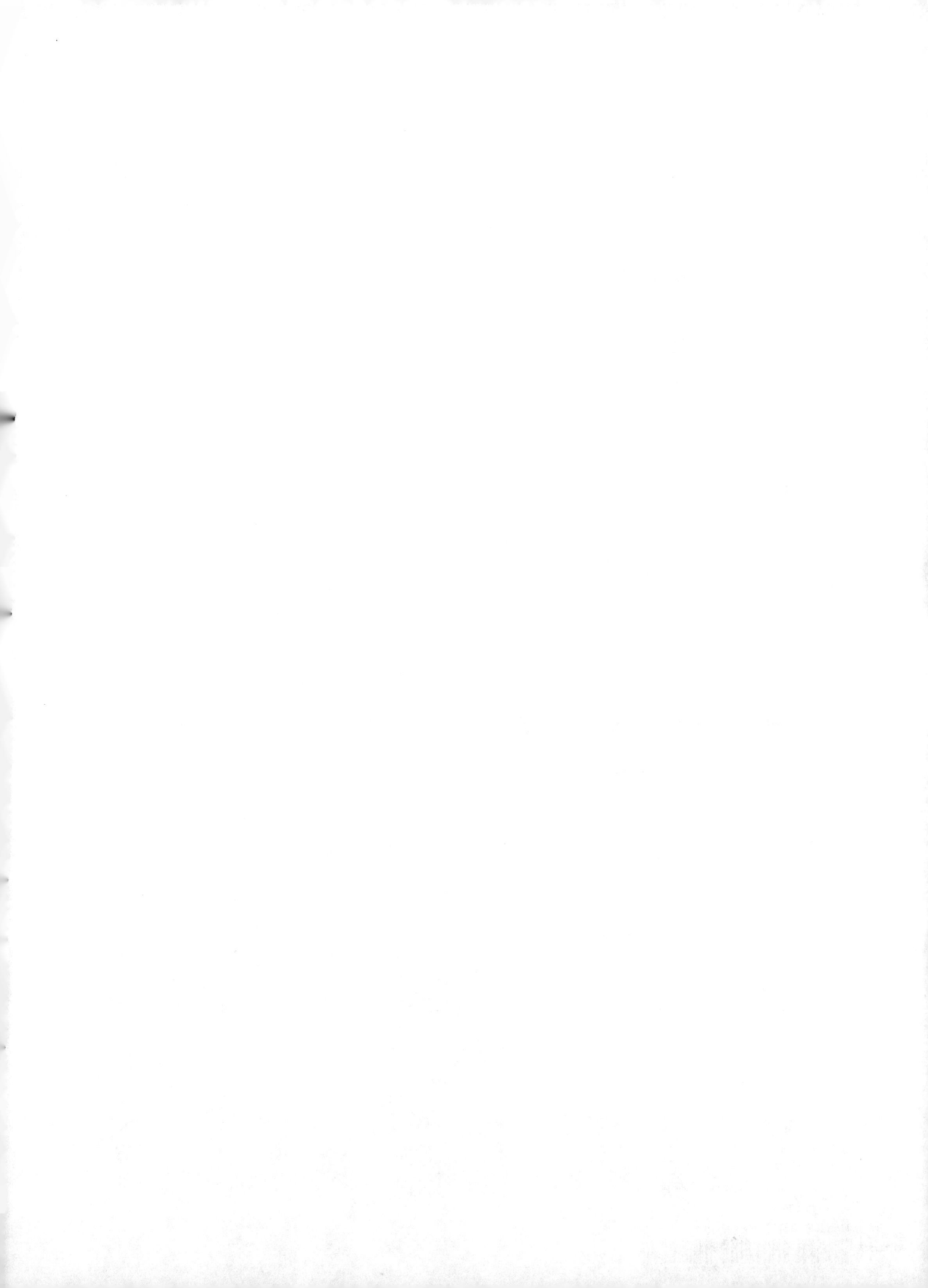

www.ingramcontent.com/pod-product-compliance
Lightning Source LLC
Chambersburg PA
CBHW080703200326

41458CB00013B/4948